Para~~medics~~
6-in-1
Handbook

Paramedics 6-in-1 Handbook

Second Edition

GD Mogli PhD MBA FHRIM (UK) FAHIMA (USA)
Visiting Professor, Medical Informatics
Mahatma Gandhi Institute of Medical Sciences
Sevagram, Maharashtra, India

Chief Executive Officer and Managing Director
Dr Mogli Healthcare Management Consultancy
Hyderabad, Andhra Pradesh, India

www.drmogliit.com
gdmogli@yahoo.com

Senior Consultant, eHealth Management
HEARTCOM INC. (USA)

Formerly served as WHO Consultant and
Senior Consultant/Adviser to the Ministries of Health of
India, Afghanistan, Iran, Kuwait, Saudi Arabia, Oman
Bahrain, Qatar and United Arab Emirates (UAE)

JAYPEE BROTHERS MEDICAL PUBLISHERS (P) LTD
New Delhi • Panama City • London • Dhaka • Kathmandu

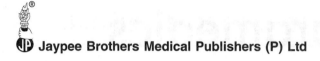

Jaypee Brothers Medical Publishers (P) Ltd

Headquarters
Jaypee Brothers Medical Publishers (P) Ltd
4838/24, Ansari Road, Daryaganj
New Delhi 110 002, India
Phone: +91-11-43574357
Fax: +91-11-43574314
Email: jaypee@jaypeebrothers.com

Overseas Offices

J.P. Medical Ltd.
83, Victoria Street, London
SW1H 0HW (UK)
Phone: +44-2031708910
Fax: +02-03-0086180
Email: info@jpmedpub.com

Jaypee-Highlights Medical Publishers Inc.
City of Knowledge, Bld. 237, Clayton
Panama City, Panama
Phone: + 507-301-0496
Fax: + 507-301-0499
Email: cservice@jphmedical.com

Jaypee Brothers Medical Publishers (P) Ltd
17/1-B, Babar Road, Block-B, Shaymali
Mohammadpur, Dhaka-1207
Bangladesh
Mobile: +08801912003485
Email: jaypeedhaka@gmail.com

Jaypee Brothers Medical Publishers (P) Ltd
Shorakhute, Kathmandu
Nepal
Phone: +00977-9841528578
Email: jaypee.nepal@gmail.com

Website: www.jaypeebrothers.com
Website: www.jaypeedigital.com

© 2013, GD Mogli

Inquiries for bulk sales may be solicited at: jaypee@jaypeebrothers.com

This book has been published in good faith that the contents provided by the author contained herein are original, and is intended for educational purposes only. While every effort is made to ensure accuracy of information, the publisher and the author specifically disclaim any damage, liability, or loss incurred, directly or indirectly, from the use or application of any of the contents of this work. If not specifically stated, all figures and tables are courtesy of the author. Where appropriate, the readers should consult with a specialist or contact the manufacturer of the drug or device.

Paramedics 6-in-1 Handbook

First Edition: 2003
Reprint: 2005
Second Edition: **2013**

ISBN: 978-93-5090-210-3

Printed at Rajkamal Electric Press, Plot No. 2, Phase-IV, Kundli, Haryana.

Preface to the Second Edition

There are quite a good number of books written by different authors available in the market related to medical field; but, to serve the professionals to grasp the exact content in a widespread approach, I have gone into efforts to prepare this book which could help to enlighten the desirable knowledge with less time and efforts. Since I have been exposed to many international organizations and countries, I have visualized the need for a concise but practical book that will be handy to very busy professionals with too many things to do in a short span of time at their disposal. Precisely, this is a cookbook for medical and allied health professionals besides other professionals who deal with medical and healthcare issues.

The important features of the book are mainly classified into three parts:

Part I: It deals with Anatomy, Physiology, Medical Terminology, Medical (History and Physical) Examination and Diagnostic Techniques and all the human body systems in combination of anatomy, physiology and medical terminology.

Part II: It includes Nursing, Allied Health Sciences (Pathology, Laboratory, Radiology, Radiation Therapy, Pharmacology, Pharmacy, Physical Therapy, Occupational Therapy, Medical Psychology, Medical Social Work, Optometry), Nutrition (Dietary), Medical Records, and Rights and Responsibilities of a Patient.

Part III: It contains Hospital Public Relations, Communication Skills, Medical Secretarial Profession, and Dictation and Transcription.

The book would be of immense use to all medical, nursing and paramedical staff dealing directly or indirectly with patient healthcare in general and to medical students, nursing and other allied healthcare professionals such as Laboratory Technicians, Radiography and Radiation Therapy Technicians, Pharmacists, Physical Therapy and Occupational Therapists, Medical Records and Healthcare Administrators, Nutritionists or Dietitians, Medical Psychologists and Medical Social Workers, apart from Public Relations, Medical Secretarial Profession, and Transcription Professionals in particular. Also, it is of significant value to health insurance companies, medical jurisprudence, consumer courts, Workmen's Compensation Settlements Organizations, healthcare research organizations, and software companies dealing with health information technology and so on.

In conclusion, this is a cookbook readymade ingredient for solving professional problems related to patient care and efficiently, swiftly, safely, improved quality with cost-contained outcome.

GD Mogli

Preface to the First Edition

The book has been written keeping the present-day requirement, serve the professionals to grasp the medical field in a comprehensive manner, absorb the concept of the human body, structure, functions, medical language other than English terms representing terms of Greek and Latin, Anglo-Saxon, German, Arabic, Indian and so on. Precisely, the book has a special feature in terms of combination of anatomy, physiology, medical terminology, medical abbreviations, medical records, medical transcribing techniques, allied health sciences and diagnostics, to serve the user with much ease. The selection of appropriate equivalent terms makes the language easy and helps the readers without background of science and biology to grab with least efforts.

I, having realized the need for the basic knowledge of medicine to other than medical professionals, had synthesized the related subjects, developed the book, to meet the facets of the requirement of the professionals such as medical records, students of paramedical including nurses, medical laboratory technologists, radiologic technologists, medical assistants, cardiovascular technicians, respiratory therapists, dental assistants, physiotherapists, occupational therapists, medical secretaries, insurance companies, law professionals, medical representatives, to serve as textbook in their academic programs, professional career building, besides reference guide throughout.

There are innumerable books available in the market with different authors related to anatomy, physiology and medical terminology. Present-day constraint of time, efforts, money at their disposal coupled with too many specialized professional books written on anatomy, physiology, medical terminology add to the confusion and makes the reader extremely difficult in selecting the appropriate material. Having realized the existing problems of learners, a special strategy has gone into my efforts to prepare a combined book, which should serve the actual need of the professionals that will enlighten the needed knowledge with least efforts and time.

The major feature of the book is descriptive illustrations, selective structural parts' names that will be grasped by the learner's mind much faster to enable him to coordinate with the structure and functions of human body, that will lead to the diagnosis or to the treatment and its related issues. Classification of systems of human body with related medical terminologies and abbreviations will add to the memory power of the learners. In simple terms this book is Six-In-One.

It was quite sometime, I was experiencing in the course of my four decade career as medical record administrator, teacher, consultant and adviser, dealing with different health professionals in different organizations, in different countries, felt that need for such a concise book, without loosing the main information part to develop a simple, practicable, handbook for the present-day users, who, with too many subjects to learn, hardly find time to scan a variety of books on single subject available in the market. With this objective, a considerable time and efforts have gone in preparing the book. It is hoped that this will serve the purpose for which it was prepared, however, there are ample scope for improvement as no book with whatever efforts one may make will ever be a complete one. I will be happy to receive any suggestions to improve the overall quality of the book.

GD Mogli

Acknowledgments

At the outset, my grateful thanks to M/s Jaypee Brothers Medical Publishers (P) Ltd, New Delhi, India, especially to Shri Jitendar P Vij (Group Chairman), Mr Ankit Vij (Managing Director) and Mr Suresh (Author Coordinator of Hyderabad Branch), for bringing out this invaluable book.

My sincere gratitude to the State Health Ministers and Deputy Ministers of Gulf Cooperation Council (GCC) Countries and other administrators, and professional colleagues of India, Afghanistan, Kuwait, Kingdom of Saudi Arabia, Sultanate of Oman, Bahrain, Qatar, and United Arab Emirates (UAE), for their support, encouragement and cooperation.

My special thanks to Mr Ramalingam Selva Kumar, formerly worked as Medical Record Officer in Saudi Arabia and Oman, currently Clinical Coder, Aberdeen Royal Infirmary Hospital, Aberdeen, Scotland, United Kingdom.

Mr Narendar Kumar Sampath, Medical Record Manager, Welcare Hospital, Dubai, United Arab Emirates (UAE).

Mrs Marie Stella Alexander, Medical Record Manager, Hamad General Hospital, Doha, Qatar.

Ms Swadhura V, working as Research Assistant in Dr Mogli Healthcare Management Consultancy, Hyderabad, Andhra Pradesh, India, for her dedicated work in bringing out the book.

Last but not least, I owe my sincere gratitude to my family.

Contents

PART–II NURSING, ALLIED HEALTH SCIENCES AND DIAGNOSTICS

PART–III HOSPITAL PUBLIC RELATIONS, MEDICAL SECRETARIAL PROFESSION, COMMUNICATION SKILLS, AND DICTATION AND TRANSCRIPTION

Plate 1

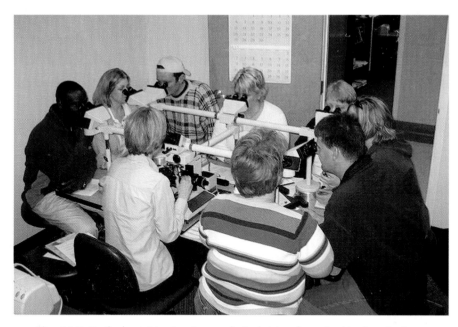

Fig. 16.1: Pathologist instructor and students of anatomical pathology

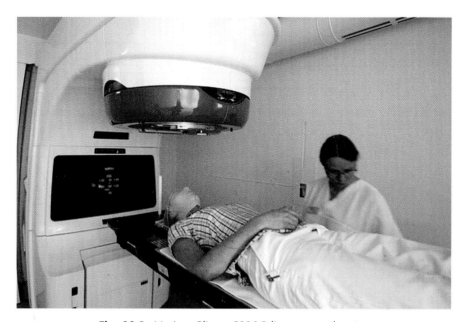

Fig. 19.1: Varian Clinac 2100C linear accelerator

Plate 2

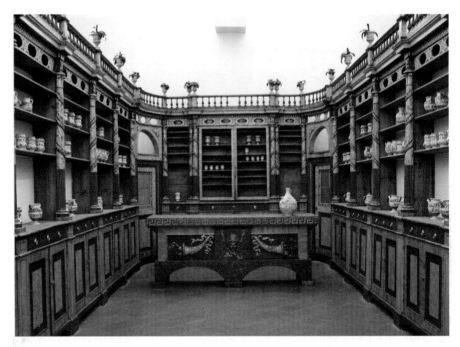

Fig. 21.1: A model of 19th century Italian pharmacy

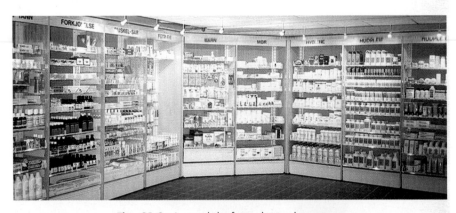

Fig. 21.2: A model of modern pharmacy

Plate 3

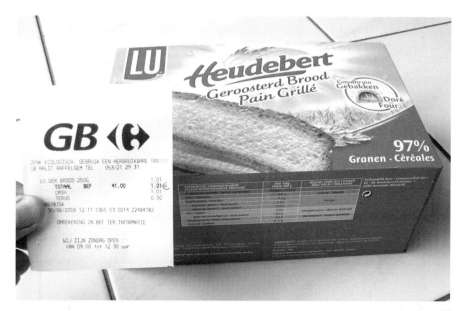

Fig. 25.1: Toasted bread is a cheap, high calorie nutrient usually unbalanced, i.e. deficient in essential minerals and vitamins, largely because of removal of both germ and bran during processing food source

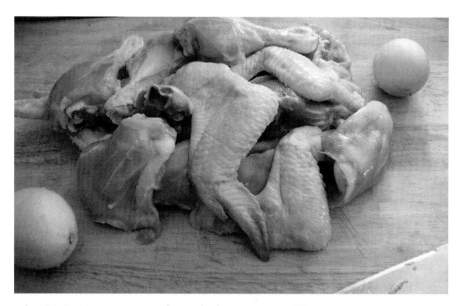

Fig. 25.2: Most meats such as chicken contain all the essential amino acids needed for humans (Protein in nutrition)

Plate 4

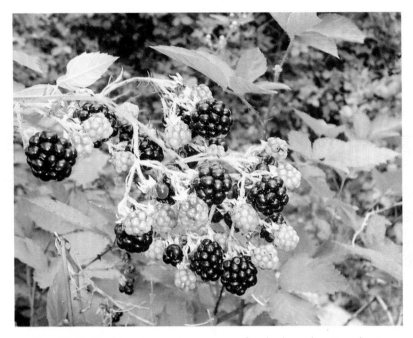

Fig. 25.4: Blackberries are a source of polyphenol antioxidants

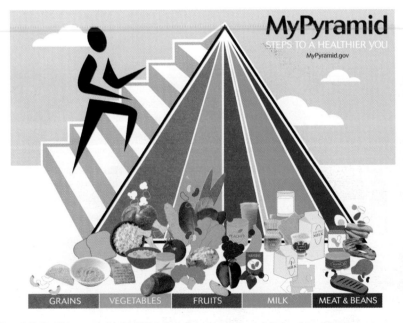

Fig. 25.5: The updated USDA food pyramid, published in 2005, is a general nutrition guide for recommended food consumption for humans

Plate 5

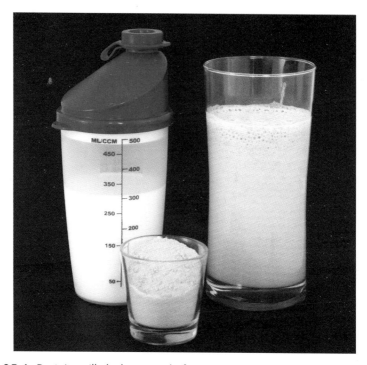

Fig. 25.6: Protein milkshakes, made from protein powder (center) and milk (left), are a common bodybuilding supplement

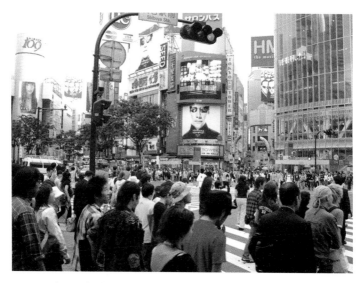

Fig. 26.2: Social psychology studies the nature and causes of social behavior

PART–I

Anatomy, Physiology, Medical Terms, and Medical Examination and Diagnostic Techniques

Human Body

CELL

INTRODUCTION

A cell is mass of a protoplasm containing a nucleus. It is the unit structure and the fundamental part of life, which carries various functions such as reproduction, respiration, excretion and adaptation to the environment. The human body is made up of a trillion number of cells of different types. The size of the cell is about 10 to 30 μm in diameter.

All cells are similar in that they contain a gelatinous substance composed of water, protein, sugar, acids, fats and various minerals. This substance is called protoplasm. Several parts of a cell are described below and pictured schematically.

STRUCTURE OF CELL (FIG. 1.1)

1. Cell membrane—covering or outer layer of the cell which protects the internal environment and determines what passes in and out of the cell.
2. Protoplasm—a white fluid, like the yolk of an egg, which consists of water, electrolytes, proteins, lipids and carbohydrates. The protoplasm forms the cytoplasm and the nucleus.
3. Cytoplasm is the protoplasmic material outside the nucleus. It triggers the work of the cell such as contraction in the muscle cell and transmitting impulses in the nerve cell. The cytoplasm contains mitochondria, endoplasmic reticulum, ribosomes, lysosomes, Golgi bodies, and the centrosome.
4. *Mitochondria:* It is responsible for the production of energy in the cell by breaking up the complex food structure into simpler substances. This process is called catabolism. It is also called as, kitchen cell (power house).

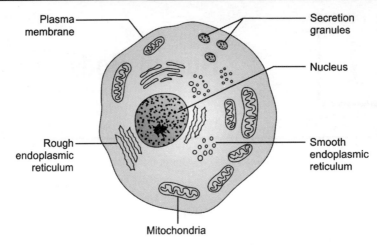

Fig. 1.1: Structure of cell

5. *Endoplasmic reticulum:* A tubule like structure. It contains small bodies called ribosomes which help to make substances (proteins) for the cells, this process is called anabolism.
6. *Nucleus:* It is the controlling structure of the cell. It controls the cell reproduction, and contains genetic material which determines the functioning and structure of the cell.
7. *Chromosomes:* There are 23 pairs of chromosomes, each chromosome consists of a chain of small units called genes made up of deoxyribonucleic acid (DNA) (hereditary information) and ribonucleic acid (RNA). Out of 23 pairs of chromosomes, 22 pairs are autosomes and 1 pair is sex chromosome which decides the sex. A female has 2 X (X,X) chromosomes whereas the male has 1X, 1Y chromosomes.

FUNCTIONS OF THE CELL

- *Absorption:* The ability of the cell to absorb or take in oxygen and food substances.
- *Nutrition:* The intake of food substances by the cell.
- *Growth:* It provides the metabolic process to enable the cell to grow to its full size and will be able to function correctly.
- *Reproduction:* On reaching maturity, the cell will divide to form two smaller cells.
- *Removal of waste products:* The removal of waste products produced during metabolism.
- *Movement:* Many cells have the power of movement.

CELL DIVISION

Division of cells are for the growth of the organism and for the replacement of damaged cells. There are two types of cell division:

Mitosis

A process of cell division which produces two new daughter cells (identical to the parent cells), e.g. plants. This involves a series of changes in which there is a rearrangement of centrioles and chromosomes so that each of the two new cells has a nucleus with 23 pairs of chromosomes. Mitosis is the common type of cell division that occurs in the body cells. It consists of four phases—prophase, metaphase, anaphase and telophase.

Prophase: The centrosome divides and the centrioles moves to the opposite poles of the cells with the spindle fibers.

Metaphase: The chromosomes align themselves at the center of the nucleus and become attached to the spindle fibers.

Anaphase: Each chromosome splits into two chromosomes. The separated chromosomes move towards the opposite poles of the cell. The centrioles are divided to form new centrosome.

Telophase: A new nuclear membrane forms around each set of chromosomes, and the spindle fiber disappear. The cytoplasm and cell membrane constrict. Finally, the cell splits into two identical cells.

Meiosis

Cell division occurring in maturation of sex cells, wherein over two successive cell division occur. Each daughter nucleus receives half the number of chromosomes typically to the somatic cells of the species.

The cell division occurring in the human reproductive system is called meiosis. Each person, male or female has 23 pairs of chromosomes comprising of 22 pairs of autosomes and 1 pair of sex chromosomes or somatic chromosomes. In the meiosis cell division, the daughter cell receives equal number of chromosomes from the parent cells, i.e. 22 pairs of autosomes from father and mother, the male has XY sex chromosomes. Whereas the mother has X and X chromosomes. The sex of a child clearly depends on whether it inherits X or Y chromosome from its father.

TISSUE FLUID

Tissue fluids are of two types: intracellular and extracellular. The fluid inside the cell is called intracellular fluid while the fluid outside the cell is called extracellular fluid. Tissue fluid acts as a sort of middle man between the blood and tissues, supplying food and oxygen to the cell and removing waste products from the cell.

TISSUES

A tissue is a group of similar cells working together to do a specific job. A histologist is one who specializes in the study of tissues.

Tissues can be classified into four major types:
1. Epithelium
2. Connective tissue
3. Muscular tissue
4. Nervous tissue.

Epithelium

The various types of epithelial tissues are as follows:

Simple Squamous Epithelium

A single layer of flat cells found in alveoli of lungs, the lining of the interior of the heart and blood vessels and the lymphatic vessels.

Stratified Squamous Epithelium

It is composed of cells which are flat and round. It is found in all parts of the body. The skin is composed of stratified squamous epithelium.

Transitional Epithelium

Cells which provide water tightness. It is found on the lining of urinary tract.

Columnar Epithelium

Cylindrical-shaped cells found in the secretory glands of the body.

Ciliated Epithelium

The free surface of each cell surrounded by fine hair like structures called cilia. It is found in the lining of (nasal cavity, trachea and bronchi) the respiratory system.

Connective Tissue

Connective tissues are fat (also called adipose tissue), cartilage (elastic, fibrous tissues attached to bones), bone, or blood tissues. They are present in different forms in the body. It is a jelly like substance and is hard.

Fibrous Tissue

There are two types of fibrous tissues:
1. White fibrous tissue
2. Yellow elastic tissue.

White fibrous tissue: It consists of bundles of white fibers which cannot stretch. It is found in tendons, ligaments, dura mater and outer layer of the pericardium.

Yellow elastic tissue: It consists of fibers which can stretch. It is found in the walls of arteries, bronchi and alveoli of lungs.

Areolar Tissue

Supporting tissue of the body. Found under the skin, mucous membrane and surrounding blood vessels and nerves.

Adipose Tissue

Found in all parts of the body where fat is deposited or stored, especially under the skin and around the eyes, heart and kidneys.

Cartilage

It is a flexible tissue found mainly in the skeleton. There are three different types of cartilage:
1. Hyaline cartilage
2. Fibrocartilage
3. Elastic cartilage.

Hyaline cartilage: It is bluish white tissue with a smooth glassy surface. It is found covering the ends of the bones, where they form joints (articular cartilage).

Fibrocartilage: It contains white fibrous tissue. It is found in intervertebral disks and semilunar cartilage of the knee joint where great strength combined with certain amount of elasticity is required.

Yellow elastic cartilage: It contains yellow elastic fibers and it is found in the epiglottis and pinna of the ear.

Muscular Tissue

The muscles are structures, which give the power of movements. Muscles are composed of thousands of elongated cells, called muscle fibers. Each contains a small nucleus. Bundles of muscle fibers lie side by side like threads. There are three different types of muscle tissue, they are voluntary, involuntary and cardiac.

Voluntary muscles are found in arms, legs and parts of the body where movement is voluntary. All the muscles attached to the skeleton are of this type and their functions are to move the bones at their respective joints and to help in maintaining the posture of the limbs and body as a whole. The microscopic structure of this muscle is striped in structure, i.e. white and black bands, hence it is also called striated muscle.

Involuntary muscles are found in the internal organs and structures of the body such as stomach, intestine, bladder, bronchi, blood vessels, and is, therefore, sometimes called visceral muscles. It cannot be consciously controlled and its nervous supply comes from the involuntary or autonomic nervous system. It is also called nonstriated or plain muscle.

The cardiac muscle is a special type of muscle found only in the heart. Although, it is an involuntary muscle, it has the form of striated muscle. It has the special property, not observed in other varieties of muscles, of automatic rhythmic contraction which can occur independently of its nervous supply.

Nervous Tissue

Nerve tissues conduct impulses all over the body. The muscles are structures which give the body the power of movements; almost every movement is governed by some portion of the nervous system which acts as a medium between brain and muscle.

ORGANS

Organs are structures composed of several types of tissues. For example, an organ like stomach is composed of muscular tissues, nerve tissues, and glandular epithelial tissues. The medical term for internal organ is viscera (singular: viscus). Examples:

Eye	Ear	Nose	Tongue
Heart	Lung	Stomach	Intestine
Hand	Leg	Liver	Spleen

SYSTEMS

Systems are groups of organs working together to perform essential fundamental functions of the individual. The different types of systems are skeletal, muscular, nervous, endocrine, circulatory, lymphatic, respiratoy, digestive, urinary, reproductive systems. Although some systems are functioning individually, the functions of various systems are very closely connected and are dependent on each other. For example, mouth, esophagus, stomach, and small and large intestines are organs which compose the digestive system.

The main systems and their organs of the body are as given in Table 1.1.

Table 1.1: The main systems and their organs

S.No.	Name of the system	Organs/parts
1.	Muscular system	There are three types of muscle tissues: a. Skeletal, voluntary or striated muscle b. Visceral, involuntary or smooth muscle c. Cardiac muscle.
2.	Skeletal system	Bones—there are 206 bones in an adult skeletal system Joints a. Fibrous or fixed joints, b. Cartilaginous or slightly movable joints c. Synovial or freely movable joints.
3.	A. Nervous system	A. The nervous system consist of: a. Brain b. Spinal cord c. Nerves.
	B. Sense organs	B. Sense organs a. Eye b. Ear c. Nose d. Tongue e. Skin or integumentary system
4.	Endocrine system (ductless gland)	a. Pituitary gland b. Thyroid gland c. Parathyroid glands d. Thymus gland e. Pancreas (islets of Langerhans) f. Adrenal gland g. Sex glands (ovaries and testes).
5.	A. Cardiovascular system or Circulatory system	A. Cardiovascular system a. Heart b. Aorta, artery, and arteriole c. Vena cava, vein, and venule d. Capillaries.
	B. Blood and blood groups	B. Blood and blood group 1. Blood composition a. Plasma b. Blood cells 1. Leukocytes or white blood cells 2. Erythrocytes or red blood cells 3. Thrombocytes or platelets 2. Blood groups a. Blood group "A" b. Blood group "B" c. Blood group "AB" d. Blood group "O" e. Rhesus factor (Rh) 1. Rhesus factor positive (+) 2. Rhesus factor negative (–).
6.	Lymphatic system	a. Lymph vessels b. Lymph nodes and other lymphatic tissues c. Spleen d. Thymus gland.
7.	Respiratory system	a. Nose b. Nasal cavities and paranasal sinuses.

Contd...

Contd...

S.No.	Name of the system	Organs/parts
		c. Pharynx
		d. Larynx
		e. Trachea
		f. Bronchi (bronchus-singular)
		g. Bronchioles
		h. Alveoli (alveolus-singular)
		i. Lung capillaries (bloodstream).
8.	Digestive system	a. Oral cavity (mouth)
		b. Pharynx
		c. Esophagus
		d. Stomach
		e. Enteron (small intestine)
		– Duodenum
		– Jejunum
		– Ileum
		f. Colon (large intestine)
		– Cecum
		– Ascending colon
		– Transverse colon
		– Descending colon
		– Sigmoid colon
		– Rectum
		g. Anus.
		B. Accessory organs
		a. Salivary glands
		b. Liver
		c. Gallbladder
		d. Pancreas.
9.	Urinary system	a. Kidneys
		b. Ureters
		c. Urinary bladder
		d. Urethra.
10.	Reproductive system	Male:
		a. Testes
		b. Scrotum
		c. Seminiferous tubules
		d. Epididymis
		e. Vas deferens
		f. Seminal vesicles
		g. Ejaculatory duct
		h. Prostate gland
		i. Penis
		j. Urethra.
		Female:
		a. Ovaries
		b. Fallopian tubes
		c. Uterus
		d. Vagina
		e. Vulva
		f. Cervix
		g. Labia majora
		h. Labia minora
		i. Hymen
		j. Mammary glands (accessory organ).

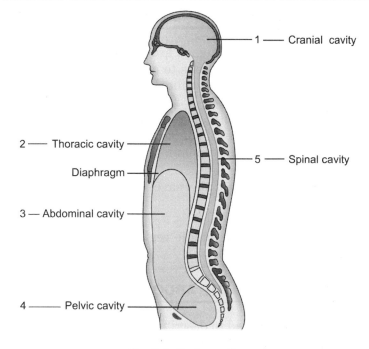

Fig. 1.2: Body cavities

BODY CAVITIES (FIG. 1.2)

A body cavity is a space within the body which contains internal organs (viscera). Some of the important viscera contained within those cavities are listed in Table 1.2.

Table 1.2: Some of the important viscera contained within those cavities

S.No.	Name of the cavity	Organs/parts
1.	Cranial cavity	Brain
2.	Thoracic cavity	Lungs, heart, esophagus, trachea, thymus gland, aorta The thoracic cavity can be divided into two smaller cavities: a. The pleural cavity—the areas surrounding the lungs. Each pleural cavity is lined with a double-folded membrane called pleura; visceral pleura is closer to the lungs, and parietal pleura is closer to the outer wall of the pleural cavity. b. The mediastinum cavity—the area between the lungs. It contains the heart, aorta, trachea, esophagus, and thymus gland.
3.	Abdominal cavity	Stomach, small and large intestines, spleen, liver, gallbladder, and pancreas.
4.	Pelvic cavity	Ureters, urinary bladder, urethra; uterus and vagina in the female.
5.	Spinal cavity	Nerves of the spinal cord runs through vertebrae

ANATOMICAL DIVISIONS OF THE BODY (FIG. 1.3)

Anatomical divisions of the abdomen are labeled in Figure 1.3. These divisions are used in anatomy texts to describe the regions in which organs and structures are found while documenting the patient care. The names of the divisions are:
1. Right hypochondriac regions (upper lateral regions beneath the ribs)
2. Epigastric region (regions of the stomach)
3. Left hypochondriac regions (upper lateral regions beneath the ribs)
4. Right lumbar region
5. Umbilical region (region of the navel or umbilicus)
6. Left lumbar region
7. Right iliac fossa
8. Hypogastric region (lower middle region below the umbilicus)
9. Left iliac fossa.

CLINICAL DIVISIONS OF THE ABDOMEN (FIG. 1.4)

The following terms are used to describe the divisions of the abdomen when a patient is examined in clinic or bedside:
1. Right upper quadrant, RUQ
2. Left upper quadrant, LUQ
3. Right lower quadrant, RLQ
4. Left lower quadrant, LLQ.

ANATOMICAL DIVISIONS OF THE BACK (SPINAL COLUMN)

See Table 1.3 and Figure 1.5.

Table 1.3: Anatomical divisions of the back (spinal column)

S.No.	Division of the back	Abbreviation	Location
1.	Cervical vertebrae	C	Neck region. There are 7 cervical vertebrae (C1-C7)
2.	Thoracic vertebrae	T or D (Dorsal)	Chest region. There are 12 thoracic vertebrae (T1-T12). Each bone is joined to a rib
3.	Lumbar vertebrae	L	Loin or flank region (between the ribs and the hip bone). There are 5 lumbar vertebrae (L1-L5)
4.	Sacral vertebrae	S	Five bones (S1-S5) are fused to form one bone, the sacrum
5.	Coccygeal	Nil	The coccyx (tailbone) is small bone composed of 4 fused pieces

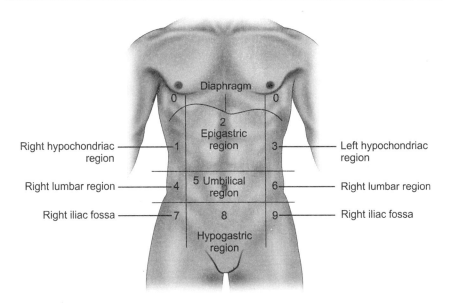

Fig. 1.3: Anatomical divisions of the body

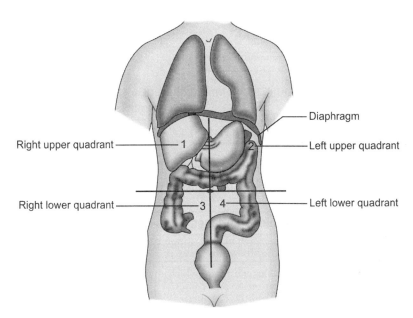

Fig. 1.4: Clinical divisions of the abdomen

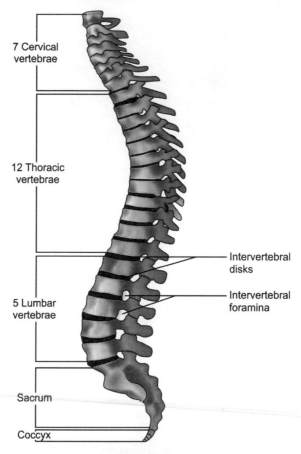

Fig. 1.5: Anatomical divisions of the back (spinal column)

PLANES OF THE BODY (FIG. 1.6)

A plane is an imaginary flat cross-section. The following terms are used to describe the planes of the body (Table 1.4):

Table 1.4: Planes of the body

S.No.	Name of the planes	Explanation
1.	Frontal	Vertical plane which divides the body or structure into anterior and posterior portions.
2.	Sagittal	Lengthwise vertical plane which divides the body or structure into right and left portions. The midsagittal plane divides the body into right and left halves.
3.	Transverse	Plane running across the body parallel to the ground (horizontal). It divides the body or structure into upper and lower portions.

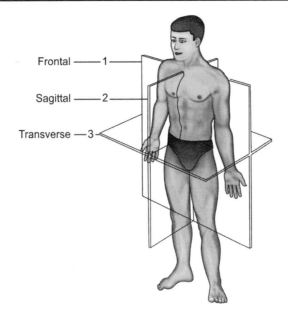

Fig. 1.6: Planes of the body

POSITIONAL AND DIRECTIONAL TERMS OF THE BODY (TABLE 1.5)

Table 1.5: Positional and directional terms of the body

Position	Description of the position
Anterior	In front of the body
Posterior	At the back of the body
Central	Pertaining to the center
Deep	Away from the surface
Superficial	Near the surface
Distal	Away from the beginning of the structure or away from the center
Proximal	Pertaining to the beginning of a structure
Inferior	Below another structure
Superior	Above another structure
Lateral	Pertaining to the sides
Medial	Near to the median of the body (structure)
Supine	Lying on the back
Prone	Lying on the belly
Afferent	Towards the structure
Efferent	Away from the structure

MEDICAL TERMINOLOGY

OBJECTIVES IN STUDYING THE MEDICAL LANGUAGE

- To analyze words structurally.
- To correlate and understand word elements with the basics of anatomy, physiology, and diseases of human body.
- To pronounce and write correct spelling of medical terms.

Basic Word Structure

Studying medical words is similar to learning of a new language. The words at first look strange and complicated although they may stand for commonly known English terms. The words gastralgia, means 'stomach ache," and ophthalmologist, means "eye doctor," are some examples.

The medical language is fascinatingly logical in each term, complex or simple, can be broken into basic components and then understood.

These basic components of medical words are:

Root:	**Foundation of the word**
Example:	gastr/ic
	↓
	root (stomach)
Suffix:	**Word ending**
Examples:	gastr/itis gastric
	↓ ↓
	suffix (inflammation) Suffix (pertaining to)
Prefix:	**Word beginning**
Examples:	epi/gastr/ic Ad/renal
	↓ ↓
	prefix (above) prefix (above)
Combining vowel:	**A vowel (usually "O") links the root with the suffix or to another root**
Examples:	cardi/o/gram electr/o/cardi/o/gram
	root ↓ suffix root ↓ root ↓ suffix
	combining vowel combining vowel

CHIEF SOURCES OF MEDICAL WORDS

ANGLO-SAXON (OLD ENGLISH)

These words are from old English, which are mostly anatomical terms.

Examples:

Arm	Back	Bladder	Blood	Cheek	Chest
Chin	Ear	Eye	Finger	Hair	Nose
Thumb, etc.					

GREECO-ROMAN (GREEK AND LATIN)

These words are from Greek and Latin languages.

Examples:
Marrow—the word marrow is derived from the Latin word medulla.
Myelitis (G) originating from the Greek word myelos. The word myelitis
is the inflammation of marrow.

Crani (G and L)	:	Skull
Cerebro (L)	:	Brain
Illi (L)	:	Ilium
Rhin (G)	:	Nose
Pneumo (G)	:	Lungs, air

ARABIC

Most of these words are used to describe chemical substances.
Examples:

Sharab	:	Sweet beverage (syrup)
Matter	:	Mother
Alcohol	:	Something subtle

MODERN GERMAN

These words are derived from French (Modern German).
Example:
Fahrenheit (German Physicist) for thermometer

Kernicterus	:	Yellow (Jaundice)

COLORS

S.No.	Color	Medical terms	Examples
1.	White	Albus	Albinism
2.	White	Leukos	Leukocyte
3.	White	Candidus	Candidiasis
4.	Black	Melan	Melanoma
5.	Black	Niger	Nigrometer
6.	Red	Erythros	Erythrocyte
7.	Red	Ruber	Rubericyte
8.	Yellow	Flavus	Flavism

Contd...

Contd...

S.No.	Color	Medical terms	Examples
9.	Yellow	Xanthos	Xathoma
10.	Green	Chloros	Chlorhydria
11.	Green	Glaucos	Glaucoma
12.	Blue	Cynos	Cyanosis
13.	Brown	Cirrhos	Cirrhosis
14.	Violet	Iodes	Iodine
15.	Purple	Porphyros	Porphyrinuria
16.	Ashy	Cinerous	Cinerea
17.	Golden	Aureus	Aueromycin

NUMERALS

S.No.	Numerals	Medical terms	Examples
1.	Half	Semi	Semilunar
2.	Half	Hemi	Hemiplegia
3.	First	Primus	Primigravida
4.	One	Unus	Unilateral
5.	Single	Monos	Monocular
6.	Two	Duo	Duodenum
7.	Second	Secundus	Secundine
8.	Two at a time	Bini	Binocular
9.	Twice	Bi, Dis, Di	Dislocation
10.	Three	Tri	Tricuspid
11.	Four	Quadri, Tetra	Quadriplegia, Tetralogy
12.	Five	Quinique	Quintuplet
13.	Six	Sex, Hex	Sexdigitate, Hexadactylism
14.	Seven	Hepta	Heptadactylia
15.	Eight	Octa	Octigravida
16.	Nine	Non	Nonipara
17.	Ten	Deca	Decameter
18.	One hundred	Centi	Centimeter
19.	One thousand	Milli	Millimeter
20.	10,000	Myri	
21.	1,00,000	Mega	
22.	1/1,00,000	Micro	

ELEMENTS OF MEDICAL TERMS

SUFFIXES AND COMPOUNDING ELEMENTS

True suffixes refer to a syllable denoting a preposition or adverb attached to the end of a word, root, or stem to modify its meaning. Many endings are adjectives or nouns added to a root to form compound words. They may be combining forms or pseudo-suffixes. To simplify learning, the modifying endings have been classified according to their meanings into diagnostic, operative and symptomatic suffixes and compounding elements.

Diagnostic Suffixes and Compounding Elements

Suffix	Medical term	Definition
-aemia (G) blood	Hyperglycemia	High blood sugar
-cele (G) hernia, tumor, protrusion	Cystocele	Hernia of the bladder
	Hydrocele	Serous tumor as of testis
	Myelocele	Protrusion of spinal cord through the vertebrae
-ectasis (G)	Atelectasis - neonatorum	Imperfect expansion of lungs at birth
expansion, dilatation	Bronchiectasis	Abnormal dilatation of a bronchus or bronchi
-graphy (G)	Electrocardiography	The recording of the electricity flowing through the heart
act of recording or writing	Echocardiography	A diagnostic procedure in which pulses of high frequency sound waves (ultrasound) are transmitted into the chest and echoes returning from the surfaces of the heart are electronically plotted and recorded.
-iasis (G)	Lithiasis	Formation of stones
	Cholelithiasis	Presence of calculi in the gallbladder
condition, formation of, presence of	Nephrolithiasis	Stones present in the kidney
-itis (G)	Carditis	Inflammation of the heart
	Gastritis	Inflammation of the stomach
inflammation	Poliomyelitis	Inflammation of the gray matter of the spinal cord
-malacia (G)	Encephalomalacia	Softening of the brain
	Osteomalacia	Softening of the bones
softening	Splenomalacia	Softening of the spleen
-megaly (G)	Cardiomegaly	Enlargement of the heart
	Hepatomegaly	Enlargement of the liver
enlargement	Splenomegaly	Enlargement of the spleen
-oma (G)	Adenoma	Glandular tumor
	Carcinoma	Malignant tumor of epithelial tissue
tumor	Sarcoma	Malignant tumor of connective tissue
-osis (G) condition, diseases,	Arteriosclerosis	Hardening of the arteries
	Dermatosis	Any skin condition
increase	Neurosis	Functional disorder of the nervous system
-pathy (G)	Adenopathy	Any glandular disease
	Myopathy	Any diseases of a muscle
disease	Myelopathy	Any pathologic disorder of the spinal cord
-ptosis (G)	Blepharoptosis	Drooping or (downward displacement) of the eyelid
	Gastroptosis	Downward displacement of the stomach
falling	Nephroptosis	Downward displacement of the kidney
-rhexis (G)	Angiorhexis	Rupture of a blood vessel or lymphatic
rupture	Cardiorhexis	Rupture of the heart

Operative Suffixes and Compounding Elements

Suffix	Medical term	Definition
-centesis (G) puncture	Paracentesis Thoracentesis	Puncture of a cavity Aspiration of the pleural cavity
-ectomy (G) excision	Myomectomy Tonsillectomy	Excision of a tumor of the muscle Removal of tonsils
-desis (G) binding fixation	Arthrodesis Spondylosyndesis	Surgical fixation of a joint Surgical fixation of the vertebrae
-lithotomy (G) incision for removal of stones	Cholelithotomy Nephrolithotomy	Incision into gallbladder for removal of stones Incision into kidney for removal of stones
-pexy (G) suspension or fixation	Hysteropexy Orchiopexy	Abdominal fixation or suspension of the uterus Fixation of an undescended testis
-plasty (G) surgical correction plastic repair of	Arthroplasty Hernioplasty	Reconstructive operation on joint Plastic repair of hernia
-rrhaphy (G) suture	Perineorrhaphy Staphylorrhaphy	Suture of a lacerated perineum Suture of a cleft palate
-scopy (G) inspection or examination	Bronchoscopy Cystoscopy	Examination of the bronchi with an endoscope Inspection of the bladder with a cystoscope
-ostomy (G) creation of a more or less permanent opening	Colostomy Cystostomy	Creation of an opening into the colon through the abdominal wall Creation of an opening into the urinary bladder through the abdomen
-otomy (G) incision into	Antrotomy Thoracotomy	Incision into the antrum for drainage Opening of the chest
-tripsy (G) crushing or friction	Lithotripsy Phrenicotripsy	Crushing of a calculus in the bladder or urethra Crushing of the phrenic nerve

Symptomatic Suffixes and Compounding Elements

Suffix	Medical term	Definition
-algia (G) pain	Gastralgia Nephralgia	Stomach pain Renal pain
-genic (G) origin	Bronchogenic Pathogenic	Originating in the bronchi Disease producing
-lysis (G) dissolution or breaking down	Hemolysis Neurolysis	A breaking down of red blood cells Disintegration of nerve tissue
-osis (G) increase or condition	Anisocytosis Lymphocytosis	Inequality of size of cells Excess of lymph cells
-penia (G) deficiency or decrease	Leukopenia Neutropenia	Abnormal decrease of leukocytes in the blood Abnormal decrease of neutrophils in the blood

Contd...

Contd...

Suffix	Medical term	Definition
-rrhage, -rrhagia (G)	Hemorrhage	The escape of blood from the vessels; bleeding
	Metrorrhagia	Uterine bleeding
excessive flow bursting forth	Otorrhagia	Hemorrhage from the ear
-rrhoea (G)	Metrorrhoea	A free or abnormal uterine discharge
flowing	Dysmenorrhoea	Painful menstruation
	Otorrhoea	Discharge from the ear
-spasm (G)	Chirospasm	A spasm as contraction of the hand (Writer's cramp)
involuntary contractions	Dactylospasm	Spasm or cramp in fingers or toes
-stasis (G)	Hemostasis	Interruption of blood flow through any vessel or to any anatomical area
stand still		
-stenosis (G)	Aorticstenosis	A narrowing of the aortic orifice of the heart
narrowing, contraction	Mitralstenosis	A narrowing of the left atrio-ventricular orifice

ROOTS

The root stem or main body of a word indicates the organ or part of which is modified by a prefix or suffix, or both. Properly, Greek combining forms or roots should be used only with Greek prefixes and suffixes, Latin with Latin. A vowel, usually a, i, or o is often inserted between the combining forms for euphony.

Root	Medical term	Definition
aden (G)	Adenectomy	Excision of a gland
gland	Adenoma	Glandular tumor
aer (G)	Aerated	Filled with air
air	Aerobic	Pertaining to organism, which lives only in the presence of air
Angio (G)	Angiotomy	Incision of blood vessels
vessel	Angitis	Inflammation of the blood vessels
arth (G)	Arthralgia	Pain in the joints
joint	Arthritis	Inflammation of the joints
blephar (G)	Blepharitis	Inflammation of the eyelid
eyelid	Blepharoptosis	Drooping of the upper eyelid
card (G)	Cardiology	The science of the heart
heart	Electrocardiogram	A graphic record of the heart beat by an electrometer
cerebro (L)	Cerebromalacia	Softening of the brain
brain	Cerebrospinal	Referring to brain and spinal cord

Contd...

Contd...

Root	Medical term	Definition
cephal (G) head	Cephalalgia Cephalic	Headache Pertaining to the head
cerv (L) neck	Cervicectomy Cervicovesical	Excision of the neck of the uterus Relating to the cervix uteri and bladder
cheil, chil (G) lip	Cheilitis Cheiloplasty	Inflammation of the lip Plastic operation of the lip
chir (G) hand	Chiromegaly Chiroplasty	Abnormal size of the hands, wrists and ankles Plastic repair of the hand
chol (G) bile	Cholangitis Cholecyst	Inflammation of bile duct Gallbladder
chondr (G) cartilage	Chondrectomy Chondroma	Excision of a cartilage A cartilaginous tumor
cost (L) rib	Costochondral Costosternal	Pertaining to a rib and its cartilage Referring to the ribs and breast bone
crani (G,L) skull	Craniotomy Cranial	Surgical opening (incision) of the skull Pertaining to the skull
cysto (G) bladder, sac	Cyst Cystoscope	A bladder; any sac containing a liquid Instrument for interior examination of the bladder
cyt (G) cell	Cytology Erythrocyte	The study of cell life Red blood cell
dacry (G) tear	Dacryocele Dacryocyst	Protrusion of the lacrimal sac The lacrimal sac
dactyl (G) finger, toe	Dactylitis Dactylomegaly	Chronic disease of bone of fingers or toe in young children Abnormal size of fingers and toes
derm (G) skin	Dermatitis Dermopathy	Inflammation of the skin Any skin disease
encephal (G) brain	Encephalitis Encephaloma	Inflammation of the brain Brain tumor
enter (G) intestine (small)	Enteritis Enterocele	Inflammation of the small intestine A hernia of the small intestine
gastr (G) stomach	Gastrectasis Gastroenteritis	Dilatation of the stomach Inflammation of the stomach and the small intestine
glyco (G) sweet	Glycemia Glycosuria	Sugar in blood Sugar in urine
hem, haemat (G) blood	Hematemesis Hemophilia	Vomiting of blood Inability of the blood to coagulate
hepat (G) liver	Hepatitis Hepatoma	Inflammation of the liver A liver tumor
hyster (G) or metr uterus	Hysterectomy Hysteropexy	Excision of the uterus Abdominal fixation of the uterus

Contd...

Contd...

Root	Medical term	Definition
ile, eile, (L-G) ileum	Ileum Ileostomy	Third part of the small intestine Creation of an opening through abdomen into the ileum
ili (L) ilium	Ilium Iliosacral	The wide, upper part of the hip bone Pertaining to ilium and sacrum
leuk (G) white	Leukocyte Leukopenia	White blood cell Abnormal decrease in number of leukocyte
lip (G) fat	Lipectomy Lipemia	Excision of fatty tissues Fat in the blood
lith (G) stone	Lithiasis Lithoscope	Presence of concretions or stones Instrument for examining stone in bladder
menig (G) membrane	Meningitis Meningioma	Inflammation of the membranes of spinal cord and brain Tumor of the meninges
metr (G) or hystr uterus	Metritis Metrorrhagia	Inflammation of the uterus Bleeding from the uterus
myel (G) marrow	Myelitis Myelosarcoma	Inflammation of spinal cord or bone marrow Malignant tumor of the bone marrow
my (G) muscle	Myitis or myositis Myocardium	Inflammation of a muscle The middle and thickest layer of the heart wall
nephr (G) kidney	Nephropexy Nephrosclerosis	Surgical attachment of a floating kidney Hardening of the kidney
ophthalm (G) eye	Ophthalmology Ophthalmoscope	The study of the eye and its diseases Instrumental examination of the eye
osteo (G) bone	Osteoma Osteomalacia	A bony tumor Softening of the bone
pneum (G) lung, or air	Pneumonia Pneumothorax	Inflammation of the lungs with consolidation and exudation Introduction of air into the pleural cavity
proct (G) rectum, anus	Proctoscopy Proctopexy	Instrumental examination of the rectum Suture of the rectum to some other part
psycho (G) soul, mind	Psychiatry Psychopathy	Medical specialty treating mental and neurotic disorders Any mental disease usually related to defective character and personality
pyel (G) pelvis	Pyelitis Pyelogram	Inflammation of the pelvis of the kidney Radiogram of the ureter and renal pelvis
pyloro (G) pylorus, gatekeeper	Pylorus Pylorostenosis	Orifice between stomach and duodenum Constriction of pylorus
pyo (G) pus	Pyogenic Pyometritis	Pus forming Purulent inflammation of the uterus
radi (L) ray	Radiology Radiotherapy	The study of X-rays in the diagnosis and treatment of disease The use of radiation of any type in treating diseases

Contd...

Contd...

Root	Medical term	Definition
spondyl (G) vertebra	Spondylitis Spondylolisthesis (olisthesis: slipping)	Inflammation of vertebrae Forward dislocation of lumbar vertebrae with pelvic deformity
trachel (G) or cervi neck	Trachelitis Tracheloplasty	Inflammation of the cervix Plastic operation of the cervix uteri
tubercul (L) tubercle	Tuberculosis Tuberculoma	An infectious disease marked by the formation of tubercles in any tissue A tuberculous abscess or tumor
viser (L) organ	Viscus Viscera	Pertaining to the internal organs Organ

PREFIXES

Prefixes are the most frequently used elements in the formation of medical terms. A prefix consists of one or two syllables placed before a word to modify its meaning. These syllables are often prepositions or adverbs. Some common prefixes are:

Prefix	Medical term	Definition
ab (L) from, away from	Abductor Abnormal	That which draws away from a common center Away from or not corresponding to rule
a, an (G) without, not	Apnea Anesthesia	Temporary absence of respiration Loss of sensation
ad (L) adherence, increase, near, toward	Adductor Adrenal	That which draws toward a common center A ductless (endocrine) gland above the kidney
ante (L) before	Antenatal Antepartum	Before birth Before the onset of labor
anti (G) against	Antisepsis Antipyretic	The exclusion of putrefactive germs A drug that reduces fever
bi (L) two, both, double	Biconvex Bilateral	Having two convex surfaces as in a lens Affecting both sides
com, con, or sym (L) together, with	Congenital defect Conjunctiva	Born with a defect, hereditary Mucous membrane which lines eyelids
contra (L) against, opposite	Contraception Contraindication	The prevention of conception A condition antagonistic to the line of treatment
dys (G) bad, difficult, painful	Dysentery	Inflammation of intestinal mucous membrane accompanied by pain

Contd...

Contd...

Prefix	Medical term	Definition
	Dysmenorrhea	Painful menstruation
	Dyspepsia	Imperfect digestion
	Dysphagia	Difficulty in swallowing
	Dysphasia	Impairment of speech
	Dyspnea	Labored or difficult breathing
	Dysuria	Pain or difficult urination
ec (G) out, ecto (G) outside	Ectopic pregnancy	Gestation outside the uterine cavity
ex-out	Ectropion of eyelid	Eversion as the edge of the eyelid
em, en (G)	Empyema	Pus in a body cavity, especially in the pleural cavity
in	Encephalopathy	Any disease of the brain
endo (G) within	Endocardium	Lining membrane of inner surface of the heart
	Endocarditis	Inflammation of the endocardium
	Endocrine gland	A ductless gland in which an internal secretion forms
	Endometrium	The mucous membrane lining the inner surface of the uterus
	Endometritis	Inflammation of the endometrium
	Endoscope	Tubular instrument for examining cavities through natural openings
	Endoscopy	Inspection of cavities by use of the endoscope
epi (G) upon, at, in addition to	Epidermis	Cuticle or outer layer of the skin
	Epigastrium	Region over the pit of the stomach
	Epiphysis	A center of ossification at both extremities of long bones
ex (G) out, away from, over	Exacerbation	Aggrevation of symptoms
	Exophthalmia	Abnormal protrusion of the eyeballs
	Expectoration	Expulsion of mucus from the lungs
	Exudate	Accumulation of fluid due to inflammatory condition
hemi (G), or	Hemiplegia	Paralysis of one-half of the body
	Hemiglossectomy	Removal of half a tongue
semi (L) half		
hyper (G) above, excessive, beyond	Hyperacidity	An excess of acid in the stomach
	Hypercalcemia	Excess of calcium in the blood
	Hyperemisis gravidarum	Excessive vomiting during early pregnancy
	Hyperemia	Congestion
	Hyperpyrexia	High fever (above 106 degree Fahrenheit)
	Hypertension	High blood pressure
hypo (G) beneath, below, deficient	Hypodermic injection	Injection under the skin
	Hypoglycemia	Low blood sugar
inter (L)	Intercostal	Between two ribs

Contd...

Contd...

Prefix	Medical term	Definition
between	Interfemoral	Between the thighs
meta (G)	Metabolism	The sum of all the physical and chemical processes by which living organized substance is produced and maintained
next, between	Metacarpal	Bone of the metacarpus
para, par (G)	Paracentesis	Puncture of a cavity with tapping
beside,	Parametritis	Inflammation of the parametrium
around, near,	Paranephritis	Inflammation of suprarenal capsules; of connective tissue above the kidney
abnormal	Parathyroid	Ductless gland near the thyroid gland
peri (G)	Pericardium	The double membranous sac enclosing the heart
around,	Pericarditis	Inflammation of the pericardium
about	Perimetritis	Inflammation of the serous membrane enveloping the uterus
	Periostitis	Inflammation of the periosteum
pre (L, G)	Precancerous	Before the development of carcinoma
before,	Pericardium	Region over the heart
in front of	Preeclampsia	Eclampsia before delivery (Eclampsia is major toxemia during pregnancy)
	Presentation	Manner of the fetus presenting itself at the cervix
pyo (G)	Pyocele	A collection of pus in the scrotum
pus	Pyocyst	A cyst containing pus
	Pyonephritis	Prulent inflammation of the kidney
post (G)	Postpartum	After delivery
	Postnatal	After birth
retro (L)	Retroflexion	A bending or flexing backward; for example of the uterus
backward, behind,	Retroperitoneal	Located behind the peritoneum
back of	Retroversion	A state of being turned back; for example, of the uterus
semi (L)	Semicoma	Mild degree of coma
half	Semilunar valves	Half-moon shaped valves of the aorta and pulmonary
sub (L)	Subclavicular	Beneath the clavicle
under,	Subcutaneous	Beneath the skin
beneath, below	Suppuration	The process of pus formation
super,	Supernatant	Floating on surface
	Supraoccipital	Situated above the occiput
supra (L) above, beyond,	Suprapubic cystotomy	Surgical opening into the bladder from above the symphysis pubis
superior	Suprarenal	Adrenal gland above the kidney

Contd...

Contd...

Prefix	Medical term	Definition
sym, sym (G) with, along, together, beside	Symphysis of pubis Synarthrosis Syndactlism	Fusion of pubic bone on midline anteriorly An immovable joint A fusion of two or more fingers or toes; webbing
toxi (G) poison	Toxicology Toxicosis Toxicophobia	The science or study of poisons Any diseased condition due to poisoning Irrational fear of being poisoned
trans (L) across, over	Transection Transfusion Transurethral prostatectomy	Incision across the long axis; cross section Injection of the blood of one person into the blood vessel of another Excision of the prostate gland through the urethra
tri (G) three	Tricuspid Trifacial Trigone	Having three cusps or points; tricuspid valve Fifth cranial nerve A triangular space, especially that of the lower part of the urinary bladder

COMMON ABBREVIATIONS

S.No.	Abbreviation	Term
1.	ACC	Adenoid cystic carcinoma
2.	AMA	Against medical advice
3.	Ant.	Anterior
4.	b.i.d.	Twice a day (bis in die)
5.	BID	Brought in dead
6.	C	Centrigrade (Centum gradus)
7.	CA(Ca)	Carcinoma
8.	CC	Chief complaint
9.	CSSD	Central sterile supply department
10.	DOA	Date of admission
11.	DOD	Date of discharge or death
12.	Dx	Diagnosis
13.	ER	Emergency room
14.	EUA	Examination under anesthesia
15.	FB	Foreign body
16.	F/U	Follow-up
17.	FUO	Fever of unknown origin
18.	GA	General anesthesia
19.	GP	General practitioner
20.	GS	General surgery
21.	GSH	Glomerulus stimulating hormone
22.	HPI	History of present illness
23.	ICD	International classification of disease
24.	IMP	Improved
25.	I and O	Intake and output
26.	IP	Inpatient
27.	IV	Intravenously
28.	LA	Local anesthesia
29.	MH	Marital history
30.	MSW	Medical social worker

Contd...

Contd...

S.No.	Abbreviation	Term
31.	NAD	Nothing abnormal detected
32.	NBM	Nothing by mouth
33.	N/C	No complaints
34.	NEC	Not elsewhere classified
35.	NED	No evidence of disease
36.	NOS	Not otherwise specified
37.	NYD	Not yet diagnosed
38.	O/A	On admission
39.	OD	Once a day
40.	OE	On examination
41.	O and E	Observation and examination
42.	OP	Out-patient
43.	OPC	Out-patient clinic
44.	OR	Operating room
45.	OT	Operation theater
46.	PH	Past history
47.	PI	Present illness
48.	PM	Postmortem
49.	PO	Postoperative
50.	PP	Postpartum
51.	q.d	Quaque die (everyday)
52.	q.d.h	Quaque duo hora (every two hours)
53.	q.h	Quaque horo (every hour)
54.	q.i.d.	Quarter in die (four times daily)
55.	q.n	Quaque nocte (every night)
56.	q.n.s	Quantum non-statis (insufficient quantity)
57.	q.q.h	Quaque quarta hora (every four hours)
58.	q.s	Quantum statis (sufficient quantity)
59.	q.t.h	Quoque tres hora (every three hours)
60.	q.v	Quantum vis (as much as desired)
61.	RAD	Radiation absorbed dose
62.	RFB	Retained foreign body
63.	RR	Recovery room
64.	RT	Radiation therapy
65.	Rx	Recipe (take)
66.	Sx	Symptoms
67.	Tx	Therapy
68.	US	Ultrasound
69.	VS	Vital signs
70.	WNL	Within normal limits
71.	XR	X-ray

Musculoskeletal System

MUSCULAR SYSTEM

INTRODUCTION

The musculoskeletal system includes the bones, muscles, and joints. The skeleton (group of bones) forms a supportive framework and consists of a series of bony levers capable, by virtue of the joints and muscles, to move upon one another. Muscles provide major support for movements of the body. Muscles and bones make up for most of the body's weight. The muscles have the special characteristics of elongation and contraction by which they produce movements of the different parts of the body. The muscle gives the posture of the human body and supports it to withstand against the gravity. The muscles, which are attached to the skeleton, are called skeletal muscles. The skeletal muscle cells have various nerve endings which produce chemical reaction during contraction and results in generation of heat. Hence, muscular activity plays an important role in maintaining the body temperature.

PROPERTIES OF MUSCLE

The power of contraction: Voluntary muscles contract as a result of stimuli reaching them from the nervous system and many nerves have their endings in muscles.

Elasticity: Muscle tissue is elastic and can be stretched by a weight, when the weight is removed, the muscle returns to its normal position.

Fatigue: When a muscle contracts, it looses energy. This energy is derived from the glucose stored in the muscle as glycogen.

Muscular tone: Even when a muscle appears to be at rest, it is always partially contracted and ready for immediate action. This state of partial contraction is called muscle tone and it is important in maintaining body posture.

CHARACTERISTICS OF MUSCULAR TISSUE

1. *Irritability or excitability:* Property of receiving stimuli and responding to them.
2. *Contractility:* Capacity of muscles to become short in response to suitable stimulous.
3. *Extensibility:* Muscle can be stretched, i.e. the property of individual cells.
4. *Elasticity:* Muscle readily returns to original shape.

Attachment of muscle: At the extremities of the muscles the connective tissue are present which form strong fibrous, non-elastic cards called tendons. Tendon attach a muscle to the bone. Sometimes they form a broad, flat expansion called as aponeurosis.

MUSCULAR TISSUE

The muscles are structures, which give the power of movement. Muscles are composed of 1000 of elongated cells, called muscle fibers, each containing a small nucleus. Bundle of muscle fibers lie side by side like threads in a skin. Three types of muscular tissues are found in the body. They are:

Voluntary or Striated or Skeletal Muscles

Voluntary muscle is attached to the skin. It is under the control of the will and is formed from long multi-nucleated cells which show a striped or striated pattern of dark and light bands in their cytoplasm. Voluntary muscles plays an important role for movement, power and strength of the body.

Involuntary or Smooth or Nonstriated or Visceral Muscles

These muscles are found in the internal organs and structures of the body such as the stomach, intestine, bladder, uterus, bronchi and blood vessels. Hence, it is also called as internal muscles or visceral muscles. It cannot be controlled by the will. It consists a series of elongated spindle-shaped cell. It has a single nucleus. Smooth muscle forms sheets of fibers as it wraps around tubes and vessels.

Cardiac Muscle

This is a special type of muscle found only in the heart. It is striated in appearance but nonstriated in action. Cardiac muscle fibers are cylindrical with centrally placed nuclei and connected strongly with adjacent fibers at intercalated disks. Its movements cannot be consciously controlled.

FUNCTIONS OF MUSCLE

Skeletal (striated) muscles are the muscles, which move the bones of body. When a muscle contracts, one of the bones to which it is joined remains virtually stationary as a result of other muscles, which holds it in place.
*   Provide the framework
*   Supports the body and gives shape
*   Give attachment to bones and tendons
*   Permit movements of the body as a whole and of parts of the body, by forming joints, that are moved by muscles.

Important muscles of upper and lower limb, head, neck and trunk are shown in Table 2.1, and their functions shown in Table 2.2. Figures 2.1 and 2.2 show anterior and posterior muscles.

DIFFERENT FUNCTIONS OF MUSCLES

Flexors	:	Muscles which bend a limb at a joint
Extensor	:	Muscle which straighten a limb at a joint
Abductor	:	Muscle which moves the limb away from the midline of the body
Adductors	:	Muscle which moves the limb towards the midline of the body
Elevators	:	Muscle which raises the part of the body
Depressors	:	Muscle which lowers a part of the body.

Table 2.1: Important muscles

Head, neck and shoulder	Trunk	Upper limb	Lower limb
• Frontalis • Orbicularis oculi • Zygomaticus major • Orbicularis oris • Masseter • Depressor anguli and depressor labii • Sternohyoid • Sternocleidomastoid • Trapezius	• Pectoralis major • Serratus anterior • Teres major and minor • Latissimus dorsi • Rectus abdominis • Transversus • External oblique • Internal oblique • External abdominis • Gluteus maximus • Gluteus medius	• Deltoid • Biceps • Triceps • Brachialis major • Carpi radialis • Carpi ulna • Long and short extensors of thumb	• Gluteus maximus • Adductor • Hamstring • Rectus femoris major • Sartorius major • Biceps • Gastrocnemius • Anterior tibial major

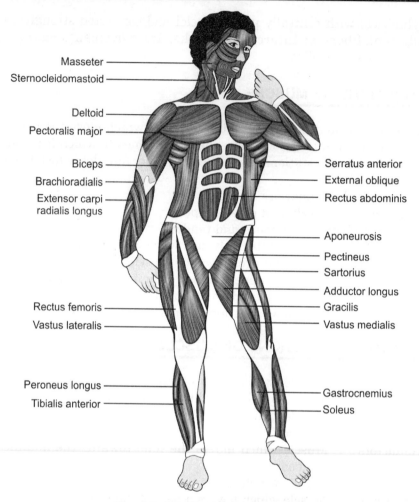

Fig. 2.1: Muscles—anterior view

Table 2.2: Muscles and their functions

S.No.	Region	Name of the muscle	Function
1.	Scalp	Epicranial or occipito frontalis	Move the scalp
2.	Head	a. Platysma	Flex head on the chest
		b. Sternomastoid Capitis (3)	Extends the head
3.	Eyes	Orbicularis oculi	Closes the eyes tightly
		Livator palpebrae superioris	Raises the eyelid
4.	Lips	Orbicularis oris	Closeslips tightly
		Buccinator	Opens the lips
5.	Mastication	Masseter	Helps in chewing
		Temporalis	

Contd...

Contd...

S.No.	Region	Name of the muscle	Function
6.	Tongue	Genioglossus	Pulls the tongue forward
		Styloglossus	Pulls the tongue backward
7.	Scapula	Serratus anterior	Abducts the scapula (extends the reach)
		Trapezius	Adducts the scapula and raises the shoulder
8.	Shoulder joint	Deltoid	Abducts the humerus (arm)
		Supraspinatus	
		Pectoralis major	Adducts the humerus (arm)
		Coracobrachialis	Pulls arm across chest (flexes arm)
		Teres major	Extends arm
		Latissimus dorsi	Rotates humerus inwards
		Teres minor	Rotates the humerus (outwards)
		Infraspinatus	
9.	Inspiration	Intercostal	Helps in inspiration
		Internal	
		External	
		Diaphragm	
10.	Expiration	Rectus abdominis	Helps in expiration
		External oblique	
		Internal oblique	
		Transverse	
11.	Back	Sacrospinalis	Holds spine erect
		Quadratus lumborum	Helps spine erect
12.	Floor of pelvis	Levator ani	Form floor of pelvis
		Coccygeus	
13.	Hip	Ilio-psoas	Flexes thigh on the trunk
		Psoas major	
		Iliacus	
		Sartorius	Flex hip knee joint
		Gracilis	
		Gluteus maximus	Extends femur
		Gluteus medius	Abduct femur
		Brevis	
		Adductor Longus	Adduct femur
		Magnus	
		Gluteus minimus	Rotates femur inwards
		Piriformis	Rotates femur outwards
14.	Knee	Hamstring	
		a. Semitendinosus	
		b. Semimembranosus	
		c. Biceps femoris	
		Sartorius	Flex the knee joint
		Gracilis	
		Quadriceps femoris	
		a. Rectus femoris	
		b. Vastus medialis	Extend the knee joint
		c. Vastus intermedius	
		d. Vastus lateralis	
15.	Forearm	Brachialis	Flexes the forearm
		Biceps brachi (Ant)	
		Triceps brachi (Post)	Extends the forearm
		Precips brachi	Supinate the hand
		Pronator teres (Upper end)	Pronate the hand
		Pronator quadratus (Lower)	
16.	Fingers	Flexors	Flex fingers
		Extensors (Post)	Extend fingers
		Forearm	

Contd...

Contd...

S.No.	Region	Name of the muscle	Function
17.	Thumb	Thenar group	
18.	Feet	Anterior tibialis	Flexes the foot
			Inverts the foot
		Gastrocnemius	
		Soleus	Extends the foot in walking
		Posterior tibialis	Extends the foot helps in invert the foot
		Peroneus (3)	Evert the foot
			Help to flex the foot
		Tibialis (Ant)	
		Tibialis (Post)	Invert the foot

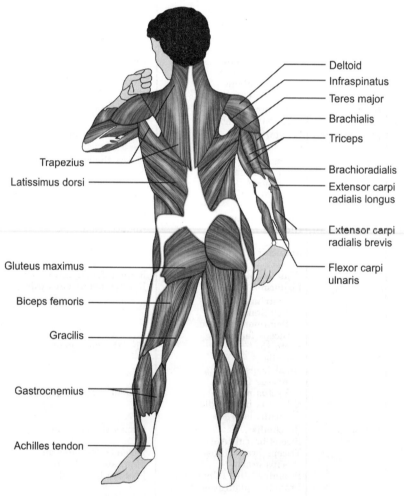

Fig. 2.2: Muscles—posterior view

SKELETAL SYSTEM

INTRODUCTION

Bones are organs composed of connective tissues called osseous (bony) tissue with a rich supply of blood vessels and nerves. Osseous tissue consists of osteocytes (bone cells), which forms bones by ossification. The inner core of bones is composed of hematopoietic tissue (red and yellow bone marrow, manufacturers of blood cells), while other parts are storage areas for minerals necessary for growth, such as calcium and phosphorus. This is the hardest of all the connective tissues. Osteology is the study of the bones.

FORMATION OF BONE

The bones are developed during the fetal stage of the human being, during that time it is made of cartilage tissue which will be less dense. Gradually, the calcium and immature bone cells are deposited on the cartilage tissues while the child grows and thus the bone becomes harder and forms the body structure. The development of bones depends on proper supply of calcium, phosphorus and vitamin D to the bone tissue. In long bones a primary center of ossification forms the shaft (diaphysis) and secondary center borns the ends (epiphysis). When the adult length of bone is reached, the epiphyseal cartilage is ossified to form strong bones.

FUNCTIONS OF BONE

- Provide the framework.
- Support the body and gives shape.
- Give attachment to muscles and tendons.
- Permit movement of the body as a whole and of parts of the body, by forming joints that are moved by muscles.
- Form the boundaries of the cranial, thoracic and pelvic cavities, protecting the organs they contain red bone marrow in which blood cells develop.
- Provide a reservoir of calcium, potassium, phosphorus and sodium.

TYPES OF BONE (FIGS 2.3 AND 2.4)

The bones of the skeleton are classified according to their shape into long, short, flat and irregular bones.

Long Bones

Long bones are found in the limbs or extremities of the body and consist of long shaft with two extremities. The bones of the arm, forearm, thigh and legs are typical examples. The shaft consists of a cylinder of compact bone containing yellow bone marrow. The extremities are formed by a thin outer shell of compact tissue with an interior network of spongy or cancellous bone containing red bone marrow.

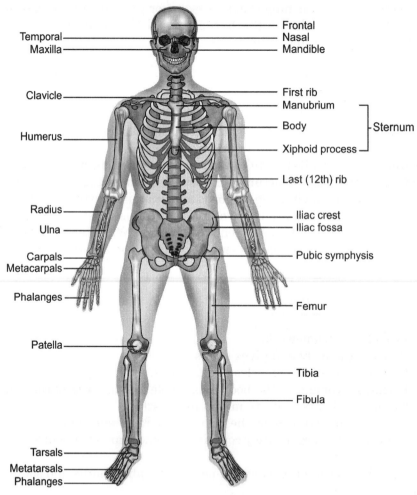

Fig. 2.3: Bones—anterior view

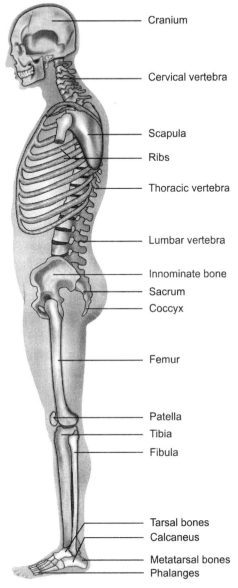

- Cranium
- Cervical vertebra
- Scapula
- Ribs
- Thoracic vertebra
- Lumbar vertebra
- Innominate bone
- Sacrum
- Coccyx
- Femur
- Patella
- Tibia
- Fibula
- Tarsal bones
- Calcaneus
- Metatarsal bones
- Phalanges

Fig. 2.4: Bones—lateral view

Short Bones

Short bones have no shaft but consist of smaller mass of spongy bones surrounded by a shell of compact bone. They are roughly box like in shape. They are found in the small bones of the wrist (carpals) and ankle (tarsal).

Flat Bones

Flat bones provide broad surfaces for muscular attachment and extensive protection for internal organs. It is made of cancellous bone sandwiched by two compact bones. Examples are bones of skull, shoulder blades (scapula) and sternum.

Irregular Bones

Irregular bones cannot be classified under any of the previous types, because of their peculiar shapes. Examples: the bones of the face and the vertebra.

Sesamoid Bones

Bones which are developed in the tendons of the muscles and are found in the vicinity of a joint. The patella is the largest sesamoid bone to quote as an example.

STRUCTURE AND TERMS USED TO DESCRIBE THE BONES

Bone process: The portion of the bone that projects is called a process.

Bone head: Rounded end of a bone separated from the body of the bone by a neck.

Tubercle: Small, rounded process which serves as a site of tendon or muscle attachment.

Trochanter: Large projection on femur which serves as a site of attachment for muscles.

Condyle: Rounded knuckle-like process at the joint.

Epicondyle: A small projection adjacent to a condyle usually giving attachments to the ligaments.

Tuberosity: Large, round process which serves as a site of muscle or tendon attachment.

Crest: An elevated ridge of the bone.

Facet: A small articulating surface of the bone.

Process: A projection from a bone.

Bone Depressions

The openings or hollow regions in a bone which help to join one bone to another and serve as passageways for blood vessels and nerves. They are:

Fossa: Depression or cavity of a bone.

Foramen: Opening for blood vessels and nerves.

Fissure: Narrow, deep, slit like opening.

Sulcus: Groove or furrow.

Sinus: Air cavity within a bone.

Articulation: A joint between two bones.

Border: The edge separating two surface of the bone.

BONES OF DIFFERENT LOCATIONS (TABLE 2.3)

The human skeleton contains 206 bones present in the adult. The classification of the bones according to the parts are listed below.

The skull consists cranium, face and lower jaw. The trunk consists spinal column, ribs and sternum. The limbs consist of upper and lower limbs together with shoulder and pelvic girdles.

Cranial Bones

The bones of the skull protect the brain and structures related to it, such as eye, ear and nose. The cranial bones of a newborn child are not completely joined. There will be gaps of unossified tissue in the skull, these are called soft spots. The bones are:

Frontal bone: Forms the forehead and bony sockets which contain the eyes.

Parietal bone: Two parietal bones which form the roof and upper part of the sides of the cranium.

Temporal bone: Two temporal bones forms the lower sides and base of the cranium. Each bone encloses an ear and contains a fossa for joining with the mandible. The mastoid process is a round process of the temporal bone behind the ear.

Occipital bone: Forms the back and base of the skull and joins the parietal and temporal bones, forming a suture. The inferior portion of the occipital bone has an opening called the foramen magnum through which the spinal cord passes.

Sphenoid bone: The bat shaped bone extends behind the eyes and forms part of the base of the skull.

Ethmoid bone: Thin delicate, spongy and cancellous bone supporting the nasal cavity and forms part of the orbits of the eyes.

Table 2.3: Table of bones

S.No.	Names of the regions/bones		Total number
1.	**Axial skeleton**		
	Skull		
	a. Frontal		
	b. Parietal 1 × 2		
	c. Temporal × 2		
	d. Occipital		
	e. Sphenoid		
	f. Ethmoid	Total 8	
	Face		
	a. Inferior nasal concha × 2		
	b. Lacrimal × 2		
	c. Maxilla × 2		
	d. Nasal × 2		
	e. Palatine × 2		
	f. Zygomatic × 2		
	g. Vomer		
	h. Mandible	Total 14	
	Ear		
	a. Malleus × 2		
	b. Incus × 2		
	c. Stapes × 2	Total 6	
	Neck		
	Hyoid	Total 1	29
2.	**Thoracic cavity**		
	Vertebral columns		
	a. Cervical 7		
	b. Thoracic 12		
	c. Lumbar 5		
	d. Sacrum 1		
	e. Coccyx 1	Total 26	
	Chest		
	a. Sternum 1		
	b. Ribs 12 × 2	Total 25	51
3.	**Upper limb**		
	Shoulder		
	Scapula 2		
	Clavicle 2	Total 4	
	Upper arm		
	Humerus 2	Total 2	
	Lower arm		
	Radius 2		
	Ulna 2	Total 4	
	Hands		
	a. Carpal 8 × 2 (16)		
	b. Metacarpal 5 × 2 (10)	Total 26	
	Fingers		
	a. Phalanges 14 × 2 (28)	Total 28	64
4.	**Lower limb**		
	Pelvis 2		
	Femur 2		
	Patella 2		
	Tibia 2		
	Fibula 2		
	Tarsal 7 × 2 (14)		
	Metatarsal 5 × 2 (10)		
	Phalanges 14 × 2 (28)	Total 62	62
		Total	**206**

Facial Bones

Most of the facial bones are immovable bones joined by sutures. The only movable bone is mandible for chewing.

Nasal bones: Two nasal bones supporting to form the bridge of the nose.

Lacrimal bones: Two paired lacrimal bones are located one at the corner of the each eye.

Maxillary bones: Two large bones compose the massive upper jaw bones.

Mandibular bone: This bone forms the lower jaw. Both the maxilla and mandible contain the sockets called alveoli in which the teeth are embedded. The mandible joins the skull at the region of the temporal bone, forming the temporomandibular joint on either side of the skull.

Zygomatic bones: Two bones, one on each side of the face, form the high portion of the cheek.

Vomer: The thin, single, flat bone forms the lower portion of the nasal septum.

Bones of Vertebral Column

The vertebral column is composed of 26 bone segments, called vertebrae, arranged in five divisions.

Cervical vertebrae: The first seven bones of the vertebral column, forming the neck bone.

Thoracic vertebrae: The second set of 12 bones which joins to the 12 pairs of ribs.

Lumbar vertebrae: The third set of five vertebral bones. They are strongest and largest of the backbones.

The sacrum: The set of four bones slightly curved, triangularly shaped bone. At birth it is composed of five separate segments, these gradually become fused in the young child.

The coccyx: This is the set of five bones and it is the tailbone of the spinal or vertebral column fused together.

Bones of Thorax, Pelvis and Extremities

Clavicle: This is collar bone, one on each side of the body, connecting the breastbone to each shoulder bone.

Scapula: Shoulder bone, two flat and triangular bones, one on each dorsal side of the thorax.

Sternum: Breast bone, a flat bone extending down the midline of the chest. The uppermost part of the sternum joins on the sides with the clavicle and ribs. The lower portion of the sternum is called the xiphoid process.

Ribs: There are 12 pairs of ribs. Out of 12 pairs, the first seven pairs (1-7) joins the sternum which are called true ribs, the ribs (8-10) are called false ribs, these ribs join the 7th rib anteriorly, instead of the sternum. Ribs 11 and 12 are the floating ribs, as they are completely free at their anterior extremity.

Bones of Arm and Hand

Humerus: Upper arm bone, the upper head joins with scapula and clavicle.

Ulna: One of the lower arm bones.

Radius: One of the lower arm bones.

Carpals: Wrist bones, composed of two rows of four bones each.

Metacarpals: Five radiating bones to the finger.

Phalanges: Finger bones each finger has three phalanges, except the thumb which has only two.

Bones of the Pelvis

Pelvic girdle: Hip bone, large bone supporting the trunk of the body and joins the thigh bone and sacrum. The ilium is the uppermost large portion, ischium is the posterior part of the pelvis. Pubis is the anterior part of the pelvis.

Differences between male and female pelvic bone depicted in Table 2.4.

Bones of the Leg and Foot

Femur: Thigh bone, this is the longest bone in the body. The head of the bone joins the socket of the hip bone. This socket is called acetabulum.

Table 2.4: Differences between male and female pelvic bone

S.No.	Name of the bone	Male	Female
1.	Ilium	Narrow and heavy	Broad and light
2.	Inlet	Round	Oval
3.	Pubic	Less than 90°	Greater than 90°
4.	Sacrum	Long and narrow	Short and broad

Patella: Kneecap, this is small, flat bone which lies in front of the joint between the femur and tibia.

Tibia: The largest of the two lower bones of the leg, it joins with femur and patella at the upper end and with ankle at lower end. The tibia is commonly called the shin bone.

Fibula: Smaller of two lower leg bones, this is thin bone.

Tarsals: Ankle bones, there are seven short bones which resemble carpal bones of the wrist but slightly larger. The calcaneus is the largest of these bones and also called as heel bone.

Metatarsals: There are five metatarsal bones, each leading to the toes.

Phalanges of the toes: Toe bones—each toe has three phalanges, except the big which has only two.

JOINTS

The joints are the places where two or more bones meet. This is also called as articulation. They are concerned with growth, rigidity and movement. There are three types of joints:
1. Fixed joints or immovable joints or synarthrosis or fibrous
2. Slightly movable joints or amphiarthrosis or cartilaginous
3. Freely movable joints or diarthrosis or synovial.

Fixed or Synarthrosis or Fibrous Joints

Synarthrosis or fibrous or fixed joint is a joint which does not permit movement at all. Bones come together and are bound, or united, by a layer of fibrous tissue which does not permit movement.

Examples of synarthrosis or fibrous or fixed joints are:
• Suture joints of the skull.
• Peg and socket—the teeth in their socket.

Slightly Movable or Amphiarthrosis or Cartilaginous Joints

Amphiarthrosis or cartilaginous or lightly movable joint is an articulation which permits slight movement. The bone surfaces of the joint are connected by elastic fibrocartilage and are partially movable.

Examples of amphiarthrosis or cartilaginous or lightly movable joints are found between the vertebrae and between the small bones of the ankle and wrist.

Freely Movable or Diarthrosis or Synovial Joints

A diarthrosis or synovial joint is a freely movable joint. Examples are ball and socket joint (hip joint) and hinge joint (elbow joint).

The bones in a diarthrotic joint are separated by a joint capsule, composed of fibrous cartilage tissue. Ligaments (fibrous bands, or sheets, of connective tissue). Often they anchor the bones together around capsule to strengthen it. The surface of the bones at the joint is covered with a smooth cartilage surface called the articular cartilage. The synovial membrane lies under the joint capsule and lines the synovial cavity which is filled with a special type of lubricating fluid called synovial fluid produced by synovial membrane.

Varieties of Synovial Joints

1. *Gliding or plane:* Two flat sufraces glide over each other, e.g. carpus and tarsus.
2. *Ball and socket:* One rounded extremity fits into a cavity in another bone, e.g. hip joint and shoulder.
3. *Hinge joint:* One rounded surfaces of the bone fits another so that movement is only possible in one place, e.g. elbow joint.
4. *Condyloid joint:* Similar to hinge joint, but moves into two planes, e.g. the wrist joint.
5. *Trochoid or pivot:* Where rotation only is possible, e.g. the head where the atlas rotates around axis.
6. *Saddle joint:* Concave-convex surface is received by another convex—concave surface, e.g. the thumb.

BURSAE

Bursae are closed sacs of synovial fluid lined within the synovial membrane. They are formed in the space between tendons (connective tissue binding muscle to the bones), ligaments (connective tissue binding bones to bones) and bones. It lubricates these areas where friction would normally develop close to the joint capsule.

MOVEMENTS OF JOINTS

- *Gliding movements:* Two flat surfaces move on each other.
- *Angular movements:* Described according to the direction in which the movement takes place.

- *Flexion:* Bending or doubling up.
- *Extension:* Stretching or straightening out.
- *Adduction:* Movement towards the medial aspect of the body.
- *Abduction:* Movement away from the medial aspect of the body.
- *Circumduction:* A combination of rotation and angular movements.

MUSCULOSKELETAL SYSTEM

Origin of Terms

S.No.	Terms	Meanings
1.	Acetabul/o	Acetabulum
2.	Acromi/o	Acromion
3.	Amphi	on both sides
4.	Ankyl/o	Stiff joint, fusion or growing together of parts
5.	Ankyle	Stiff joint
6.	Arthr	Joint
7.	Arthron, Articul	Joint
8.	-blast	Germ cell, primitive, embryonic
9.	Brachi/o	Arm
10.	Bursa	Purse, sac
11.	Calc/o	Calcium
12.	Calcane/o	Calcaneum, heel bone
13.	Carp/o	Wrist, carpus
14.	Cartilage	Gristle
15.	Cavus	Hollow
16.	Cephal	Head
17.	Cervi	Neck
18.	Chondr/o	Cartilage
19.	-clast	To break
20.	Clavicul/o	Clavicle
21.	Condyl/o	Rounded projection on a bone
22.	Condylos	Knuckle
23.	Cost/o	Ribs
24.	Coxa	Hip
25.	Crani	Skull bones
26.	Crani/o	Skull bones, cranium
27.	Dactyl/o	Digit
28.	-desis	Binding, stabilization
29.	Fascia	Band
30.	Femor/o	Femur
31.	Fibros	Fibrous
32.	Fibul/o	Fibula
33.	Genu	Knee
34.	Hallux	Great toe

Contd...

Contd...

S.No.	Terms	Meanings
35.	Humer/o	Humerus
36.	Ili/o	Ilium
37.	Ischi/o	Ischium
38.	Kyphos	Hump
39.	Lamin	Part of vertebral arch
40.	Leios	Smooth
41.	Ligament	That which ties
42.	Lordosis	Bending backbone with forward curvature
43.	Lumb/o	Loins
44.	Luxatio	To dislocate
45.	-malacia	Softening
46.	Malleol/o	Malleolus
47.	Malleus	Hammer
48.	Mandibulum	Lower jaw
49.	Maxilla/o	Upper jaw bone
50.	Meniskos	Cresent
51.	Metacarp/o	Metacarpals
52.	Myel/o	Bone marrow, spinal cord
53.	Myo	Muscle
54.	Oesteo	Bone
55.	Olecran/o	Elbow
56.	Patell/o	Patella, kneecap
57.	Ped/I, pod/o	Foot
58.	Pelv/I	Pelvi
59.	Pelv/I	Pelvic bone
60.	Phalang/o	Phalanges
61.	Phragm	Fence, wall
62.	-physis	to grow
63.	Planus	Flat
64.	Plasty	Formation, surgical repair, plastic repair
65.	-porosis	Pores or cavities
66.	Pub/o	Pubis anterior
67.	Radi/o	Radius; ray
68.	Rhabdo	Rod, striated
69.	Scapula/o	Scapula
70.	-schisis	To split
71.	Scoli/o	Crooked, bent
72.	Spondyl, Vertebr/o	Vertebra
73.	Spondylos	Vertebra
74.	Stern/o	Sternum, breastbone
75.	Submaxill/o	Lower jaw bone
76.	Syn	Together
77.	Taliped	Club footed
78.	Talus	Heel, ankle
79.	tendo, teno	Tendon
80.	Thorac/o	Chest
81.	Tibi/o	Tibia
82.	Uln/o	Ulna
83.	Valgus	Bentout, or twisted

SYMPTOMATIC AND DIAGNOSTIC TERMS

S.No.	Terms	Meanings
1.	Ankylosing spondylitis	Chronic, progressive arthritis with stiffening of joints, primarily of the spine
2.	Ankylosis	Stiff joint
3.	Arthritis	Inflammation of joints
4.	Arthrocentesis	Surgical puncture of the joint space with a needle
5.	Arthropathy	Any disease of the joints
6.	Arthroscopy	Visual examination of the inside of a joint with an endoscopy
7.	Bunion	Swelling of the bursal sac at the metatarsophalangeal joint near the base of the big toe
8.	Bursitis	Inflammation of a bursa
9.	Capsulitis	Inflammation of joint capsule
10.	Carpal tunnel syndrome	Soreness, tenderness, and weakness of the muscles of the thumb caused by pressure on the median nerve at the point at which it goes through the carpal tunnel of the wrist
11.	Carpoptosis	Wrist drop
12.	Cervicitis	Painful neck
13.	Chondritis	Inflammation of a cartilage
14.	Chondroblastoma	Benign, vascular, cartilaginous tumor arising from the epiphysis of a long bone
15.	Chondroma	Benign neoplasm arising from cartilage
16.	Chondrosarcoma	Malignant tumor derived from cartilage
17.	Claudication	Limping, intermittent type due to ischemia of leg muscles
18.	Contracture	Permanent shortening of one or more muscles caused by paralysis, spasm or scar formation
19.	Crepitation	A dry, crackling sound or sensation, such as that produced by the grating of the ends of a fractured bone
20.	Coxarthrosis	Arthrosis of hip
21.	Diaphysis	A shaft of long bone
22.	Dislocation	Displacement of a bone from its joint
23.	Electromyography	The process of recording the strength of muscle contraction as a result of electrical stimulation
24.	Exostoses	Bony growths arising from the surface of the bone
25.	Fascitis	Inflammation of the fascia
26.	Fracture	Sudden breaking of a bone
27.	Genu valgus	Knock-knee
28.	Genu varus	Bowleg
29.	Gouty arthritis	Inflammation of joints caused by excessive uric acid in the body
30.	Graphospasm	Writer's cramp
31.	Greenstick fracture	Fracture in children, especially due to rickets

Contd...

Contd...

S.No.	Terms	Meanings
32.	Gonarthrosis	Arthrosis of the knee due to degeneration or trauma
33.	Hematoma	Collection of blood under skin (bruise)
34.	Hemarthrosis	Bloody effusion in a joint cavity.
35.	Hyperkinesia	Abnormally increased muscular movement and physical activity
36.	Kyphosis	Hunchback; abnormal posterior curvature of thoracic spine
37.	Lumbago	Pain in the lumbar region.
38.	Multiple myeloma	A primary malignant tumor of plasma cells usually arising in bone marrow, usually progressive, and generally fatal.
39.	Muscular dystrophy	Progressive disease of unknown etiology, marked in infants by enlarged calves, waddling gait, sway back and winged shoulders. As the disease advances there is extensive wasting of muscles and development of bizarre deformities.
40.	Myasthenia gravis	Chronic neuromuscular disorder, characterized by weakness, usually first manifested in ocular muscles resulting in bilateral ptosis of eye lids and sleepy appearance. The myasthenic facies is apathetic and expressionless. There may be involvement of the muscles of speech, mastication and swallowing. When the chest muscles are affected, dyspnea may develop. Infrequently weakness of the legs inter-feres with walking. Symptoms fluctuate in severity ranging from exacerbations to remissions.
41.	Myoma	Benign muscular tumor
42.	Myositis	Inflammation of muscle
43.	Ossification	Bone formation
44.	Osteitis fibrosa cystica	Inflammation of bone with fibrous changes in the bone tissue
45.	Osteoarthritis	Chronic inflammation of bones and joints due to degenerative changes in cartilage.
46.	Osteoblasts	Bone forming cells
47.	Osteoclasia, osteolysis	Breaking plus absorption and destruction of bony tissue.
48.	Osteocytes	Bone cells lying in lacunae within intercellular substance
49.	Osteodystrophy	Abnormal development of bone
50.	Osteogenic sarcoma	Highly malignant, vascular tumor usually involving the upper part of long bones, the pelvis or knee. Metastases are common and life-threatening.
51.	Osteoid osteoma	A benign, small, very painful tumor, found in almost any bone of the skeleton but most frequently in the lower extremities

Contd...

Contd...

S.No.	Terms	Meanings
52.	Osteomalacia	Softening of bone caused by deficiency in calcium or phosphorus or both needed for ossification of mature bone in adults. In children the primary cause is lack of vitamin D and sunlight necessary for the normal absorption of the vitamin
53.	Osteomyelitis	Inflammation of the bone and bone marrow. Infective agents may be pyogenic bacteria, Brucella, *Salmonella* or other organisms.
54.	Osteoporosis	Loss of bone density
55.	Osteitis	Inflammation of bone
56.	Paget's disease	Osteitis deformans
57.	Polyarthritis	Inflammation of periosteum
58.	Polymyalgia rheumatica	Muscle pain, primarily of the shoulder and pelvis, with absence of arthritis and signs of muscle distress
59.	Polymyositis	A primary myopathy characterized by muscle weakness in pelvic and shoulder girdles, distal lower and upper extremities, muscle pain or tenderness. It may be associated with connective tissue disease.
60.	Protrusion of an intervertebral disk (disc), disk prolapse	Abnormal extension of a cartilaginous intervertebral pad into the neural canal
61.	Quadriplegia	Paralysis of all four limbs
62.	Rhabdomyoma	A striated muscle tumor
63.	Rheumatoid arthritis	Chronic disease in which joints become inflamed and painful. It is believed to be caused by an immune reaction against joint tissues.
64.	Rickets	Calcium and vitamin D deficiency or early childhood which leads to demineralization of bones and deformities.
65.	Sciatia	Painful condition most commonly caused by prolapse of the intervertebral disk associated with sciatic nerve
66.	Sequestrum	A piece of dead bone separated from the surrounding bone in necrosis.
67.	Spondylitis	Inflammation of one or more vertebrae
68.	Spondylosis	Ankylosis of vertebrae; also any degenerative lesion of the spine.
69.	Sprain	Twisting of a joint, with partial rupture of its ligaments.
70.	Subluxation	A partial or incomplete dislocation
71.	Synovitis	Inflammation of synovial membrane
72.	Systemic lupus Erythematosus	Chronic inflammatory disease involving joints, skin, kidneys, nervous system, heart and lungs.
73.	Talipes	Deformities of the foot, especially those occurring congenitally, club foot
74.	Tenosynovitis	Inflammation of synovial lining of tendon sheath

OPERATIVE TERMS

S.No.	Medical terms	Description
1.	Amputation	Partial or complete removal of limb
2.	Arthroclasia	Surgical breaking of a stiff joint
3.	Arthrocentesis	Puncturing of a joint, to remove accumulated fluid
4.	Arthrodesis	Surgical fixation of a joint to immobilize the joint
5.	Arthrolysis	Freeing the joining fibrous bands or excess cartilage to restore its mobility
6.	Arthroplasty	Surgical repair of a joint. The hip, knee, elbow and temporomandibular joints are best suited for reconstruction
7.	Arthroscopy	Endoscopic visualization of a joint
8.	Arthrotomy	Surgical opening of a joint
9.	Bone grafting	Transplantation of bone
10.	Bunionectomy	Removal of bony prominence (bunion) from medial aspect of first metatarsal head
11.	Bursectomy	Excision of bursa
12.	Closed reduction	Repair of fracture by manipulation and application of cast, or application of splint or traction apparatus in selected cases when the fractured ends are not in alignment
13.	Decompression	Relief of pressure, e.g. on nerve
14.	Disarticulation	Amputation or separation at a joint
15.	Keller's operation	Removal of bunion
16.	Laminectomy	Surgical excision of the posterior arch of a vertebra
17.	Menisectomy	Removal of semi-lunar cartilage of knee joint
18.	Myoplasty	Surgical repair of a muscle, e.g. by free muscle graft or pedicle graft
19.	Myorrhaphy	Suture of a muscle
20.	Myotosis	Stretching of a muscle
21.	Open reduction	Surgical repair of fracture; manipulation and insertion of plate, screws or nail with occasional prosthesis for severe fractures of the upper or lower end of the humerus or femur.
22.	Osteoplasty	Plastic surgery of the bones
23.	Spinal fusion	Fusion of spinal vertebrae
24.	Suture	Juncture line where two bones form a synarthrosis
25.	Sympathectomy	Removal of sympathetic nerve tissue
26.	Synovectomy	Excision of synovial membrane
27.	Tenodesis	Surgical fixation of a tendon
28.	Tenoplasty, tendoplasty	Surgical repair of a tendon
29.	Tenosynovectomy	Resection or removal of a tendon sheath
30.	Coccygectomy	Excision of the coccyx
31.	Prosthesis	Replacement of a missing part by an artificial substitute, such as an artificial extremity, knee, hip, etc.
32.	Rachiocentesis, rachicentesis	Puncture into the spinal column
33.	Sequestrectomy	Excision of a piece of dead bone separated from the sound bone in necrosis

COMMON ABBREVIATIONS

S.No.	Abbreviation	Term
1.	AC	Acromioclavicular (joint)
2.	AE	Above the elbow
3.	AJ	Ankle jerk
4.	AK	Above the knee
5.	AKA	Above knee amputation
6.	AP	Anteroposterior
7.	BE	Below the elbow
8.	BJM	Bones, joints, muscles
9.	BK	Below the knee
10.	BKA	Below knee amputation
11.	C-1	First cervical vertebra
12.	C-2	Second cervical vertebra
13.	Ca	Calcium
14.	CDH	Congenital dislocation of the hip
15.	CK	Creatine kinase
16.	DTR	Deep tendon reflexes
17.	EMg	Electromyography
18.	ESR	Erythrocyts sedimentation rate
19.	HD	His disarticulation
20.	HNP	Herniated nucleus pulposus (herniated disk)
21.	HP	Hemipelvectomy
22.	IDK	Internal derangement of knee
23.	IDKJ	Internal deranagement of knee joint
24.	IM	Intramuscular
25.	IS	Intracostal space
26.	KD	Knee disarticulation
27.	KJ	Knee jerk
28.	L-1	First lumbar vertebra
29.	L-2	Second lumbar vertebra
30.	L-3	Third lumbar vertebra
31.	LAT, Lat	Lateral
32.	LE cell	Lupus erythematosus cell
33.	MD	Muscular dystrophy
34.	NBI	No bone injury
35.	NSAID	Nonsteroidal anti-inflammatory drug
36.	OA	Osteoarthritis
37.	ORTH, Ortho	Orthopedics, orthopaedics
38.	P	Phosphorus
39.	PIVD	Prolapse intervertebral disk.
40.	PMA	Progressive muscular atrophy
41.	PMR	Physical medicine and rehabilitation
42.	POP	Plaster of paris
43.	RA	Rheumatoid arthritis
44.	RF	Rheumatoid factor
45.	RIF	Right iliac fossa
46.	SD	Shoulder disarticulation
47.	SI	Sacroiliac joint
48.	SLE	Systemic lupus erythematosis
49.	TEV	Talipes equiovarus
50.	T-1	First thoracic vertebra
51.	T-2	Second thoracic vertebra
52.	T-3	Third thoracic vertebra
53.	THA	Total hip arthroplasty
54.	THR	Total hip replacement
55.	TKA	Total knee arthroplasty
56.	TKR	Total knee replacement

3

Cardiovascular System

INTRODUCTION

The various organs in the body need energy from the food substances which reach them after being taken into the body. Food contains stored energy which can be converted into the energy for movements and work. This conversion of stored energy into active energy of work occurs when food and oxygen combine in cells during the chemical process of catabolism. It is obvious then that each cell of each organ is dependent on a constant supply of food and oxygen in order to receive sufficient energy to work well. The cardiovascular system plays a vital role in transporting food and oxygen to all organs and cells of the body through the fluid called blood vessels to carry the blood and the muscular pump called the heart. In addition to this, these blood vessels are used to transport cellular waste materials such as carbon dioxide and urea to the lungs and kidneys respectively, where it is removed from the body. Thus the cardiovascular system is one of the important systems of the human body.

The cardiovascular system is the transport system, carrying oxygen, nutrition, hormones and other substances to the tissues and conveying carbon dioxide to the lungs and other waste products to the kidney.

Arteries, arterioles, veins, venules and capillaries, together with the heart form cardiovascular system for the flow of blood.

ARTERIES

Arteries are the blood vessels which carry oxygenated blood from the heart to the various parts of the body. The microscopic structure of arteries has three layers:

1. Tunica adventia   –   Outer layer
2. Tunica media   –   Middle layer
3. Tunica intima   –   Inner layer

Table 3.1: Important arteries

Head and brain	Upper limb	Lower limb	Chest	Thigh
• Occipital • Cerebellar • Basilar • Temporal • Supraorbital • Supratrochlear • Maxillary • Carotid • Common carotid • Deep cervical • Vertebral • Thoracic • Subclavian	• Cervical • Vertebral • Common carotid • Suprascapular • Deltoid • Brachial • Radial • Ulnar • Interosseous • Palmar • Digital	• Genicular • Popliteal • Femoral • Tibial • Fibular • Calcaneal	• Subclavian • Brachiocephalic • Axillary • Pulmonary • Aorta • Ascending aorta • Arch of aorta • Descending aorta • Intercostal • Renal • Inferior mesenteric • Common iliac • Thoracic • Clavicular • Pectoral	• Abdominal aorta • Common iliac • Middle sacral • Inguinal • Femoral • Perineal • Urethral • Penis • Rectal

Tunica adventia is composed of fibrous tissue which gives protection and strength to the vessels. Tunica media is composed of smooth muscle with yellow elastic fibers which are arranged in circular manner. It contracts and relaxes to maintain the blood pressure. Tunica intima consists of a layer of endothelial cells. Arterioles, a minute arterial branch, one just proximal to a capillary.

Important Arteries (Fig. 3.1)

Generally, the names of the arteries mostly coincide with the names of the bone, organs, or cavity, etc. it passes through. However, some of the important arteries are listed in Table 3.1.

VEINS

Veins are the blood vessels which carry deoxygenated blood from various parts of the body to the heart. It also possesses three layers same as that of arteries, but they are much thinner. The smooth muscle inside their walls are under the control of the autonomic nervous system. Small veins are called as venules.

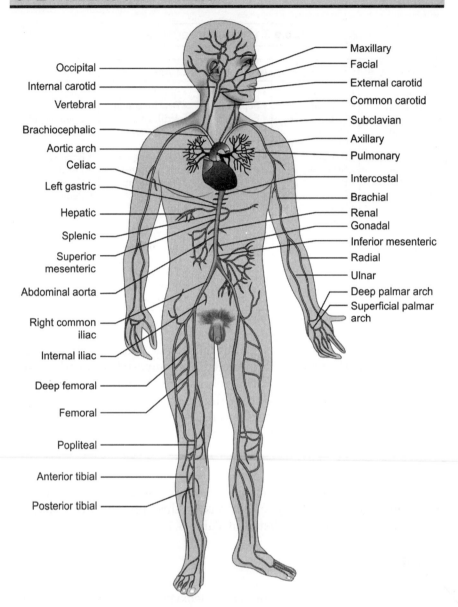

Fig. 3.1: Important arteries

Important Veins (Fig. 3.2)

See Table 3.2.

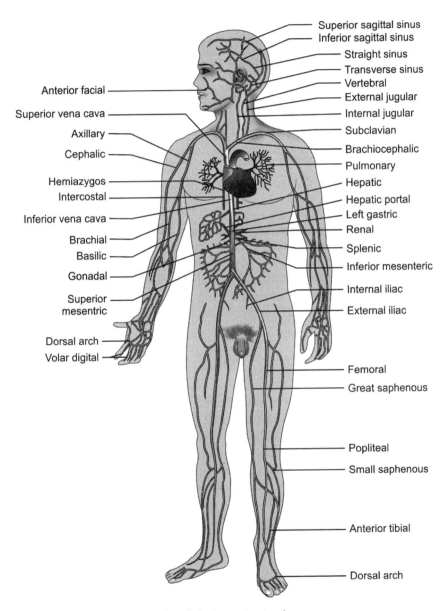

Fig. 3.2: Important veins

Table 3.2: Important veins

Head and neck	Upper limb	Lower limb and thigh	Thoracic cavity
• Sagittal sinus • Straight sinus • Transverse sinus • Facial • External jugular • Internal jugular • Subclavian • Brachiocephalic	• Axillary • Brachial • Cephalic • Basilic • Palmar digital	• Superior iliac • Superior epigastric • Femoral • Great saphenous • Popliteal • Small saphenous • Anterior tibial • Dorsal venous arch • Dorsal digital	• Superior vena cava • Left subclavian • Portal • Splenic • Mesenteric • Inferior vena cava • Colic • Superior mesenteric • Ileocolic • Rectal • Deep femoral

CAPILLARIES

Capillaries are only one cell thick and are just large enough to allow red blood cells to pass through. It is in the capillaries that the nutrient/gas exchange (diffusion) takes place. They act as a very important link in the circulatory system because it is the capillaries that serve all the tissues in the body, by absorbing the energy (glucose) from the blood of the arteries, and transporting the waste materials through the venules to the kidneys.

THE HEART

Heart is a conical shaped hollow muscular organ situated in the mediastinum, in between the two lungs in the thoracic cavity. It is slightly tilted towards left side. The heart is made of a special type of muscle called the cardiac muscle, composed of striated muscle fibers. The heart has a base above and an apex below and its size will be almost equal to the owner's fist. The heart is divided into two sides the right and left. The right side of the heart receives the deoxygenated blood and pumps into the lungs for purification and the left side of the heart receives the oxygenated blood from the lung and pumps into the various parts of the body through the aorta and arteries. Each side of the heart is further divided into two chambers which communicate by means of valves. The upper chambers are the thin walled atria or atrium or auricle. The lower chambers are the thick walled ventricles. Usually they are represented as right atrium and left atrium and right ventricle and left ventricle (Fig. 3.3).

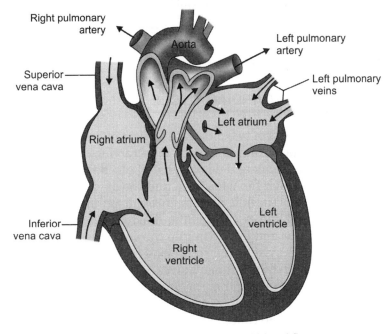

Fig. 3.3: Structure of heart and blood flow

The four chambers of the heart are separated by partitions called septa (singular septum). The interatrial septum separates the two upper chambers (atria), and the interventricular septum is a muscular wall which comes between the two lower chambers.

The heart wall is composed of three layers. They are:
1. *Endocardium:* Smooth layer of cells which lines the interior of the heart.
2. *Myocardium*: Middle muscular layer of the heart wall and is the thickest layer.
3. *Pericardium:* Delicate, double-folded membrane which surrounds the heart like a sac.

VALVES OF THE HEART

The valves of the heart play an important role to prevent the backflow of the blood into the chambers.

Mitral valve: Bicuspid valve is situated between the left atrium and ventricle (left side of the heart).

Tricuspid valve: Lies between the right atrium and right ventricle.

Semilunar valves: Lies on the mouth of the pulmonary artery, which arises from the right ventricle and on the mouth of the aorta which arises from the left ventricle.

HEART CYCLE OR CARDIAC CYCLE

The heart cycle consists of two phases. The first phase is called diastole (relaxation) and the second is systole (contraction). During diastolic phase the ventricles relax and deoxygenated blood flows into the right atrium of heart through the vena cava and the oxygenated blood from the lungs pours into the left atrium through pulmonary veins. The tricuspid and mitral valves are open in diastolic phase and the blood passes from the right and left atria into the ventricles.

The next phase is systolic phase. During this phase the walls of the ventricle contract and the semilunar valves open and the blood is pumped into the pulmonary artery and aorta from the right and left ventricles respectively. The diastole-systole cardiac cycle last about 0.8 seconds and occurs between 70 and 80 times per minute. The cardiac cycle consists of atrial systole—contraction of the atria, ventricular systole—contraction of ventricles, complete cardiac diastole—relaxation of atria and ventricles. Thus, the heart pumps about 70 ml of blood with each contractions. This can be picturized to understand easily as follows:

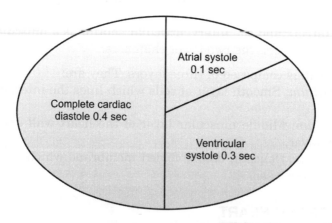

PULMONARY AND SYSTEMIC CIRCULATION

The circulation of blood through the vessels from the heart to the lungs and then back to the heart again is known as the **pulmonary circulation.** The circulation of blood from the body organs (except the lungs) to the heart and back again is called the **systemic circulation.**

Systemic Circulation (Fig. 3.4)

Deoxygenated blood enters the heart through the two largest veins in the body, the superior vena cava and inferior vena cava to the right atrium. The right atrium contracts to force the blood through the tricuspid valve into the right ventricle. As the right ventricle contracts to pump deoxygenated blood to the lungs through the pulmonary artery, the tricuspid valve is closed to prevent any blood from pushing back into the right atrium. The pulmonary (semilunar) valve, between the right ventricle and pulmonary artery opens as the blood is pumped into the pulmonary artery.

Similarly, the newly oxygenated blood enters into the left atrium through the pulmonary vein. The walls of the left atrium contract to force blood through the mitral valve into the left ventricle. The left ventricle pumps blood with great force so that the blood is pumped through the aortic valve, into the aorta which have three branches ascending aorta, arch of aorta and descending aorta and the blood is pumped to all parts of the body through the arteries. The aortic valve prevents the return of aortic blood to the left ventricle once it has been pumped out.

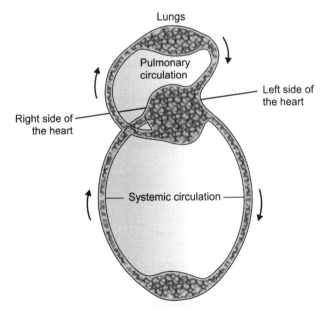

Fig. 3.4: Systemic circulation

Pulmonary Circulation

During the contraction of the ventricle, the deoxygenated blood is pumped into the pulmonary artery through the pulmonary (semilunar) valve from the right ventricle. This blood when reaches the capillaries of the lung, the exchange of the carbon dioxide and oxygen occurs and the the blood is purified. The newly purified blood is brought back to the heart through the pulmonary vein to the left atrium. This is called pulmonary circulation. The important point to be noted is that in pulmonary circulation, the arteries carry deoxygenated blood, whereas the veins carry oxygenated blood, which is reverse in the the systemic circulation.

Note: The reader should keep in mind, the differences between the systemic arteries and veins and pulmonary arteries and veins. For instance, the sytemic arteries carry oxygenated blood, whereas the pulmonary arteries, carried deoxygenated blood, similarly, the systemic veins carry deoxygenated blood, whereas the pulmunary veins carry oxygenated blood.

Portal Circulation (Flow chart 3.1)

Portal circulation is an important sub-division of the general circulation. Blood from the stomach, pancreas and spleen is collected by the portal

Flow chart 3.1: Block diagram representing the functioning of the heart and blood circulation

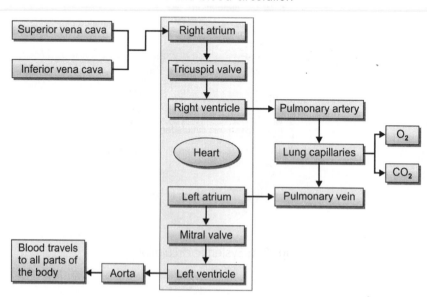

vein and passed to the liver. Here the capillary network unites with the capillary network of the hepatic artery. This double blood supply is collected by the hepatic vein and passed to the inferior vena cava.

BLOOD PRESSURE

The force exerted by the blood against the arterial walls during the systole and diastole of heart is called blood pressure. The blood pressure is expressed as systolic pressure/diastolic pressure separated by a slash. The normal BP is 120/80 but it may vary due to the influence of age, emotional stress, constriction of blood vessels, etc.

The diastole (dilation) and systole (contraction) cardiac cycle last about 0.9 seconds and occurs between 70 and 80 times per minute (100,000 times a day).

THE PULSE

The arterial pulse is a wave of increased pressure felt in the arteries when blood is pumped out of the heart. The pulse is most readily felt where an artery passes over a bone and lies near the surface, e.g. the radial pulse at the wrist. The pulse rate is usually described as the number of heart beats per minute. The adult range is between 60 and 80 beats per minute. In children the rate is higher.

ELECTRICAL CONDUCTION OF THE HEART PULSES

An electrical impulse originates from small muscle tissue, in the right atrium called the sinoatrial node (SA node), this is called the pacemaker of the heart. The impulse from the pacemaker radiates to the posterior portion of the interatrial septum (AV node). The AV node sends electrical impulses to the bundle of His, which further divides into right and left branches and carries the impulse to the right and left ventricles, resulting them to contract. Thus systole of ventricles occurs and the blood is pumped away from the heart. After a short duration, the way of excitation is initiated by the pacemaker again. Electrocardiogram is the instrument to record the electrical impulse of the heart, commonly called as ECG.

CARDIOVASCULAR DISORDERS

Origin of Terms

S.No.	Terms	Meanings	S.No.	Terms	Meanings
1.	Angi/o	Vessel	12.	Oxy/o	Oxygen
2.	Aort/o	Aorta	13.	Phleb/o	Vein
3.	Arteriol/o	Little artery	14.	Pulsus	Stroke, beat
4.	Artery	Air duct	15.	Sphygm/o	Pulse
5.	Cardi/o, cardiac,	Heart	16.	-stenosis	Narrowing
	cardium, cor		17.	Systole	Contraction
6.	Cuspid	Point, cusp	18.	-tension	Pressure
7.	Diastole	Expansion	19.	Thromb/o	Clot (of blood)
8.	Embol/o	Embolus, plug	20.	Varix	Swollen vein
9.	Hemangi/o	Blood vessel	21.	Vas/o	Vessel
10.	Luna	Moon	22.	Vena	Vein
11.	Corona	Crown	23.	Venul/o	Venule

Symptomatic and Diagnostic Terms

S.No.	Terms	Meanings
1.	Acrocyanosis	Bluish discoloration of finger tips and toes especially extremities
2.	Aneurysm	A dilation or bulging out of the wall of the heart, aorta or any other artery
3.	Angina pectoris	Short attacks of substernal pericardial pain which radiates to the shoulder provoked by exercise and relieved by rest
4.	Angiospasm, vasospasm	Involuntary contraction of the muscular coats of the blood vessels
5.	Arrhythmia	Variation from normal rhythm of the heart by tachycardia or bradycardia
6.	Ascites	Fluid in peritoneal cavity
7.	Atrial septal defect	Abnormality resulting in a shunting of oxygenated blood from the left into the right atrium
8.	Blood pressure	Pressure of blood flow felt on blood vessels
9.	Bradycardia	Slow heart action
10.	Cardiac arrest	Cessation of effective heart action usually caused by a systole or ventricular fibrillation
11.	Cardiac edema	Retention of water and sodium in congestive heart failure due to circulatory impairment
12.	Cardioversion	Conversion of a pathological cardiac rhythm such as ventricular, fibrillation to normal sinus rhythm usually accomplished by use of a device called cardiac averter, which administers counter shock to the heart through electrodes placed on the chest wall
13.	Carditis	Inflammation of the heart
14.	Claudication	Limping due to occlusive arterial disease
15.	Coarctation	Narrowing of a vessel, especially the aorta (coarctation of aorta)
16.	Congestive cardiac failure (CCF)	Condition in which the heart is unable to pump adequate amounts of blood to tissues and organs

Contd...

Contd...

S.No.	Terms	Meanings
17.	Cor pulmonale/ Pulmonary heart disease	Heart lung disease characterized by the right ventricular hypertrophy due to pulmonary disorders resulting in pulmonary hypertension
18.	Coronary occlusion	Complete obstruction of coronary artery
19.	Cyanosis	Bluish discoloration of skin due to reduced hemoglobin in blood.
20.	Diastole	Resting time of heart or period of dilatation of heart
21.	Dyspnea	Pain on breathing or difficulty in breathing
22.	Embolism	Obstruction of blood vessels by blood clot or foreign body
23.	Endocarditis	Acute or sub-acute disease of the lining of the heart and especially valve leaflets marked by inflammation of endocardium
24.	Fibrillation	Small, local, involuntary muscular contraction due to spontaneous activation of single muscle cells or muscle fibers.
25.	Flutter	Rapid regular cardiac action of beats 200 to 400 per minute
26.	Heart block	Loss of conduction through the atrioventricular junction tissue due to pathologic factors, with atrioventricular disassociation in which a sinus or atrial beat excites the atria. Condition of prolonged impulses transmitted may result in cardiac stand still
27.	Hemopericardium	Effusion of blood into the pericardium
28.	Hypertension	High blood pressure
29.	Hypotension	Low blood pressure
30.	Hypothermia	Having a body temperature below normal
31.	Ischemia	Lack of blood supply to a part due to functional constriction or obstruction
32.	Ischemic heart disease	Cardiac disease marked by reduced blood supply to the heart muscle due to coronary atherosclerosis, which may lead to myocardial infarction, heart failure or angina pectoris
33.	Mitral regurgitation or Mitral insufficiency	Back flow of blood from the left ventricle into the left atrium due to inadequate functioning (insufficiency).
34.	Mitral stenosis	A very common sequel of rheumatic fever marked by thrombi which narrow the orifice of the mitral valve leaflets
35.	Murmur	A soft blowing sound heard on auscultation; may result from vibrations associated with the movement of blood and or valvular action
36.	Myocardial	Relating to the myocardium
37.	Myocardial infarction	Clinical syndrome manifested by persistent usually intense cardiac pain, unrelated to exertion and often constrictive nature followed by diaphoresis, pallor. The underlying disease is usually coronary artherosclerosis, which progressed to coronary thrombosis and occlusion and resulted in a sudden curtailment of blood supply to the heart muscle and myocardial ischemia. Gross necrosis of myocardium may occur due to interruption of blood supply to that area, commonly called as heart attack.

Contd...

Contd...

S.No.	Terms	Meanings
38.	Myocarditis	Inflammation of heart muscle which may result in myocardial fibroses followed by cardiac enlargement and congestive heart failure
39.	Palpitation	Subjective sensation of skipping, pounding or racing heart beats.
40.	Paroxysmal	Sudden rapid regular heart beat or sudden intensification of symptoms
41.	Pericarditis	Inflammation of the covering membranes of the heart
42.	Phlebitis	Inflammation of the veins
43.	Phlebosclerosis	Hardening of the walls of the veins
44.	Rheumatic heart disease	Clinically manifested by rheumatic fever, damaging the myocardium, pericardium and endocardium, with the valvular endocardium as the site of predilection.
45.	Subacute bacterial endocarditis (SBE)	Infectious endocarditis caused by various bacteria including streptococci, staphylococci, enterococci, gonococci, gram negative bacilli.
46.	Syncope	Faint
47.	Systole	Contraction of ventricles/atria to propel blood
48.	Tachycardia	Rapid heart action
49.	Tetralogy of Fallot	A combination of four factors of congenital defects of heart: 1. Pulmonary stenosis 2. Interventricular septal defect 3. Dextra position of aorta 4. Ventricular hypertrophy
50.	Thrombophlebitis	Inflammatory reaction of the walls of the veins associated with intravascular clotting
51.	Thrombosis	Formation of blood clot
52.	Varicose veins, varicosity	Distended veins
53.	Vasoconstriction	Narrowing of vascular lumen resulting in decreased blood supply
54.	Vasodepression	Collapse due to vasomotor depression
55.	Vasodilation	A widening of vascular lumen increasing the blood supply to a part
56.	Rheumatic heart disease	Involvement of the heart occurring in the course of rheumatic fever attacking layers of the heart with endocardium most commonly
57.	Valvular heart disease	Disorder referring to any permanent organic deformity of one or more valves.
58.	Hypertensive heart disease	Hypertension causing heart disease.
59.	Dilated cardiomyopathy	Disease condition of the dilation of heart vessels marked by enlargement of the cavities of the heart with thinning of its wall
60.	Bundle branch block (Left) – LBBB	Obstruction of wave of excitation in either branch of the atrioventricular bundle.

Operative Terms

S.No.	Terms	Meanings
1.	Aneurysmectomy	Removal of an aneurysm
2.	Atriotomy	Incision of the atrium
3.	Cardiac massage	Emergency thoracotomy and manual compression of the heart, 40 to 60 times a minute, to reinstate and maintain blood circulation.
4.	Cardiolysis	Freeing pericardial adhesions to surrounding tissues, involving resection of ribs and sternum
5.	Cardiotomy	Incision of the heart
6.	Catheterization	The passage of a catheter into the heart through arm vein and blood vessels leading into the heart for the purpose of obtaining cardiac blood samples, detecting abnormalities and determine intercardiac pressure anomalies
7.	Embolectomy	Removal of an embolism
8.	Open heart surgery	Correction or reconstruction of septal defects removal of aneurysm thrombus, tetralogy of Fallot, myocardial infarction, congenital anomaly, replacement of valves, etc. which involves incision into one or more chambers of the heart through sternotomy and thoracotomy along with extracorporeal circulation by a heart lung machine
9.	Pericardiectomy	Excision of a portion of the pericardium
10.	Phleborrhaphy	Suturing of a vein
11.	Phlebotomy	Opening or piercing of a vein for removal of blood, or for the introduction of fluids or medications
12.	Shunt	A passage between two blood vessels or between two sides of the heart
13.	Valvotomy	Surgical incision of a valve to increase the size of the orifice; more frequently mitral valvotomy is done to treat mitral stenosis
14.	Venotomy	Surgical incision of a vein
15.	Anastomosis	End to end union of two different blood vessels after excision of the lesions (making communication between vessels)
16.	Endarterectomy	Removal of inner coat of artery for occlusive vascular disease
17.	Phlebotomy	Incision of a vein or opening of a vein
18.	Venesection/ Phlebotomy	Incision into a vein
19.	Bypass graft	Implantation of an autograft usually a segment of a saphenous vein to bypass a vascular obstruction of the coronary or carotid-subclavian arteries
20.	Valve replacement	Removal of incompetent or stenotic valve and its replacement with a prosthetic valve

COMMON ABBREVIATIONS

S.No.	Abbreviation	Term
1.	A_2	Aortic second sound
2.	AAA	Abdominal aortic aneurysm
3.	AAS	Aortic arch syndrome
4.	ABE	Acute bacterial endocarditis
5.	ABP	Arterial blood pressure
6.	ACG	Angiocardiography
7.	ACVD	Acute cardiovascular disease
8.	AH	Arterial hypertension
9.	AHA	American heart association
10.	AHD	Arteriosclerotic heart disease
11.	AI	Aortic insufficiency
12.	AI	Aortic incompetence
13.	AMI	Acute myocardial infarction
14.	AR	Aortic regurgitation
15.	AS	Aortic stenosis
16.	ASD	Atrial septal defect
17.	ASH	Asymmetrical septal hypertrophy
18.	ASHD	Arteriosclerotic heart disease
19.	ASO	Arteriosclerosis obliteran
20.	AST	Aspartate aminotransferase
21.	AV	Atrioventricular
22.	AVF	Arteriovenous fistula
23.	BBB	Bundle-branch block
24.	BP	Blood pressure
25.	CAD	Coronary artery disease
26.	CAHD	Coronary atherosclerotic heart disease
27.	CC	Cardiac catheterization
28.	CCF	Congestive cardiac failure
29.	CCU	Coronary care unit
30.	CHB	Complete heart block
31.	CHD	Coronary heart disease
32.	CHD	Congestive heart disease
33.	CHF	Congestive heart failure
34.	CK	Creatine kinase
35.	CLBBB	Complete left bundle branch block
36.	CPB	Cardiopulmonary resuscitation
37.	CPR	Cardiopulmonary resuscitation
38.	CRBBB	Complete right bundle branch block
39.	CRP	C-reactive protein
40.	CV	Cardiovascular
41.	CVA	Cereberovascular accident
42.	CVP	Central venous pressure
43.	DM	Diastolic murmur
44.	DVT	Deep vein thrombosis
45.	ECG, EKG	Electrocardiogram
46.	EH	Essential hypertension
47.	ESR	Erythrocyte sedimentation rate
48.	HBP	High blood pressure
49.	HCVD	Hypertensive cardiovascular disease
50.	HD	Heart disease
51.	HDL	High-density lipoprotein
52.	HF	Heart failure

Contd...

Contd...

S.No.	Abbreviation	Term
53.	HHD	Hypertensive heart disease
54.	HVD	Hypertensive vascular disease
55.	IASD	Interatrial septal defect
56.	ICC	Intensive coronary care
57.	ICCU	Intensive coronary care unit
58.	ICU	Intensive care unit
59.	IHD	Ischemic heart disease
60.	IHSS	Idiopathic hypertrophic subaortic stenosis
61.	IMF	Idiopathic myelofibrosis
62.	IVC	Inferior vena cava
63.	IVSD	Interventricular septal defect
64.	LA	Left atrium
65.	LBB	Left bundle branch
66.	LBBB	Left bundle brach block
67.	LD	Lactic dehydrogenase
68.	LDL	Low-density lipoprotein
69.	LHF	Left heart failure
70.	LV	Left ventricle
71.	LVF	Left ventricular failure
72.	LVH	Left ventricular hypertrophy
73.	MI	Myocardial infarction
74.	mm Hg	Millimeter of mercury
75.	MS	Mitral stenosis
76.	MVP	Mitral valve prolapse
77.	OHS	Open heart surgery
78.	OMI	Old myocardial infarction
79.	PA	Pulmonary artery
80.	PAC	Premature atrial contraction
81.	PAT	Paroxysmal atrial tachycardia
82.	PDA	Patent ductus arteriosus
83.	PHT	Pulmonary hypertension
84.	PVC	Premature ventricular contraction
85.	PVP	Portal venous pressure
86.	PVT	Paroxysmal ventricular tachycardia
87.	RVH	Right ventricular hypertrophy
88.	RA	Right atrium
89.	RBBB	Right bundle branch block
90.	RCA	Right coronary artery
91.	RCU	Respiratory cardiac unit
92.	RF	Rheumatic fever
93.	RHD	Rheumatic heart disease
94.	RHF	Rheumatic heart failure
95.	RPA	Right pulmonary artery
96.	RV	Right ventricle
97.	RVF	Right ventricular failure
98.	SA	Sinoatrial (node)
99.	SBE	Subacute bacterial endocarditis
100.	SBP	Systolic blood pressure
101.	SGOT	Serum glutamic-oxaloacetic transaminase
102.	SGPT	Serum glutamic pyruvic transaminase
103.	SVC	Superior vena cava
104.	SVG	Sapheneous vein graft
105.	SVT	Supraventricular tachycardia

Contd...

Contd...

S.No.	Abbreviation	Term
106.	TAO	Thromboangitis obliterans
107.	TS	Thoracic surgery
108.	VV	Varicose veins
109.	VF	Ventricular fibrillation
110.	VHD	Valvular heart disease
111.	VLDL	Very low density lipoproteins
112.	VSD	Ventricular septal defect
113.	VT	Ventricular tachycardia

4

Blood and Lymphatic System

INTRODUCTION

Blood and lymph are the specialized liquid tissues of the body; each is composed of cells that are suspended in a liquid medium. Both these tissues play a vital role in defending the body against infection. They also act as the transportation system for body cells, since they are movable throughout the entire body.

BLOOD

The blood is red and viscid, alkaline in reaction and it is divided into a fluid part and a solid part as follows:

Fluid part	Plasma, which is straw-colored fluid and contains essential substances.
Solid part	Three major blood cells:

        a. Red blood cells   (Erythrocytes)
        b. White blood cells   (Leukocytes)
        c. Platelets   (Thrombocytes)

Plasma accounts for about 55 percent and blood cells accounts for about 45 percent of the total blood volume (Fig. 4.1).

The main functions of the blood are to:
- Convey oxygen to the tissues by means of hemoglobin in the red blood cells
- Remove waste products from the tissue
- Carry nutrients to all parts of the body
- Carry hormones or chemical messengers of the body
- Aid in defence of the body by phagocytic action

- Participate in the circulation of lymphocytes required for immune response
- Carry antibodies to the sites of infection.

PLASMA

Plasma is the liquid portion of the blood in which the corpuscles are suspended. It is composed of about 92 percent water and solid materials, which are mainly proteins with lesser amounts of sugar, wastes, salts, hormones and other substances. The four major proteins presents in the plasma are:
1. Albumin
2. Globulin
3. Fibrinogen
4. Prothrombin.

Plasma makes it possible for the chemical communication between all the body cells by carrying these products to different parts of the body.

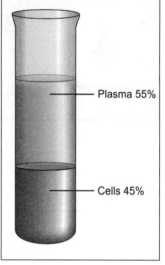

Fig. 4.1: The blood in the test tube shows the per-centage composition of plasma and cells

Albumin and globulin are the serum proteins that help to maintain the proper water content of the blood by holding water in the blood, opposing its tendency to leak out into the tissue spaces, which would cause edema (swelling). The globulin portion of plasma contains antibodies which can fight off foreign antigens. There are three different kinds of globulins in plasma. They are called alpha, beta, and gamma and they are distinguished by the process of electrophoresis. Immunoglobulins are a specific type of gamma-globulin which are capable of acting as antibodies. Examples of immunoglobulin antibodies are IgG and IgA. When free of corpuscles, plasma is thin and colorless. The fibrinogen helps in clotting of blood.

Blood serum is a product of blood plasma. It differs from plasma in that serum does not contain fibrinogen. This can be represented as follows:

Plasma – Fibrinogen = Serum

The composition of the plasma is as follows:
- Water 90 to 92 percent
- Plasma proteins 60 g/l
  Albumin 35 to 50 g/l
  Globulin 20 to 37 g/l
  Gibrinogen 2 to 4 g/l
  Prothrombin 100 to 150 mg/l
- Mineral salts
- Nutrient materials
- Organic waste products

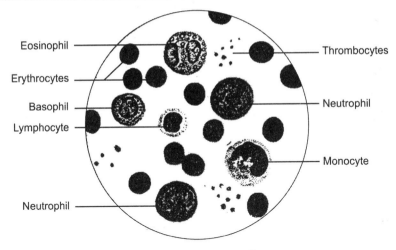

Fig. 4.2: Blood cell

- Hormones
- Enzymes
- Antibodies and antitoxins
- Gases.

The solid part of the blood is composed of (Fig. 4.2):
- Erythrocytes or red blood cells
- Leukocytes or white blood cells
- Thrombocytes or platelets or clotting cells.

ERYTHROCYTES (RED BLOOD CELLS)

Erythrocytes are formed in the red bone marrow of the spongy bones that are at the ends of the long bones. The development of red blood cells is called erythropoiesis. During their development, RBCs develop a special compound called hemoglobin, which is rich in iron-containing pigment, that gives the erythrocyte its red color. It is the hemoglobin in the erythrocytes that enable the cell to carry oxygen all through the body. The combination of oxygen and hemoglobin (oxyhemoglobin) produces the bright red color of blood. Normally, 13 to 18 gm/100 ml of hemoglobin is present in male and 12 to 16 gm/100 ml hemoglobin is present in female.

The average life of the erythrocytes is about 120 days in the circulating bloodstream. After this time, the wornout erythrocytes are destroyed by the cells of spleen, liver and bone marrow. These cells called macrophages, set the hemoglobin free from the erythrocyte and break the hemoglobin down into its haem and globin portions. The haem decomposes into bilirubin and iron. Iron is used to form new red cells or is stored in the spleen, liver, and bone marrow for later use. Bilirubin is carried to the liver and excreted through the intestine with bile.

The process of breakdown of the wornout cells is called hemolysis, which is carried out by the cells of the reticuloendothelial system. These cells are called phagocytic, i.e. capable of engulfing and destroying foreign bodies such as micro-organisms and worn erythrocytes.

LEUKOCYTES (WHITE BLOOD CELLS)

The leukocytes play a vital role in the body's immune system by protecting it against the invasion by bacteria and other foreign substances. It also plays a vital role in tissue repair, but this activity is still not fully understood.

White blood cells (WBC) can be classified into two categories, the granulocytes (with granules in the cytoplasm) and the agranulocytes (without granules). Each of these categories can be further subdivided as follows:
1. Granulocytes
   • Neutrophils
   • Eosinophils
   • Basophils.
2. Agranulocytes
   • Monocytes
   • Lymphocytes.

Granulocytes

Granulocytes are the most numerous leukocytes (about 60%). The granulocytes are formed in the red bone marrow from stem cells, which give rise to myeloblasts. Myeloblasts differentiate into:
• Neutrophils
• Eosinophils
• Basophils.
   These names were derived from the dye used to stain blood smears in the laboratory.
• *Neutrophils:* They compose 57 percent of the leukocytes. The neutrophils are motile and highly phagocytic. They fight disease by engulfing and swallowing up germs. They also increase in a number of pyrogenic (fever-producing) infections and in some types of leukemia.
• *Eosinophils:* It protects body by releasing many substances that are capable of detoxifying foreign protein and other material. Eosino-

phils are increased in allergic conditions and parasitic infections. They are also capable of destroying antigen/antibody complexes.

- *Basophils:* The exact functions are not known. It releases histamines and heparin in the area of damaged tissues. Histamines, causes inflammatory reaction, ultimately increasing the blood flow. Therefore, additional neutrophils or phagocytes are brought to the damaged area.

Agranulocytes

Agranulocytes cells contain single large nucleus and therefore they are called mononuclear cells. These form 33 percent of the leukocytes. It is composed of:
- Lymphocytes
- Monocytes.
- *Lymphocytes:* They play a vital role in the immune system of the body. They are capable of making antibodies which can neutralize and destroy foreign antigens (bacteria and viruses) that may enter the body. The harmful invader is called antigen; the defense provided by the body is called the antibody. This reaction is called antigen – antibody reaction.
- *Monocytes:* Monocytes provide protection to the body, in the same manner as neutrophils, by phagocytes. They dispose dead and dying cells and other debris by engulfing and swallowing the cells.

Thrombocytes (Platelets)

The thrombocytes are the smallest elements within the blood. Platelets are formed in the red bone marrow from giant multinucleated cells called megakaryocytes. The main function of platelets is to help in the clotting mechanism of the blood.

BLOOD CLOTTING MECHANISM

Blood clotting or coagulation, is a complicated process involving many different chemical reactions as follows:
- Prothrombin activator (thromboplastin) is released when there is a break in the tissue or at the site of injury or when platelets rupture.
- The thromboplastin acts on prothrombin and converts prothrombin into thrombin.
- The thrombin acting on the fibrinogen converts it into fibrin which is insoluble, which trap red blood cells to form the clot.
  The period of time, taken by fibrin to form the blood clot is known as the coagulation time. Normally, it will be less than 15 minutes. The

time taken for the platelets to plug up a small puncture of the skin is called bleeding time and it is normally less than 8 minutes.

BLOOD GROUP

Blood is divided into four groups namely A, B, AB and O based on the presence or absence of blood antigens in the RBCs. Table 4.1 illustrates the presence of the antigen and antibodies for the four different types of blood group and the possible donor:

Table 4.1: Blood groups

S.No.	Blood group	Antigen present	Antibody present	Can receive blood from	Can donate blood to
1.	A	A	Anti-B	A and O group	A and AB groups
2.	B	B	Anti-A	B and O group	B and AB groups
3.	AB	A and B	No antibody present	A, B, O, AB (Universal recipients)	AB group only
4.	O	No antigent present	Both Anti-A and Anti-B	O	A, B, AB, and O groups (Universal donors)

Besides grouping by classifying A and B antigen, there are many other antigens located on the surface of the RBC. One of these is called the Rh factor (named because it was first found in the blood of a rhesus monkey). The term Rh-positive refers to a person who is born with Rh antigen on his or her red blood cells, and the Rh-negative person does not have the Rh antigen.

LYMPHATIC SYSTEM

The lymphatic system consists of lymph a tissue fluid, which is found all over the body through a network of transporting structure called lymph vessels, lymph nodes and the spleen, thymus and tonsils. Other noncellular constituents of lymph are water, salts, sugar and wastes of metabolism, such as urea and creatinine. The primary functions of the lymphatic system are:
- To drain fluid from tissue spaces and return it to the blood
- . Transporting materials to body cells
- Carrying waste products from body tissues back to the bloodstream
- To convey lipids or fats, away from the digestive organs
- To control infection by providing lymphocytes and monocytes, which are used to defend against infections caused by micro-organisms.

Lymph originates from the blood plasma. As blood circulates through the capillaries, some of the plasma steps out of these thin-walled vessels.

This fluid, now called interstitial, or tissue fluid, resembles plasma, except it contains less protein. When the fluid enters into the capillaries, it is called as lymph. Lymph capillaries are thin-walled tubes, same like blood capillaries. These capillaries carry lymph from the tissue space to the large lymphatic vessels and finally to lymph nodes, which serve as depositories for cellular debris. The lymph nodes are present all over the body (Fig. 4.3). As lymph passes through the nodes it is filtered and replenished with lymphocytes, globulins, and anitbodies. Bacteria and debris are engulfed by macrophages that line the nodes.

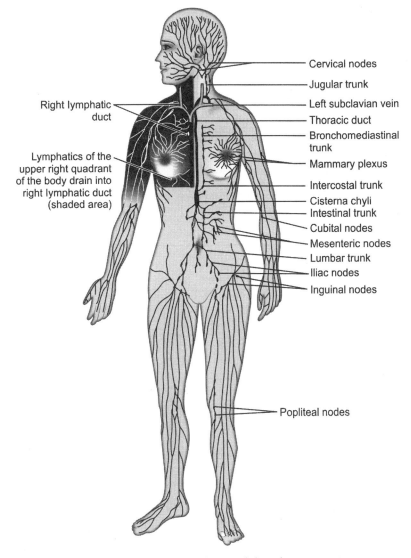

Fig. 4.3: Lymph nodes and their location

The thoracic duct acts as the major duct to drain the lymph from all parts of body except the right chest and arm, which drains into the left subclavian vein. Whereas the lymph vessels of the right chest and arm join the right lymphatic duct, which drains into the right subclavian vein. Thus, the lymph is recycled into the circulating blood in order to begin the cycle, once again, throughout the body.

LYMPH NODES (FIG. 4.3 AND TABLE 4.2)

The lymph node is bean shapped and has afferent (away from lymph node) lymphatics at the convex border and efferent (towards the lymph node) lymphatics at the hilum. Each lymph node has a capsule, an outer cortex containing mostly lymphatic nodules, and an inner medulla containing lymphatic sinuses. Lymph nodes are placed along the lymphatics. When a part of the body is infected and inflamed, the lymph nodes drain, hence that part become enlarged and palpable.

Table 4.2: Lymph nodes and their locations

S.No.	Lymph nodes	Location
1.	Superficial and deep cervical nodes	Neck
2.	Parotid, submandibular, mastoid and occipital nodes	Head
3.	Bronchomediastinal, brochopulmonary and tracheobronchial nodes	Thorax
4.	Gastric, hepatic, splenic, mesenteric and lumbar	Abdomen
5.	Axillary nodes	Axilla
6.	Inguinal nodes	Groin

RELATED LYMPHATIC ORGANS

The organs composed of lymphatic tissue are:
• Spleen
• Thymus
• Tonsils.

Spleen

Spleen is the biggest lymphatic organ. It is located in the left upper quadrant of the abdomen, adjacent to the stomach. The main functions of the spleen are:
• Destruction of old RBC, by which bilirubin is formed and added to the bloodstream.
• Filtration of micro-organisms and other foreign materials from the blood.
• Production of antibodies and immunity, chiefly by leukocytes.
• Storage of blood, especially RBC. Blood is released by the spleen when the body needs it.
• Production of blood cells such as lymphocytes and monocytes.
• Stimulates the production of blood cells from the bone marrow.

Thymus

Thymus is located in the mediastinum, posterior to the breastbone and between the lungs. It plays a vital role in the body's immunologic system. It produces special lymphocytes called T cells, which migrate to the site of antigens and to destroy the antigen by the process of phagocytosis. Other types of lymphocytes are called B-cells, these cells are produced in the bone marrow and they destroy antigen by producing antibody.

Tonsils

Three sets of tonsils, the palantine, pharyngeal and lingual tonsils, contain T and B lymphocytes which protect against infection at the entrance of the digestive and respiratory tracts.

IMMUNITY

The study of the body's defense mechanism against the foreign organisms is called immunology. Immunity is a capacity to resist all types of organisms and toxins. Natural immunity is one's own ability to fight against disease. Acquired immunity is the protection against, invasive organisms to which the body does not have natural immunity. Vaccination is a process of injecting antibodies against the foreign organisms and then remain in the body to protect against subsequent infection. Many diseases can be prevented by artificial immunization.

Example:
- Poliomyelitis
- Smallpox
- Tetanus
- Tuberculosis
- Typhoid fever
- Diptheria
- Measles
- Hepatitis B.

Acquired active immunity involves two major disease fighters, B-cell lymphocytes (humoral immunity) and T-cell lymphocytes (cell mediated immunity). B-cells originate from bone marrow stem cells and migrate to lymph nodes and other lymphoid tissue. When a B-cell is confronted with a specific type of antigen, it transforms into an antibody-producing cell called a plasma cell. The antibodies that are made by plasma cell are immunoglobulins, such as IgM, IgG, IgD, IgE and IgA. Immunoglobulins travel to the site of an infection to react with and neutralize antigens.

T-cell lymphocytes originate from stem cells in the bone marrow and are processed in the thymus gland where they are acted upon by thymic hormones. Then they migrate to lymph nodes and lymphoid organs. When an antigen encounters a T-cell, the T-cell multiplies rapidly and can engulf and digest the antigen (bacterium, virus, cancer cell, or fungus) T-cell also react to foreign tissues, such as skin grafts and transplanted organs.

Some T-cells are cytotoxic or killer (called T8 cells), whereas other T-cells produce chemicals (interferon's and interleukins) that destroy cells or bacteria. One special class of T-cells, called helper cells or T4 cells, stimulates antibody production. CD4 + T cells (CD4 + is the name of the protein on the cell) are attacked by the HIV (human immunodeficiency virus) in AIDS. Suppressor cells are other T-cells that regulate the amount of antibody produced by inhibiting the activity of the B-cell lymphocytes.

DISORDERS OF THE BLOOD AND LYMPHATIC SYSTEM

Origin of Terms

S.No.	Terms	Meanings	S.No	Terms	Meanings
1.	plasma	Anything formed	18.	reticulum	Network
2.	bas	Basic or alkaline	19.	neutr	Neutral dye
3.	heme, -emia,	Blood	20.	kary	Nucleus
4.	-phoresis	Borne, carried	21.	-globin	Protein
5.	-cyto	Cell	22.	eythro	Red
6.	thromb	Clot	23.	-eosin	Red, rosy, dawn-colored
7.	-penia	Decrease	24.	immune	Safe, protected
8.	heter	Different	25.	hom	Same
9.	is	Equal	26.	morph	Shape, form
10.	-poiesis	Formation, production	27.	splen	Spleen
11.	blast	Germ	28.	-stasis	Standing still
12.	granul	Granule	29.	thym	Thymus gland
13.	-osis	Increase, abnormal Condition	30.	phage	To eat
14.	sider	Iron	31.	-phil	To love
15.	lymph	Lymph	32.	poikil	Varied irregular
16.	lymphaden	Lymph gland	33.	leuko	White
17.	polymorph	Many forms	34.	agranulo	Without granules

Diagnostic and Symptomatic Terms

S.No.	Terms	Meanings
1.	Anemia	Lack of hemoglobin
2.	Anisocytosis	Variation in size of red cells, seen in pernicious anemia
3.	Aplastic	Cells destroyed in bone marrow
4.	Asplenia	Absence of spleen
5.	Blood dyscrasia	Morbid blood condition
6.	Dyscrasia	Any blood abnormality
7.	Elephantiasis	Hypertrophy and fibrosis of the skin and subcutaneous and lymphoid tissue due to long-standing obstructed circulation in the blood or lymphatic vessels, chiefly by the presence of the filarial worms *Wuchereria bancrofti*
8.	Eosinophila	Increased count of eosinophils in the blood, during allergic conditions
9.	Erythrocytosis	Abnormal increase in red blood cells
10.	Erythropenia	Abnormal decrease in red blood cells

Contd...

Contd...

S.No.	Terms	Meanings
11.	Fibrinolysis	Dissolution of fibrin, blood clot becomes liquid
12.	Granulocytosis	Abnormal increase in granulocytes in the blood
13.	Hemophilia	Inherited disease passed from mother to son, where blood does not clot in the normal time
14.	Hemochromatosis	Excessive deposits of iron throughout the body
15.	Hemolysis	Destruction of RBC and subsequent escape of hemoglobin into blood plasma
16.	Hemolytic anemia	Anemia due to rapid destruction of red blood cells
17.	Hemophilia	Excessive bleeding caused by a congenital lack of a substance necessary for blood clotting
18.	Hodgkin's disease	Malignant tumor arising in lymphatic tissue such as lymph nodes and spleen
19.	Hypersplenism	A syndrome with splenomegaly associated with destruction of blood cells in spleen resulting in anemia, leukopenia and thrombocytopenia.
20.	Hypersplenism	Excessive splenic activity associated with highly increased blood cell destruction leading to anemia, leukopenia and thrombocytopenia.
21.	Iron deficiency anemia	Lack of iron in blood
22.	Leukocytes	White blood cells
23.	Leukocytosis	Transient increased condition of white blood cells
24.	Leukopenia	Decrease in white blood cells
25.	Leukemia	Cancerous condition characterized by distorted proliferation and development of leukocytes and their precursors in the blood and bone marrow
26.	Leukopenia	Abnormally low white cells count
27.	Lymphadenitis	Inflammation of lymph nodes, usually due to infection
28.	Lymphocytopenia	Deficient number of lymphocytes in the blood
29.	Lymphocytosis	Increased number of lymphocytes in the blood and bone marrow
30.	Lymphosarcoma	Malignant tumor of lymph nodes which closely resembles Hodgkin's disease
31.	Macrocytosis	Abnormally large erythrocytes in the blood
32.	Megaloblastosis	Large, usually oval shaped embryonic red corpuscles found in the bone marrow and blood.
33.	Microcytosis	Abnormally small erythrocytes present in the blood
34.	Mononucleosis	Acute infectious disease with enlarged lymph nodes and spleen and increased numbers of lymphocytes and monocytes in bloodstream
35.	Myeloma (multiple)	Malignant tumor of bone marrow
36.	Neutropenia	Excessively low neutrophils count
37.	Neutrophilia	Increased neutrophils including immature forms, seen in Rh pyogenic infections

Contd...

Contd...

S.No.	Terms	Meanings
38.	Pancytopenia	Abnormally decrease in RBC, erythrocytes, leukocytes and platelets
39.	Poikilocytosis	Irregular shaped red cells in the blood seen in pernicious anemia
40.	Polycythemia	An increase in the total red cell mass of the blood
41.	Proliferation	Increase in reproduction of similar forms or cells
42.	Purpura	Hemorrhages into the skin tissues
43.	Reticulocytosis	Increase in reticulocytes in the peripheral blood
44.	Rouleaux formation	False agglutination in which erythrocytes look like stakes of coin.
45.	Sarcoidosis	Abnormal growth of small tubercles in lymph
46.	Serology	The study of blood serum especially on antigen-antibody reactions
47.	Sickle cell anemia	Hereditary condition characterized by abnormal shape of erythrocytes and by hemolysis
48.	Splenomegaly	Enlargement of spleen
49.	Splenoptosis	Downward displacement of the spleen
50.	Splenorrhexis	Rupture of spleen due to injury or advanced disease condition
51.	Thalassemia (thalass = sea)	An inherited defect in the ability to produce hemoglobin, usually seen in persons of Mediterranean background
52.	Thrombocytopenia	Deficiency of thrombocytes or platelets in the circulating blood
53.	Thrombocytosis	Excess of thrombocytes or platelets in the circulating blood.

Surgical Procedures

S.No.	Terms	Meanings
1.	Lymphadenectomy	Excision of lymph node
2.	Lymphoidectomy	Excision of lymphoid tissue
3.	Splenectomy	Excision of spleen
4.	Splenopexy	Surgical fixation of a movable spleen
5.	Splenorrhaphy	Suture of a ruptured spleen
6.	Splenotomy	Incision into the spleen
7.	Lymphadenotomy	Incision and drainage of lymph gland
8.	Bone marrow transplantation	Grafting and transplantation of donor's bone marrow to the patients of congenital blood disorders like thalassemia and sickle cell disease.

COMMON ABBREVIATIONS

S.No.	Abbreviation	Term
1.	A/B	Acid-base ratio
2.	AAR	Antigen antiglobulin reaction
3.	Ab	Antibody
4.	ABO	Three main blood types
5.	ACD	Acid citrate dextrose
6.	ACM	Albumin-calcium-magnesium
7.	ACS	Antereticular cytotoxic serum
8.	ACT	Activated coagulation time
9.	Ad lib	As desired (Ad libitum)
10.	ADA	Anterior descending artery
11.	ADS	Antibody deficiency syndrome
12.	AGL	Acute granulocytic leukemia
13.	AHA	Acquired hemolytic anemia
14.	AHF	Antihemophilic factor VIII
15.	AHG	Antihemophilic globulin factor VIII
16.	AIHA	Autoimmune hemolytic anemia
17.	ALL	Acute lymphoblastic leukemia
18.	Alt Hor	Every other hour (Alternis Horos)
19.	Alt dieb	Every other day (Alternis Diebus)
20.	Alt noc	Every other night
21.	AML	Acute myeloplastic leukemia
22.	AMOL	Acute monocytic leukemia
23.	ANA	Antinuclear antibodies
24.	APC	Aspirin, phenacetin, caffeine
25.	APTT	Activated partial thromboplastin time
26.	ATS	Antitetanic serum
27.	B_{12}	Vitamin B_{12}
28.	BB	Blood bank
29.	BCG	Bacille calmette guerin (Vaccine)
30.	BSR	Blood sedimentation rate
31.	BT	Bleeding time
32.	CBC	Complete blood count
33.	CBC and diff	Complete blood count and differential
34.	CEA	Carcinoembryonic antigen
35.	CF	Christmas factor
36.	CHA	Congenital hypoplastic anemia
37.	CLL	Chronic lymphocytic leukemia
38.	CML	Chronic myeloblastic leukemia
39.	CMR	Cerebral metabolic rate
40.	CT	Cerebral thrombosis
41.	DIC	Diffuse/Disseminated intravascular coagulation
42.	diff	Differential count (WBC)
43.	DTP	Diptheria, tetanus and pertussis
44.	eos	Eosinophils
45.	ESR	Erythrocytic sedimentation rate
46.	G/S	Glucose and saline
47.	Hb	Hemoglobin
48.	Hb A	Hemoglobin adult
49.	Hb F	Hemoglobin fetal
50.	Hb S	Sickle cell hemoglobin
51.	Hct, HT	Hematocrit
52.	HDN	Hemolytic disease of newborn

Contd...

Contd...

S.No.	Abbreviation	Term
53.	HHA	Hereditary hemolytic anemia
54.	IgA, IgD, IgG	Immunoglobulins
55.	ITP	Idopathic thrombocytopenic purpura
56.	LAG	Lymphangiography
57.	Lymph	Lymphocyte
58.	MCH	Mean corpuscular hemoglobin
59.	MCHC	Mean corpuscular hemoglobin concentration
60.	MCT	Mean corpuscular time
61.	MCV	Mean corpuscular volume
62.	MON; mon	Monocytes
63.	PA	Pernicious anemia
64.	PCV	Packed cell volume
65.	PK	Pyruvate kinase
66.	PMN	Polymorphonuclear neutrophil
67.	poly	Polymorphonuclear leukocyte
68.	PPH	Postpartum hemorrhage
69.	PPU	Perforated peptic ulcer
70.	PT	Prothrombin
71.	PTT	Partial thromboplastin time
72.	RBC	Red blood count
73.	RNA	Ribo nucleic acid
74.	SCA	Sickle cell anemia
75.	SPC	Serum protein electrophoresis
76.	SPE	Serum protein electrophoresis
77.	TT	Tetanus toxoid
78.	TTP	Thrombotic thrombocytopenic purpura
79.	VPRC	Volume packed red cells
80.	WBC	White blood count
81.	WCC	White cell count
82.	X-match	Cross match

5 Nervous System

INTRODUCTION

The nervous system is one of the most complexed of all human body systems. This system communicates between the various parts of the body. More than 10 billion nerve cells are operating all over the body. Some of the important and day-to-day activities such as speaking, moving, hearing, tasting, seeing, thinking, emotions, secreting hormones, responding to dangerous situations such as pain, heat, cold, touch, etc. are composed of small number of many activities which are controlled by the nervous system.

Microscopic nerve cells collected into bundles are called nerves, which carry electrical message all over the body. External stimuli, as well as internal chemicals such as acetylcholine activates the cell membranes of nerve cells so as to release stored electrical energy within the cells. This energy when released and passed through the length of the nerve cells are called nerve impulses. Thus the external receptor like sense organs (eye, ear, tongue, skin, nose) as well as internal receptors in muscles and blood vessels receive and transmit these impulses to the complex network of the nerve cells in the brain and the spinal cord. Within the central part of the nervous system impulses are recognized, interpreted and finally relayed to other nerve cells which extends to all parts of the body, such as muscles, glands and internal organs.

The nervous system is made up of innumerable number of nerve cells called neurons and it is the basic unit of the nervous system. A neuron is an individual nerve cell, a microscopic structure through which impulses are passed along the path of the nerve cell in a definite manner and direction. The nerve cells collectively form the gray matter of the brain, and the nerve fibers are grouped together to form the white matter.

A bundle of nerve fibers is a nerve, bound together by connective tissue and the interbranching of nerves is known as plexus. Nerves are classified into two types, namely sensory or afferent nerves and motor or efferant nerves.

STRUCTURE OF NERVOUS SYSTEM

The nervous system may be divided into two main portions namely, the central nervous system (CNS) consisting of brain and spinal cord. The peripheral nervous system or autonomic nervous system consist of spinal nerves between the central nervous system, muscles and various organs.

The peripheral nervous system is further divided into two nervous systems, such as somatic nerves (voluntary) and autonomic nerves (involuntary). The autonomic nerves are further branched into sympathetic and parasympathetic nerves (Flow chart 5.1).

CENTRAL NERVOUS SYSTEM

The central nervous system (CNS) controls voluntary muscles and the nerves supplied to the limbs, etc. The main parts of the CNS are brain and spinal cord.

Flow chart 5.1: Structure of nervous system

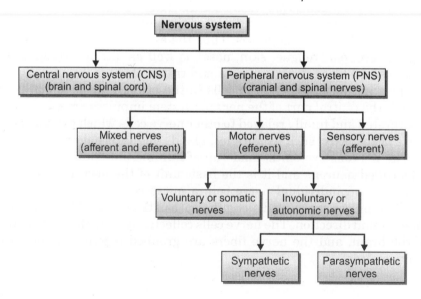

Brain

Brain is the major part of central nervous system. The brain is composed of billions of neurons and nerve endings. It looks like a giant wrinkled walnut crammed inside the skull. It integrates almost every physical and mental activity of the body. This organ is also the center for memory, emotion, thought, judgment, reasoning and consciousness.

The brain is covered by a three layer membrane collectively called as meninges, to protect the delicate nerve tissue, to secrete cerebrospinal fluid which protect the spinal cord from any concussion and to carry the blood vessels to the brain. Approximately, the weight of the brain is 1.3 kg. The three layers of the meninges are:

1. Dura mater—dense and tough and lines the skull
2. Arachnoid mater—fine middle layer
3. Pia mater—inner layer covering the fissures of the brain and spinal cord. The space between the arachnoid mater and pia mater is called as subarachnoid space.

Parts of Brain (Fig. 5.1)

Brain is divided as three portions namely, fore brain, mid brain and hind brain.

Fore brain	Cerebrum
Hind brain	Cerebellum
Mid brain/Brainstem	Pons varolii and medulla oblongata

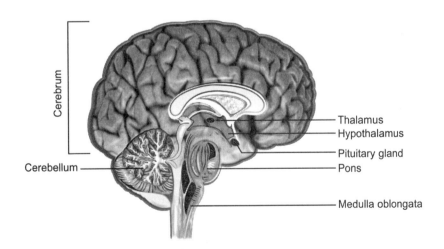

Fig. 5.1: Parts of brain

Cerebrum

The cerebrum is the largest part of the brain which is divided into right and left cerebral hemispheres connected by corpus callosum. Each lobe is covered by outer covering of gray matter known as the cortex and an inner part made up of white matter. Each cerebral hemisphere has frontal, parietal, temporal and occipital lobes. It is arranged in folds to form elevated portion known as convolutions or Gyri and depressions known as fissures or sulci. These divide the cerebrum into lobes such as frontal, temporal parietal and occipital lobes. The cerebral cotrex has important functional areas like motor areas in frontal lobe, general sensory and gustatory areas in parietal lobe, olfactory and auditory areas in temporal lobe and visual area in occipital lobe.

The main functions of cerebrum are memory, association, judgement, discrimination and thought. In addition to that sensory impulses and motor impulses are registered and controlled. The spaces or canals in the middle region of the cerebrum are called ventricles which contain a watery fluid flowing throughout the brain and spinal cord called cerebrospinal fluid (CSF). The cerebrospinal fluid can be withdrawn for diagnosis and relief of pressure from the brain. This is called spinal puncture or lumbar puncture.

Cerebrospinal Fluid

The cerebrospinal fluid is a clear, slightly alkaline fluid, consisting of water, mineral salts, glucose, protein, creatinine, and urea. Its specific gravity is 1.005. The main functions of the CSF are:

1. To protect brain and spinal cord from any shock and acts as a cushion
2. To maintain uniform pressure around these delicate structures
3. To keep the brain and spinal cord moist.

Cerebellum (Small Brain)

It is located beneath the posterior part of the cerebrum. The internal structure and functional organization of the cerebellum is complex but the general principle of its function are easily understood. The main function of the cerebellum is to maintain the balance, posture and co-ordination of voluntary movements and muscle tone. To perform this task it requires information and it receives this from the motor area of the cerebral cortex, and sensory receptors, namely vestibular and auditory receptors, visual receptors, proprio receptors (detecting sensation from within the body, e.g. as to the position of its parts, tactile touch), and visceral receptors.

The brainstem is composed of mid brain, pons varoli and medulla oblongata. The mid brain forms the upper part of the brainstem. The reflex areas of sight and hearing and from its base, to continue below through the pons and medulla oblongata to the spinal cord.

Pons

The pons is the part of the brain which literally means "Bridge". It lies between mid brain and medulla oblongata. Trigeminal, abducent, facial and vestibulo cochlear nerves arise from it. It is part of the brain containing nerve fibers, which connect the cerebellum and cerebrum with the rest of the brain.

Medulla Oblongata

It is located at the base of the brain which connects the spinal cord and the brain. Nerve tracts cross over in medulla oblongata. Hence, the nerves that control the movement of left side of the body are found in the right of the cerebrum and vice versa. In addition, it contains vital centers which control the rate and depth of breathing, rate of heart beat, swallowing and vomiting.

Thalamus and Hypothalamus

The thalamus is the large mass of gray matter which is situated below the cerebrum thalamus is predominantly a sensory relay station, with incoming fibers from the spinal cord and brainstem and onwards to the cerebral cortex. Lesions of the thalamus may cause pain, often continuous and of a burning nature, in the opposite side of the body.

The hypothalamus is composed of a number of nuclei and is the areas below the thalamus, at the base of the brain. The hypothalamus has neural connections to the posterior lobe of the pituitary gland (hypophysis) and vascular connections (known as portal hypophyseal vessels) to the anterior lobe of that gland.

The functions of hypothalamus are:
1. Synthesis of vasopressin
2. Control of anterior pituitary secretion
3. Control of appetite
4. Control of thirst
5. Regulation of body temperature
6. Emotional feeling and expression
7. Sexual behavior
8. Control of cardiac rhythms.

Spinal Cord

Spinal cord is the major part of the CNS, which lies in the vertebral canal. It extends from the medulla oblongata to second lumbar vertebra within the vertebral column. It ends as the cauda equina (horse tail), a fan of nerve fibers found below the second lumbar verterbra of the spinal column. Spinal cord is 45 cm long and 2 cm thick. It has two wider parts namely the cervical and lumbar enlargement from where the nerves of limbs originate. These nerves are called spinal nerves.

Bones protect both the brain and the spinal cord against injury. The brain is enclosed within the skull and the spinal cord is enclosed within the vertebral column. In addition, both the brain and the spinal cord receive limited protection from a set of three coverings called meninges.

The outer most coat, the dura mater is tough and fibrous. Immediately beneath the dura mater is the cavity called subdural space. The next layer of meninges is the arachonoid mater. The space beneath the arachnoid mater is called subarachnoid space, which is filled with cerebro-spinal fluid, which provides additional protection for the brain and spinal cord by acting as shock absorbers. The inner most layer, the pia mater contains numerous blood vessels and lymphatics which provides nourishment for the underlying tissues.

Functions of spinal cord are to relay impulses:
1. In and out at the same level
2. Up and down to other levels of the cord
3. To and from the brain.

PERIPHERAL NERVOUS SYSTEM

The peripheral nervous system (PNS) consists of cranial and spinal nerves. The PNS includes 12 pairs of cranial nerves, emerging from the base of the skull, and 31 pairs of spinal nerves, emerging from the spinal cord. All of these nerves consist of fibers that may be either sensory or motor or a mixture of both. Sensory or afferent nerves, carry impulses from the tissues to the brain for interpretation and give rise to sensations such as cold, heat, pain, etc. Motor or efferent nerves carry impulses away from the brain and spinal cord, to the tissues. Nerves composed of both sensory and motor fibers are called mixed nerves. An example of this is facial nerve, as it transmits the taste through the tongue and it supplies facial muscles impulses for smiling or masticating, etc.

Spinal Nerves

There are 31 pairs of spinal nerves namely; 8 cranial, 12 thoracic, 5 lumbar, 5 sacral, 1 coccygeal. Each spinal nerve is attached to the spinal cord by an anterior and a posterior root and divides into an anterior and a posterior ramus. The anterior root consists of motor fibers. The posterior root consists of a sensory fiber and has a posterior root (spinal) ganglion. The anterior ramus supplies the skin and muscles of the front and sides of the trunk and the limbs. The posterior ramus supplies the skin and muscles of the back of the trunk. Each spinal nerve consists of sensory and motor fiber. A nerve fiber branches and terminates in nerve endings, e.g. of sensory nerve endings, free nerve endings for pain, Meissner's corpuscles for touch, pacinian corpuscles for pressure, Krause end organs for cold, Ruffini end organs for warmth, and muscle spindles for proprioception (sensivity); e.g. for motor nerve endings, motor end plates on a muscle fiber.

The PNS is divided into two specialized nerves such as somatic nerves and autonomic nerves.

Somatic Nerves

The somatic nerves are under the direct control of the individual. It innervates the extremities and the body wall, including skeletal muscles and the skin. It is under the conscious control, and therefore it is voluntary, e.g. voluntary activity include walking, talking, etc.

Autonomic Nerves

The autonomic nerves comprises the sympathetic and parasympathetic nerves, producing actions that balance one another. The sympathetic and parasympathetic nerves function quite opposite to each other. The sympathetic nerves produce vasoconstriction, increase heart rate, elevate blood pressure and depress gastrointestinal activity. While parasympathetic nerves decrease blood pressure, dialate the pupil, slower heart rate, etc. The autonomic functions are evident in fight or flight situations. In either way the blood flow increases in skeletal muscles to prepare the individual to either fight or run away from a threatening situation.

Cranial Nerves

There are 12 pairs of cranial nerves connecting with the brainstem at different levels; some of them are motor nerves, some sensory and some mixed nerves (Table 5.1 and Fig. 5.2). They are:

Table 5.1: Names of cranial nerves and their functions

Position of cranial nerve	Name of the cranial nerve	Function
1.	Olfactory	Sensory nerves of smell from the nose
2.	Optic	Sensory nerves of sight from the eye
3.	Oculomotor	Motor nerves to the various muscles of eye
4.	Trochlear	Motor nerves to the various muscles of the eyeball
5.	Trigeminal	Has three branches—sensory nerves from the skin of the head and face, membrane of the mouth and nose and teeth and motor supplying the muscles of mastication (chewing)
6.	Abducent	Motor to one muscle of the eyeball
7.	Facial	• Sensory nerves of taste from the front part of the tongue • Motor nerves to the muscles of expression and the scalp
8.	Auditory/accoustic/ Vestibulocochlear	Sensory nerve of hearing and balance
9.	Glossopharyngeal	Sensory nerve of taste from back part of tongue
10.	Vagus	Sensory from many of the internal organs of the thorax and abdomen and blood vessels
11.	Spinal accessory	Motor joining the vagus to supply the larynx and pharynx and motor to the muscles of the neck
12.	Hypoglossal	Motor to the muscles of the tongue

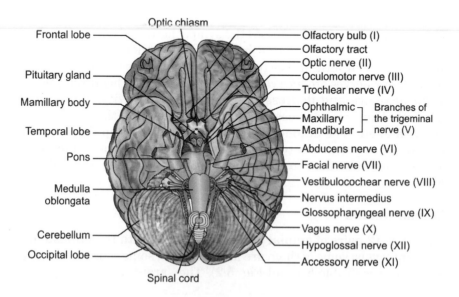

Fig. 5.2: Cross-section of brain with cranial nerves

NERVOUS SYSTEM

Origin of Terms

S.No.	Terms	Meanings	S.No.	Terms	Meanings
1.	-algesia, algia, algos	Pain	21.	Narc/o	Sleep
2.	-asthenia	Without strength	22.	Neur/o	Nerve, neuron
3.	Axon	Axis	23.	Nucleus	Little kernel
4.	Blephar/o	Eyelid	24.	Occiput	Back of head
5.	Cerebello	Cerebellum	25.	-paresis	Partial or incomplete paralysis
6.	Cerebrum, encephalon	Brain	26.	Phas/o	Speech
7.	Cord	String	27.	-plegia	Paralysis
8.	Cortex	Rind, bark	28.	Plexus	Braid, network or tangle
9.	Crani/o	Skull	29.	Polio-	Gray matter of the brain and spinal cord
10.	Dendron	Tree	30.	Pons	Bridge
11.	-esthesia	Feeling, sensation	31.	-praxia	Action
12.	Ganglion	Knot	32.	Radicle	Root
13.	Gli/o	Glue	33.	Spina	Thorn
14.	Gyrus	Convolution	34.	Synapse	Clasp
15.	Kinesi/o	Movement	35.	-taxia	Muscular coordination
16.	Lamina	Thin plate	36.	Thalamo	Chamber
17.	Lemma, Thec/o	Sheath	37.	Ton/o	Tone
18.	-lepsy	Seizure	38.	-trophy	Nourishment, development
19.	Medulla, myelo	Marrow	39.	Ventricle	Little belly or cavity
20.	Meninges	Membranes			

Symptomatic and Diagnostic Terms

S.No.	Terms	Meanings
1.	Amnesia	Loss of memory of recent events
2.	Analgesia	Loss of normal sense of pain
3.	Anesthesia	Loss of sensation with unconsciousness
4.	Aphasia	Difficulty in speech or understanding words
5.	Apoplexy	Stroke
6.	Astrocytoma	Slowly growing brain tumor consisting of astrocytes, that infiltrate widely into neighboring brain tissue and may undergo cystic degeneration
7.	Ataxia	Motor in coordination
8.	Aura	Warning signal or patient's awareness of onset of epileptic seizure
9.	Aural vertigo	Severe dizziness due to non-suppurative disease of labyrinth in ear
10.	Automatic bladder	Passing urine at regular intervals due to injury to spinal cord
11.	Autonomous bladder	Lack of bladder control characterized by urinary leak and residual urine

Contd...

Contd...

S.No.	Terms	Meanings
12.	Bell's palsy	Facial paralysis of unknown etiology or infection due to functional disorder of facial nerve (7th) resulting in unilateral paralysis of facial muscles and perceptions
13.	Causalgia	Burning pain often accompanied by tropic skin changes due to injury of a peripheral nerve
14.	Cerebral aneurysm	Ballooning of cerebral artery
15.	Cerebral arterial sclerosis	Hardening of the cerebral arteries
16.	Cerebral concussion	Transient unconsciousness following head injury as a result of injury to brainstem
17.	Cerebral embolism	Clot of blood or fat that travels in blood vessels (cerebral artery)
18.	Cerebral infarction	Local necrosis of brain tissue due to loss of blood supply in obstruction
19.	Cerebral ischemia	Anemia of the brain as a result of diminished blood flow
20.	Cerebral palsy	Paralysis due to pathology of brain characterized by in coordination and aberrations of motor and sensory functions
21.	Cerebral thrombosis	Thrombus formation within an intracranial artery leading to occlusion and necrosis of the one supplied by the thrombosed vessel
22.	Cerebrospinal otorrhea	Escape of CSF from ear following craniocerebral trauma due to fistula between ventricles or subarachnoid space and ear
23.	Cerebrospinal rhinorrhea	Escape of CSF from nose following cerebrospinal trauma due to fistulous communication between ventricles and subarachnoid space and the nose
24.	Cerebrovascular accident	Neurologic disorder caused by pathologic changes in the extracranial or intracranial blood vessels primarily by atherosclerosis, thrombosis, embolic episodes, hemorrhage, or by arterial hypertension resulting in hemiplegia (stroke)
25.	Cervical spondylitis	Inflammation of the cervical spine
26.	Chorea	Nervous disorder characterized by bizarre, abrupt involuntary movement
27.	Coma	State of unconciousness which cannot be aroused by external stimulation
28.	Concussion	An injury (usually to the brain) resulting from impact with an object
29.	Convulsion	Paroxysms of involuntary muscular contractions and relaxations
30.	Diplegia	Paralysis on both sides of the body
31.	Dysarthria	Incoordination of speech muscles joint defect in mandible
32.	Dyskinesia	Impairment of power of voluntary movements postures due to brain lesion

Contd...

Contd...

S.No.	Terms	Meanings
33.	Encephalitis	Inflammation of brain
34.	Encephalocele	Protrusion of the brain substance through a fissure of the skull
35.	Enuresis	Involuntary discharge (or) incontinence of urine druing sleep at night
36.	Ependymoma	Tumor arising from the line of the ventricular valve composed of ependymal cells
37.	Epilepsy	Convulsive disorder, recurrent seizures may occur
38.	Euphoria	Exaggerated feeling of wellbeing
39.	Fasciculation	Involuntary twitching of group of muscle fibers
40.	Festination	Quick shuffling steps in Parkinson's disease
41.	Frequency of urination	Voiding at close in intervals, more often at even 2 hours. It is normal in children
42.	Ganglioneuroma	True neuroma made up of nerve cells
43.	Glioblastoma multifoma	Rapidly growing malignant glioma causing edema and necrosis of brain tissue
44.	Glioma	Malignant tumor or brain
45.	Glycosuria	Sugar in urine
46.	Grand mal epilepsy	A serious form of epileptic seizure with or without coma
47.	Hematuria	Blood in urine
48.	Hemiparesis	Slight degree of paralysis affecting one side of the body
49.	Hemiplegia	Paralysis affecting one side of the body
50.	Hydrocephalus	Dilation of the cerebral ventricles occurring secondarily to obstruction of the cerebrospinal fluid pathways marked by enlargement of the head
51.	Hyperesthesia	Increased sensibility to sensory stimuli .
52.	Intention tremor	Trembling when attempting voluntary movements
53.	Intracranial hematoma	Local mass of extravasated blood forming subsequent to intercranial hemorrhage
54.	Intracranial hemorrhage	Rupture of vessel beneath the skull with leakage of blood in the brain may be due to stroke injury or ruptured of aneurysm. Brain damage depends upon the location and extent of lesion involved.
55.	Meningioma	A hard, usually vascular tumor
56.	Meningitis	Inflammation of the meninges due to bacteria, fungi, virus, etc.
57.	Meningocele	Protrusion of the meninges through the defect in spinal cord
58.	Meningomyelocele	Herniation of cord at meninges through the defect of spinal cord (vertebral column).
59.	Microcephalus	Abnormally small head associated sometimes with ideally, mental deficiency

Contd...

Contd...

S.No.	Terms	Meanings
60.	Migraine	Left/right sided headache or one sided headache
61.	Myelitis	Inflammation of the spinal cord
62.	Myelopathy	Disease of the spinal cord
63.	Myasthenia gravis	Muscle weakness marked by progressive paralysis
64.	Nystagmus	Constant involuntary movements of eyeballs
65.	Oligodendroglioma	Tumor of the cerebral hemispheres similar to astrocytoma in behavior, different in histological studies
66.	Papilledema	Swelling of the optic disc
67.	Paraparesis	Slight paralysis of lower limbs
68.	Paraplegia	Paralysis of lower limbs and lower trunk
69.	Paresis	Partial paralysis
70.	Paresthesia	Abnormal sensation heightened sensory response to stimuli
71.	Parkinsonism	Hardening of brain tissue
72.	Petit mal epilepsy	Mild form of epileptic seizure lasting 10–30 seconds
73.	Poliomyelitis	Viral disease with lesions in CNS and causing varying disabilities including paralysis and deformity of the limbs, atrophy of muscles, stiffness of neck and back.
74.	Quadriplegia	Paralysis of upper spine; paralysis of all four extremities and usually the trunk
75.	Radiculitis	Inflammation of spinal nerve roots accompanied by pain and hyperesthesia
76.	Sciatic neuritis, sciatica	A syndrome characterized by radiating pain from the back into the buttock, thigh and running inside of the leg
77.	Subarachnoid hemorrhage	Bleeding into subarachnoid space due to injury or intracranial aneurysm, rupture associated with excreting headache, convulsions and coma
78.	Syncope	Fainting due to in adequate blood flow to brain
79.	Syringomyelocele	Protrusion of cord and meninges through the defect in spinal cord
80.	Tic	Spasmodic muscular contraction commonly in face, neck, and shoulder
81.	Torticollis	Stiff neck
82.	Tremor	Involuntary shaking or trembling
83.	Vertigo	Dizziness
84.	Paralysis	Loss of sensation and voluntary movements, either temporary or permanent a. Flaccid lower motor neuron involvement b. Spastic upper motor neuron involvement
85.	Paraplegia	Paralysis of lower part of the body

Operative Terms

S.No.	Terms	Meanings
1.	Cordectomy	Removal of a portion of spinal cord to convert a spastic paralysis (of lower extremities) to a paralysis
2.	Cordotomy, chordotomy	Section of a nerve fiber tract within the cord for relief of pain
3.	Craniectomy	Excision of part of the skull
4.	Craniotomy	Opening of the skull (Burrhole or Trafilination) in order to prepare bone flap
5.	Cryoneurosurgery	Operative use of cold in the destruction of neurosurgical lesions
6.	Cystostomy	Surgical creation of cutaneous bladder fistula for urine drainage
7.	Encephalopuncture	Puncture into brain substance
8.	Ganglionectomy	Excision of ganglion (sympathectomy)
9.	Laminectomy	Excision of one or more posterior arch of vertebra method of approach to spinal cord postevacuated part of each side of vertebra
10.	Meatotomy	Incision of urinary meatus (opening) to increase its caliber
11.	Microneurosurgery	Use of the surgical binocular microscope which provides powerful light source with 25 times magnification, employed for cerebral aneurysm pituitary tumor and spinal cord tumors
12.	Neurectomy	Dissection of a nerve partial or total
13.	Neuroanastomosis	Surgical communication between nerve fibers
14.	Neurolysis	Freeing a nerve from adhesions (breaking up of peripheral nerve adhesions)
15.	Neuroplasty	Plastic repair of the nerve
16.	Neurorrhaphy	Suture of the injured nerve
17.	Neurotomy	Surgical cutting of a nerve
18.	Sympathectomy	Excision or resection of part of the sympathetic nervous pathways
19.	Thalamotomy	Partial destruction of the thalamus in order to treat psychosis or intractable pain
20.	Tractotomy	Transaction of a fiber tract of the CNS, sometimes restored for relief of intractable pain
21.	Trephination	Boring with hole into skull, a method of approach into the brain "circular opening"
22.	Vagotomy	Transection of vagus nerve

COMMON ABBREVIATIONS

S.No.	Abbreviation	Term
1.	Ach	Acetylcholine
2.	AEG	Air encephalogram
3.	ANS	Autonomic nervous system
4.	BIH	Benign intracranial hypertension
5.	CA	Chronologic age
6.	CAT	Computerized axial tomography
7.	CBF	Cerebral blood flow
8.	CBS	Chronic brain syndrome
9.	CNS	Central nervous system
10.	CP	Cereberal palsy
11.	CSF	Cerebrospinal fluid
12.	CST	Convulsive shock therapy
13.	CT Scan	Computerized tomography scan
14.	CVA	Cerebrovascular accident
15.	CVD	Cerebrovascular disease
16.	DT	Delirium tremens
17.	ECS	Electroconvulsive shock
18.	ECT	Electroconvulsive therapy
19.	EEG	Electroencephalogram
20.	EJ	Elbow jerk
21.	EST	Electric shock therapy
22.	HNP	Herniated nucleus pulposus (herniated disk)
23.	ICT	Insulin coma therapy
24.	IQ	Intellegence quotient
25.	JBE	Japanese B encephalitis
26.	KJ	Knee jerk
27.	LP	Lumbar puncture
28.	MA	Mental age
29.	MS	Multiple sclerosis
30.	NS	Neurosurgery
31.	OBS	Organic brain syndrome
32.	PEG	Pneumoencephalogram
33.	PMI	Point of maximum impulse
34.	PNS	Peripheral nervous system
35.	REM	Rapid eye movement
36.	SCI	Spinal cord injury
37.	SLE	St. Louis encephalitis
38.	SNS	Sympathetic nervous system
39.	SR	Stimulus response
40.	TBM	Tuberculosis meningitis
41.	TIA	Transient ischemic attack
42.	UCR	Unconditional reflex
43.	VMR	Vasomotor rhinitis
44.	WPWS	Wolf-Parkinson-White (syndrome)

Digestive System

INTRODUCTION

The digestive system is one of the important systems of the body, through which the energy is supplied externally as food, which is converted into the required chemicals for the nutrition of the cells, tissues, etc. The digestive system is also called the alimentary or gastrointestinal system.

Food is one of the essential needs of the body and good health depends on proper nutrition. There are six essential nutrients with which the body must be constantly supplied. They are proteins, vitamins, carbohydrates, mineral salts, fats and water. When food is ingested, the digestive system plays a vital role in the conversion process of complex food substance such as proteins to simple amino acids, complex sugars to simple sugars (glucose) and large fat molecules are broken down to fatty acids and glycerol, which can be absorbed by the cells as nutrients. Finally, the unwanted materials are eliminated through the anus.

Digestion can be defined as the complete process of changing the chemical and physical compositions of food in order to facilitate assimilation of the nourishing ingredients of food by cells of the body.

The primary functions of the organs of the digestive system can be explained simply in three stages:

1. *Digestion:* Breaking down of the complex food materials mechanically or chemically, into simpler amino acids, glucose, fatty acids and triglycerides as it travels through the gastrointestinal tract (passageway).
2. *Absorption*: Absorption of the digested foods into the bloodstream by entering into the walls of small intestine.
3. *Elimination:* The third and final function of the digestive system is to eliminate, the solid waste materials which are unable to be absorbed into the bloodstream. This process is called as defecation.

ORGANS OF THE DIGESTIVE SYSTEM (FIG. 6.1)

The organs of the digestive system are:
• Oral (or) buccal cavity or mouth
  – Lips
  – Cheeks
  – Palate
  – Uvula
  – Tongue
  – Teeth
  – Gums
  – Tonsils
  – Epiglottis
  – Salivary glands
• Pharynx
• Esophagus
• Stomach
• Small intestine
• Large intestine
• Colon
• Rectum
• Anus.

Oral Cavity (Fig. 6.2)

The gastrointestinal (GI) tract is a continuous tubular passageway that begins at the oral cavity or mouth.

Lips

Lips form an opening for the oral cavity. The lips are a highly muscular, vascular and motile organ, which also serves as the organ for speech.

Cheeks

Cheeks are the walls of the oval-shaped oral-cavity. It acts as the temporary reservoir for food substances during the mastication process.

Palate

Palate forms the bottom and roof of the mouth (oral cavity). There are two palates, viz hard palate forms the anterior portion of the roof of the oral cavity and the muscular soft palate lies in its posterior portion and it separates the mouth from the pharynx.

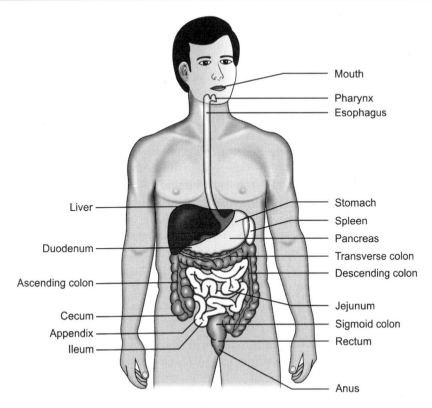

Fig. 6.1: Parts of the digestive system

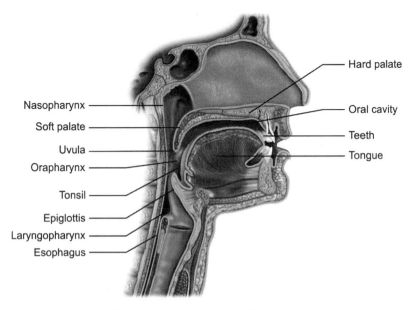

Fig. 6.2: Cross-section of oral cavity

Uvula

A small V-shaped soft tissue hanging from the soft palate. The main function of the uvula is producing sounds and speech while the other is to guide the downward movement of the food after chewing into the pharynx.

Tongue

Tongue extends across the floor of the mouth. Tongue acts as a sense, speech and digestive organ. The main functions of the tongue are to move the food around during mastication (chewing), deglutition (swallowing), speech production and determination of taste. The surface of the tongue is covered by small projections called papillae, which contain cells, called taste buds, which are sensitive to the chemical reaction. These taste buds respond to the brain through the 7th cranial nerve (facial nerve) and 9th cranial nerve (glossopharyngeal nerve) to determine the taste and nature of the substance in contact.

Teeth

Teeth are situated in the front of the oral cavity. They play an important role in the initial stages of digestion. A tooth consists of a crown, which is above the gum and a root, which is embedded in the body tooth socket. The outmost protective layer of the crown is called the enamel. Enamel is a dense, hard white substance. The dentine is the root, covered by a protective and supportive layer called cementum. A periodontal membrane surrounds the cementum and holds the tooth in its place of the tooth socket. Below the dentine, the pulp is present which contains blood vessels, nerve endings, connective tissue and lymph vessels.

For an adult, normally there will be 16 pairs (32 teeth) of teeth situated at the upper and lower jaw. The teeth located in the front of the oral cavity are called incisors, which cut and tear the food into smaller pieces. The teeth located in the rear of the oral cavity are called molars, they further crush and grind the food into finer particles.

The following are the names of the teeth of one-half of either lower or upper jaw. Thereby 4 times of the 8 teeth collectively form 32 permanent teeth in any adult:

1. Central incisor
2. Lateral incisor
3. Canine
4. First bicuspid
5. Second bicuspid
6. First molar
7. Second molar
8. Third molar or wisdom tooth

In general, there will be 2 incisors (1 and 2), 1 canine (3), 2 premolars (4 and 5), 3 molars (6 to 8).

Gums

The gums are made of pink fleshy tissue and are surrounded by the sockets in which the teeth are planted.

Tonsils

The tonsils are the organs made-up of lymphatic tissue. They are situated in depressions of the mucous membranes in the wall of the pharynx. They act as filters to protect the body from the invasion of microorganisms and produce lymphocytes, which are white blood cells able to fight diseases.

Epiglottis

A small flap of tissue that covers the trachea. It acts as a gatekeeper to prevent the inflow of food through the trachea (wind pipe) and allows all food to be channeled to stomach through the esophagus.

Salivary Glands

There are three pairs of salivary glands situated in the oral cavity. They are parotid gland in the posterior part of the oral cavity, submaxillary gland under the maxillary bone or beneath the jaw and sublingual gland below the tongue on either side in the mouth. Narrow ducts carry the saliva into the oral cavity. The salivary glands are exocrine glands producing saliva, which contain digestive enzymes. The saliva is released when the food is smelt or during the thought of the food. It contains 90 percent of water and the enzyme ptyalin, which begins the digestion of carbohydrates. It also contains a thick slippery lubricant called mucin and small amount of calcium salts.

Pharynx

The pharynx is a muscular membrane. It is the common passage for air and food. The walls of the pharynx are composed of muscles arranged in thin overlaping sheets, these form the constrictor muscles which contract during the act of swallowing. The pharynx is divided into three major sections:
1. Nasopharynx—behind the nose and throat
2. Oropharynx—behind the mouth
3. Laryngopharynx—part of the throat above the larynx. It is further divided into two tubes, one leads to lungs called trachea (wind pipe) and other leads to stomach called esophagus.

Esophagus

The esophagus is a tube like structure called as food pipe, which extends from the laryngopharynx to the stomach. It is about 9 to 10 inches long. The main function of the esophagus is to move the food from the pharynx cavity to the stomach by the process called Peristalsis. Peristalsis is progressive, wavelike contractions which propels the food through the system.

Gastrointestinal Tract

The stomach, small intestine, and large intestine together form the gastrointestinal (GI) tract.

Stomach

The stomach is an elastic sac like structure located in the abdominal cavity, below the diaphragm which separates the abdominal and thoracic cavity. It is a muscular organ and its shape and size vary according to the amount and type of its contents.

The stomach is divided into three parts 1. Fundus (the upper part), 2. Body (the middle part), 3. Antrum (the end part). The openings of the stomach are governed by the sphincters, the cardiac sphincter between the esophagus and fundus (the upper part of the stomach) preventing the backflow of the food into the esophagus, and the pyloric sphincter between the antrum (the end part of stomach) and the small intestine. Within the stomach, there is considerable number of folds called rugae. These rugae appear when stomach is empty and when it is full, it disappears and the inner wall becomes smooth. The stomach is lined by mucous membrane, which secretes mucus that protects the stomach walls and food from the acid secretions. The interior wall of the stomach is composed of mucous membrane and contains the glands that secrete hydrochloric acid (HCl) and gastric juices.

Gastric juice is a clear and slightly acidic fluid, containing HCl, enzymes, minerals and salts. A total quantity of 1½ to 2 liters is secreted every day. The three enzymes play an important role in digestion by converting food into nourishing ingredients absorbed by the cells of the body.

Beginning the chemical digestion, **Pepsin** reduces proteins to peptones and polypeptides; a further stage of protein digestion takes place in the small intestine.

Rennin converts the soluble milk proteins caseinogen to the insoluble form, casein, which is then reduced to peptones by pepsin.

Gastric Lipase is an enzyme produced in small amounts, and it begins the digestion of fats.

The intrinsic factor (protein compound) is necessary for the absorption of vitamin B_{12}. Vitamin B_{12} is also called the anti-anemic factor. It is present in food and is absorbed through the walls of the small intestine and stored in the liver until required in the red bone marrow for the normal development of erythrocytes.

Food entering into the cardiosphincter is mixed with the gastric secretions such as gastric juice, HCl and mucus by churning. Once the food is mixed with gastric juices and HCl, it forms semicreamy fluid called chyme. When it is sufficiently digested, the chyme leaves the stomach through the pyloric sphincter to enter into the small intestine.

Functions of stomach:
- Physical digestion
- Changing solid food into semisolid
- Chemical digestion begins here.

Small Intestine

The small intestine is the continuation of the gastrointestinal tract from the pyloric sphincter to the large intestine. It is about 20 feet long and has three parts:
1. *The duodenum:* Upper most division about 1 foot long
2. *Jejunum:* The second part of the intestine which is about 8 feet long
3. *Ileum:* The third part of the intestine which is about 11 feet long.

The small intestine has four layers:
1. An outer serous layer
2. Muscular middle layer
3. Submucous layer
4. Innermost mucous membrane layer.

The functions of the small intestine are completion of digestion of food, and to absorb the essential nutrients (end products) of digestion.

The secretion of the acid chyme in the duodenum distends the intestinal wall and causes the mucosa to secrete mucus and intestinal juice which contain the enzyme enterokinase. At the same time the hormones such as secretin, and cholecystokinin are secreted and stimulate the pancreas to secrete the fluid containing sodium bicarbonate that reacts with the acid in the chyme and neutralize it. This process prevents the ulceration of duodenum.

Cholecystokinin causes the pancrease to secrete digestive enzymes: Amylase for digesting carbohydrates, trypsinogen and chymotrypsionogen for digesting proteins, lipase for digesting fats. Cholecystokinin also stimulates the gallbladder to empty bile, (which is essential for the digestion of fats) into duodenum through the bile duct and the ampula of vater.

In the walls of the entire small intestine, there are tiny projects called villi. Through the tiny capillaries in the villi, the nutrients such as monosaccharides and aminoacids are absorbed into the bloodstream, in addition to this, iron, vitamins and calcium, any fluids that are ingested, and almost all the secretion of the alimentary tract are also reabsorbed which is approximately 8 liters a day. Only about 800 ml is passed to the large intestine.

Functions of small intestine:
- Complete physical and chemical digestion
- Secreting digestive juice which contain enzymes
- Provides a large surface area for absorption of food
- Passes waste material to large intestine by peristalsis
- Protection by screening bacteria.

Large Intestine

The large intestine is a continuation of the gastrointestinal tract and is attached to ileum of the small intestine and ends at the sigmoid colon. The large intestine is divided into two major divisions cecum and colon. The large intestine has 4 layers, they are serous, muscular, submucous and mucous layers.

The cecum or the first part of the large intestine is about 2 to 3 inches long and it is connected to the ileum by ileocecal sphincter. The vermiform appendix suspends from the cecum. The appendix is the only organ which has no anatomy.

The colon is about 5 feet long and has three divisions:
1. *Ascending colon*: Extending from the cecum to the lower border of the liver.
2. *Transverse colon*: Extending the ascending colon and passing horizontally to the left towards the spleen.
3. *Descending colon*: Extending from the transverse colon and being downwards and bending in the S-shape, at the distal end to form the sigmoid colon.

The major function of large intestine is to receive the waste products from the small intestine after the digestion and store them until these are released from the body. The water in the waste products is absorbed here and the solid feces (stools) are formed.

Functions of large intestine:
- Absorption of water from the fecal matter
- Secretion of mucus
- Passes the fecal by mass peristalsis into rectum
- Rectum expels the fecal known as defecation.

Rectum

The rectum extends from the sigmoid colon and it ends in the lower opening of the GI tract called the anus. It serves as a storage area for the waste products.

Anus

The anus is the end part of the GI tract. It has internal and external sphincters or muscles, which is closed, except during the process of defecation.

ACCESSORY ORGANS OF DIGESTION

The important accessory organs of the digestive system are:
- Liver
- Pancreas
- Gallbladder.

Liver

The liver is the largest gland in the body and weighs around 1 to 1.5 Kg. It lies under the diaphragm on the right hand side of the abdomen. It has a large right lobe and a small left lobe. The vital functions of the liver are:
- Produces bile, which is used in the small intestine to break and absorb fats
- Removes glucose (sugar) from blood, which it synthesizes and stores as glycogen
- Stores vitamins such as B_{12}, A, D, E, and K
- Removal of poisons from the blood
- Destroys old erythrocytes and releases bilirubin
- Produces various blood proteins, such as prothrombin and fibrinogen, which helps in the clotting of blood.

The liver substance consists of hepatic lobules, which are composed of hepatic cells arranged as sheets called hepatic laminae. Between the laminae are hepatic sinusoids. Blood enters the sinusoids from hepatic artery and portal vein and leaves by hepatic veins, which join the inferior vena cava.

Bile

Bile is the external secretion of the liver and is produced in a diluted form, which is then concentrated by gallbladder to a greenish viscous fluid. It is composed of water, bile salts, bile pigments, and mucus. Bile salts play an important role in assisting the digestive action of pancreatic enzymes and in aiding the absorption of fat and fat-soluble vitamins from the small intestine. Bile pigments are derived from the breakdown of hemoglobin of worn-out red blood cells and give the bile its characteristic color. If there is an obstruction to the excretion of bile, the bile accumulates in the blood, giving the skin and mucous membrane a yellow color (jaundice). At the same time they appear in the urine, which turns into dark brown.

Bile is continuously released from the liver, travels down to the hepatic duct, cystic duct, and gallbladder where it is stored and concentrated for later use.

Gallbladder

The gallbladder is a small pear-shaped organ situated below (underneath) the liver and acts as resorvior for the bile from the liver and to concentrate it. It is capable of storing 60 ml of bile. The hepatic duct connects the liver and gallbladder through which the bile is passed and stored in the gallbladder. The gallbladder has three layers:
1. An outer serous peritoneal coat
2. A middle muscular layer
3. An inner lining of mucous membrane continuous to the lining of the bile ducts. This membrane secretes mucin and absorbs water and electrolytes thus concentrating the bile.

Gallbladder is connected to the duodenum by cystic duct with which the hepatic duct becomes the common bile duct. Whenever any fatty substance is identified in the duodenum, hormone cholecystokinin is released and when it reaches the gallbladder, the bladder contracts, to release bile through the cystic duct into the common bile duct, which joins the pancreatic duct before entering into the duodenum.

Pancreas

The pancreas is a leaf like structure situated behind the stomach between the loop of duodenum and spleen. It acts as both endocrine and exocrine gland. In the digestive system, it provides digestive juices that pass through the pancreatic duct, thus it becomes an exocrine gland and also releases hormones directly into the bloodstream and functions as endocrine or ductless gland. The exocrine part secrets three enzymes: trypsin which acts on protein, amylase which acts on maltose, lipase which acts on fat. The endocrine part of the pancreas is related to islets of Langerhans, whose beta cells secrete the hormone insulin and alpha cells secrete the hormone glucagon, which regulate the blood sugar level.

Functions of Pancreas

Exocrine pancreatic juice contains three enzymes:
1. Trypsin   acts on protein
2. Amylase   acts on maltose
3. Lipase   acts on fats
   Endocrine secretes insulin, necessary for metabolism of glucose and fat.

METABOLISM

Metabolism is the chemical reaction, which occurs, in the whole body. It is divided into two major processes anabolism and catabolism.

Anabolism is building or synthesis of new compound and this process is energy consuming. Catabolism is the breaking down of large molecules to smaller units to release energy and heat. In healthy adults, there will be a balance between anabolism and catabolism, which is called energy balance. Both processes occur continuously and simultaneously in regulating chemical reactions in series.

DIGESTIVE SYSTEM

Origin of Terms

S.No.	Terms	Meanings	S.No.	Terms	Meanings
1.	Celi	Abdomen	33.	Colon	Large intestine
2.	Laparo	Abdominal wall	34.	Cheilos, Labio, Labium	Lip
3.	—iasis	Abnormal condition	35.	Uvula	Little grape
4.	Tonsilla	Almond, tonsil	36.	Hepato	Liver
5.	Ano, Procto	Anus	37.	Mandible	Lower Jaw
6.	Append	Appendix	38.	Omentum	Membrane enclosing bowel
7.	Fundus	Base	39.	Os, ora, Stoma	Mouth
8.	Parotid	Beside the ear	40.	Palatum	Palate
9.	Cholangi	Bile duct	41.	Pancreat	Pancreas
10.	Choledoch	Bile duct	42.	-prandial	Pertaining to a meal
11.	Bile, Chole	Bile, gall	43.	Pylor	Pylorus, gatekeeper
12.	Sphincter	Binder	44.	Rect/o	Rectum
13.	Cecum	Blind gut	45.	Ptyalin, Sialon	Saliva
14.	Emulsification	Breaking up of large fat molecules	46.	Sialangi	Salivary duct
15.	Staphyle	Bunch of grapes	47.	Sialaden	Salivary gland
16.	-lith	Calculus, stone	48.	Vermiform	Shape of worm
17.	Cec/o	Cecum	49.	Sigmoid	Sigmoid colon
18.	Bucca	Cheek	50.	Spleen	Spleen
19.	Enterolith	Concretion of feces due to constipation	51.	Gaster	Stomach, belly
20.	-rrhea	Discharge, flow	52.	Sigm	Straight
21.	Jejunum	Empty	53.	Peritoneum	Stretching over
22.	-ase	Enzyme	54.	Glyc/o	Sugar
23.	Lip/o steat/o	Fat, lipids	55.	-phagia	Swallowing, ingesting, eating
24.	Ruga	Fold crease	56.	Pharynx, pharyng/o	Throat
25.	Esophagus	Food carrier	57.	-crine	To secrete
26.	Cholecyst	Gallbladder	58.	Ileum	To twist
27.	Glycogen/o	Glycogen	59.	Glosso, Lingua	Tongue
28.	Gingiva	Gum	60.	Dent, Odent	Tooth
29.	Herni/o	Hernia	61.	Duodenum	Twelve
30.	-chlorhydria	Hydrochloric acid	62.	-emesis	Vomit
31.	Ile/o	Ileum	63.	Cirrho	Yellow, tawny
32.	Enteron, enter/o	Intestine			

Symptomatic and Diagnostic Terms

S.No.	Terms	Meanings
1.	Achlorhydria	Lack of hydrochloric acid in the stomach
2.	Aerophagia	Swallowing of air
3.	Ankyloglossia	Immovable tongue or tongue tie

Contd...

Contd...

S.No.	Terms	Meanings
4.	Anorexia	Loss of appetite
5.	Aphagia	Inability or absence from eating or swallowing
6.	Appendicitis	Inflammation of appendix
7.	Ascites	Collection of ascitic fluid in the peritoneal cavity
8.	Borborygmus	Gurgling, splashing sound heard over the large intestine
9.	Bulimia	An eating disorder characterized by binge eating following by purging in girls/young women
10.	Cheilitis	Inflammation of the lip
11.	Cholangitis	Inflammation of bile duct
12.	Cholecystitis	Inflammation of gallbladder frequently associated with gallstones
13.	Choledocholithiasis	Presence of calculi in the common bile duct
14.	Cholelithiasis	Presence of calculi in the bile duct
15.	Cholemia	Abnormal amount of bile in the blood which results in hepatic coma
16.	Cirrhosis (liver)	A chronic disease of the liver
17.	Colic	Spasm in any hollow or tubular soft organ accompanied by pain
18.	Colitis	Inflammation of the colon (large intestine)
19.	Constipation	Infrequent or difficult evacuation of the feces
20.	Deglutition	Swallowing
21.	Dental caries	Disease of the calcified tissues of the teeth, resulting by the action of microorganisms on carbohydrates, characterized by decalcification and disintegration of the organic portion
22.	Diabetes mellitus	The most significant pathogenic alternation of the islets cell cause a depression in the insulin storage resulting in polyuria, glycosuria, elevated blood sugar level
23.	Diaphragmatic hernia	Herniation of the abdominal wall through the diaphragm
24.	Diarrhoea	Frequent discharge of watery and fluid stool due to infection, allergy, increase of temperature and seasonal changes
25.	Digestant	An agent capable of aiding digestion
26.	Diverticulosis	Herniation in the colon
27.	Duodenal ulcer	Circumscribed erosion of duodenal walls which may involve its full thickness and usually located near the pylorus
28.	Dysentery	Painful inflammation of the intestinal mucosa characterized by frequent stool with blood and mucous due to infection
29.	Dyspepsia	Poor digestion
30.	Dysphagia	Inability or difficulty in swallowing
31.	Enteritis	Inflammation of small intestine
32.	Enterocolitis	Inflammation of small intestine and large intestine

Contd...

Contd...

S.No.	Terms	Meanings
33.	Enterolysis	Freeing of intestinal adhesions disease
34.	Eructation	Producing gas from the stomach, belching
35.	Esophagitis	Inflammation of the esophagus
36.	Fecalith	Fecal concretion
37.	Femoral	The organ passes through the femoral canal
38.	Fissure-in-ano	Tear in anal mucosa which may become ulcerated, infected, spastic and painful
39.	Fistula in ano	Abnormal communication between anal canal or lower rectum and skin near anus
40.	Flatus	Gas in the digestive tract
41.	Gastric ulcer	Ulceration or localized erosions of gastric mucosa with burning sensation
42.	Gastritis	Inflammation of the stomach
43.	Gastroenteritis	Inflammation of stomach and intestine due to infection or food poisoning with vomiting and diarrhea, sometimes ulcer may occur
44.	Gastroptosis	Downward displacement of the stomach commonly seen in old age. In women it may be due to giving birth to too many children or standing for a long-time
45.	Gingivitis	Inflammation of the gum
46.	Glossitis	Inflammation of the tongue
47.	Glycosuria	Presence of sugar in urine
48.	Halitosis	Bad or offensive odour of breath due to infection in the stomach, intestine, excess hydrochloric acid, ulcer infection in the gum or tooth
49.	Harelip (cleft lip)	Congenital anomaly of the upper lip consisting of vertical fissure, often associated with cleft palate
50.	Hematemesis	Vomiting blood
51.	Hepatic coma	Terminal stage of hepatic cirrhosis characterized by slow or rapid bizarre disorientation, trauma, hyperactive reflexes due to the failure of liver
52.	Hepatitis	Acute or chronic inflammation of liver caused by virus A or virus B. It is of three types as infective hepatitis, viral hepatitis and serum hepatitis
53.	Hepatomegaly	Enlargement of liver
54.	Hernia	Protrusion or descending of part, from its normal position
55.	Hyperglycemia	High blood sugar
56.	Hyperperistalsis	Excessive worm like movement of small intestine or exacerbated muscular spasm of intestine causing discomfort on account of rapid contractions
57.	Hypertrophy of adenoids and tonsils	Increase in size of tonsils and adenoids due to increased cell constituency
58.	Ileocolitis	Inflammation of ileum and colon due to ischemia and results in ulceration
59.	Incisional hernia	Postoperative hernia through an open scar
60.	Intussusception	The slipping of one part of an intestine into the immediate adjacent part just below it (telescoping)

Contd...

Contd...

S.No.	Terms	Meanings
61.	Irritable bowel syndrome (IBS)	Inflammatory condition marked by large amount of mucous in stool
62.	Jaundice	Yellow discoloration of the skin and sclera due to excess bilirubin in the blood circulation
63.	Ketosis	Condition of having excessive amount of ketone in body tissues and fluids
64.	Leukoplakia of mouth	Disease marked by the development of white patches upon the mucous membrane of the cheeks, gums and teeth. Sometimes with fissure common in smokers which may become malignant
65.	Melanuria	Presence of melanin in the urine
66.	Melena	Black stool and sometimes with black color vomiting
67.	Obstipation	Extreme constipation due to obstruction
68.	Pancreatitis	Inflammation of the pancreas
69.	Parotitis	Inflammation of the parotid gland due to obstruction in salivary duct or viral and bacterial infection
70.	Peptic ulcer	Overall name for ulcer of stomach
71.	Peristalsis	A progressive wavelike movement that occurs involuntarily in hollow tubes of the body, especially the alimentary canal
72.	Peritonitis	Inflammation of the peritoneum
73.	Polyphagia	Excessive food intake
74.	Portal hypertension	A portal venous pressure above 20 mm Hg. Associated with splenomegaly increased collateral circulation varicosity, bleeding, and ascites
75.	Proctitis	Inflammation of rectum
76.	Ptyalism	Excessive secretion of saliva
77.	Pyloric stenosis	Congenital or acquired condition marked by obstruction of the pyloric orifice of the stomach
78.	Quinsy	Sore throat or peritonsilar abscess
79.	Regurgitation	Return of solids or fluids to the mouth from the stomach
80.	Sialoadenitis	Inflammation of salivary gland
81.	Sialolithiaisis	Formation of calculi in the salivary gland
82.	Steatorrhea	Excessive amount of fat in the feces, as in the malabsorption syndromes
83.	Stomatitis	Inflammation of mucosa of the mouth due to systemic disease, allergy or toxic drug effect, ulcers and fissures in the corners of the mouth may be present
84.	Thrush	Whitish spots in the mouth and tongue. It is common in infants and rare in adults with fever and gastroenteritis
85.	Ventral hernia	Hernia through the anterior abdominal wall
86.	Visceroptosis	Prolapse or downward displacement of the viscera especially the abdominal organs
87.	Xerostomia	Dry mouth condition or dryness of the mouth due to lack of normal salivary secretions.

Operative Terms

S.No.	Terms	Meanings
1.	Anastomosis	Surgical formation of a passage of opening between two hollow viscera or vessels
2.	Adenoidectomy	Removal of adenoids
3.	Anorexia	Loss of appetite
4.	Appendectomy	Surgical removal of appendix
5.	Biopsy of liver	Removal of piece of liver tissue for microscopic study
6.	Cecectomy	Removal of cecum
7.	Cheiloplasty	Plastic repair of the lip
8.	Cholecystectomy	Removal of gallbladder
9.	Choledocholithotomy	Incision into the bile duct for removal of gallstones
10.	Clipping of franum linguae	Clipping of membraneous fold below the tongue to relieve the tongue tie
11.	Colectomy	Excision of the infected part of colon and end to end anastomosis
12.	Diverticulectomy	Excision of diverticulum
13.	Dysphagia	Difficulty in swallowing
14.	Enteroenterostomy	Anastomosis or connection between two parts of intestine
15.	Eructation	Belching (bringing of gas out of stomach)
16.	Esophagectomy	Removal of a part of the esophagus
17.	Esophageotomy	Incision of the esophagus for diverticulum in the esophagus
18.	Esophagogastrostomy	Surgical operation of making an artificial communication between the stomach and esophagus
19.	Esophagojejunostomy	Formation of a communication between the esophagus and jejunum
20.	Exodontist	A person who extracts the tooth
21.	Exploratory laparotomy	Incision of the abdomen that allows the surgeon to explore the abdominal cavity to determine the extent of disease
22.	Gastrectomy	Removal of stomach due to ulcer or cancer Partial 50% of stomach is removed Subtotal 75% of stomach is removed Radical 100% of stomach along with adjacent part is removed
23.	Gastrojejunostomy	Anastomosis or creation of communication between stomach and jejunum
24.	Gastrostomy	Surgical creation of an artificial gastric fistula for feeding
25.	Gingivoplasty	Surgical repair of gum
26.	Glossectomy	Removal of tongue may be partial or total
27.	Glossodynia	A painful tongue due to chronic inflammatory process of lingual papilla
28.	Hematemesis	Vomiting of blood

Contd...

Contd...

S.No.	Terms	Meanings
29.	Hemorrhoidectomy	Removal of hemorrhoid
30.	Hepatic lobectomy	Removal of a lobe of the liver
31.	Hepatotomy	Incision into the liver
32.	Hernioplasty, herniorrhaphy	Surgical repair of a hernia
33.	Herniorrhaphy	Repair of hernia or hernioplasty
34.	Hyperchlorhydria	Increased amount of hydrochloric acid in the gastric juice
35.	Ileostomy	Surgical creation of an opening into the ileum with a stoma on the abdominal wall
36.	Laparotomy	Incision and inspection of abdomen for diagnostic purpose
37.	Mesopexy	Operation and fixing of a torn or ruptured mesentry
38.	Odynophagia	Painful swallowing
39.	Esophagogastrectomy	Excision of esophagus and stomach
40.	Esophagogastrostomy	Surgical anastomosis between the esophagus and the jejunum
41.	Esophagoscopy	Endoscopic examination of esophagus
42.	Orthodontist	Dentist who practices prevention and correction of irregularities of tooth
43.	Pancreatectomy	Partial or total removal of pancreas for tumors of islet cells
44.	Pancreatoduodenostomy	Anastomosis of pancreas to duodenum
45.	Parotidectomy	Excision of parotid gland
46.	Proctectomy	Removal of rectum
47.	Proctoplasty	Plastic repair or reconstruction of rectum
48.	Pyloromyotomy	Incision of the longitudinal and circular muscles of the pylorus
49.	Pyloroplasty	Revision of pylorus for pyloric stenosis
50.	Pyrosis	Heart burning sensation due to ulcer
51.	Regurgitation	Back flow of gastric contents into the mouth
52.	Sialolithotomy	Incision into salivary gland for removal of calculus
53.	Sialadenectomy	Removal of salivary gland
54.	Staphylorrhaphy	Repair of cleft palate
55.	Stomatoplasty	Surgical reconstruction of the mouth
56.	Tonsillectomy and Adenoidectomy	Surgical removal of tonsil and adenoid

COMMON ABBREVIATIONS

S.No.	Abbreviation	Term
1.	AC, a.c	Ante cebum (before meals)
2.	ALP	Alkaline phosphatase
3.	AVH	Acute viral hepatitis
4.	BID, b.i.d	Bis in die (twice a day)
5.	Ba	Barium
6.	BaE	Barium enema
7.	BM	Bowel movement
8.	CBD	Common bile duct
9.	D and V	Diarrhea and vomiting
10.	DU	Duodenal ulcer
11.	FBS	Fasting blood sugar
12.	GB	Gallbladder
13.	GI	Gastrointestinal
14.	GIT	Gastrointestinal tract
15.	GTT	Glucose tolerance test
16.	GU	Gastric ulcer
17.	h.s.	at bed time
18.	HCl	Hydrochloric acid
19.	IVC	Intravenous cholangiography
20.	LFT	Liver function test
21.	LIH	Left inguinal hernia
22.	LKS	Liver, kidney and spleen
23.	NG	Nasogastric tube
24.	NPO	Nothing per oral (mouth)
25.	OCG	Oral cholecystogram
26.	PC, p.c	After meals (post cebum)
27.	PO	Orally (per ora)
28.	p.r.n.	as required (proreneta)
29.	PD	Postprandial (after meals)
30.	PU	Peptic ulcer
31.	q.d	Every day (quaque die)
32.	QID, q.i.d	Quantum in die (four times a day)
33.	RIIH	Right indirect inguinal hernia
34.	ROIH	Right oblique inguinal hernia
35.	RDH	Registered dental hygienist
36.	RIH	Right inguinal hernia
37.	SGOT	Serum glutamic oxaloacetic transminase
	SGPT	Serum glutamic pyruvic transminase
38.	SH	Serum hepatitis
39.	SOS	Slopus sit (If necessary)
40.	Stat	Immediately
41.	TID, t.i.d.	Three times a day (Ter in die)
42.	TPN	Total parenteral nutrition
43.	UC	Ulcerative colitis
44.	UGI	Upper gastrointestinal
45.	V and D	Vomiting and diarrhea

7 Endocrine System

INTRODUCTION

The endocrine system is composed of endocrine glands that release hormones, a chemical substance, which regulate the basic metabolic activities of the body. For example, the growth hormone regulates the growth of bones. Glands, which secrete their hormones directly into the bloodstream rather than into ducts leading to the exterior of the body are called endocrine glands, in short, they are ductless glands. The glands which transport hormones through ducts are called exocrine glands, e.g. lacrimal glands, sweat glands and mammary glands.

HORMONES

A chemical substance produced by the cells and transported through bloodstream to the cells and organs on which it has to act. Hormones are secreted in minute but effective quantities. In structure, they are either steroids or proteins. Most of the hormones are excreted by the pituitary gland, liver and kidneys.

DIFFERENT ENDOCRINE GLANDS PRESENT IN THE HUMAN BODY (FIG. 7.1)

Different endocrine glands present in the human body are as follows:
1. Thyroid gland
2. Parathyroid gland (four glands)
3. Adrenal gland (one pair)
4. Pancreas
5. Pituitary gland
6. Ovaries in female (one pair)
7. Testes in male (one pair)

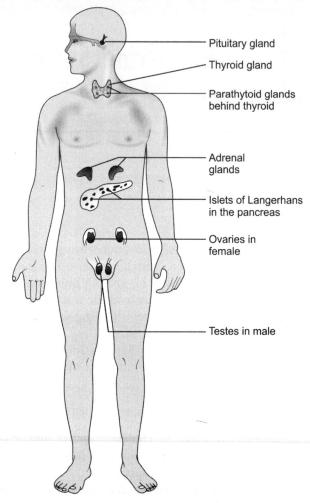

Pituitary gland

Thyroid gland

Parathytoid glands
behind thyroid

Adrenal
glands

Islets of Langerhans
in the pancreas

Ovaries in
female

Testes in male

Fig. 7.1: Endocrine glands of human body

8. Pineal gland
9. Thymus gland.

THYROID GLAND

The thyroid gland is the largest gland of the endocrine system. It is a H-shaped organ located in the neck just below the larynx. This gland is composed of two fairly large lobes left and right lobes, that are separated by a tissue called as isthmus. The major function of the thyroid gland is to produce, store and release two hormones: Thyroxine (T_4) and Triiodothyronine (T_3). Recent research indicate that a new hormone by name calcitonin is also secreted by thyroid gland.

Hormones Secreted by Thyroid Gland and its Functions

Thyroxine (T_4) and Triiodothyronine (T_3)

- Increase the oxygen consumption and metabolism of all cells
- Increase the rate of fat utilization
- Both work with the growth hormone to stimulate the nervous system.

Calcitonin

- Regulates the calcium level in blood, when the calcium level is high, it inhibits the production of calcium by the bones.

Hyposecretion of the Thyroid Hormone

The condition of hyposecretion of the thyroid is called hypothyroidism. In infants, the condition of hypothyroidism is called **Cretinism**. It may lead to mental retardation, impaired growth, low body temperatures and abnormal bone formation. When hypothyroidism is developed in adults it is known as **myxedema**. The indication of this disease are edema, low level of T_3 and T_4, mental retardation, weight gain and sluggishness.

Hypersecretion of Thyroid Hormone

The condition of hypersecretion of the thyroid is called hyperthyroidism. The most common disorders of this condition are Graves' disease and toxic goiter.

Graves disease is marked by elevated metabolic rate, abnormal weight loss, excess perspiration, muscular weakness, and emotional instability. In severe conditions, the eye may protrude, because of edematous swelling in the tissue behind the eye, called as exophthalmos.

Toxic goiter: When the TSH of the pituitary gland secretes more, the thyroid cells are likely to enlarge, and secrete extra amounts of hormones.

PARATHYROID GLANDS

The parathyroid glands are four small oval bodies, located on the posterior surface (behind) of the thyroid gland. It secretes only one hormone called parathyroid hormone (PTH). This hormone is also known as parathormone. The functions of the PTH are:

- Regulates the calcium metabolism by influencing three types of organs—the bones, the intestine, and the kidneys.

- Mobilizes calcium from bones into the bloodstream, where the calcium is necessary for proper functioning of body tissues, especially muscles.
- Enhances the absorption of calcium and phosphates from food in the intestine.
- Causes kidneys to conserve blood calcium and to increase the excretion of phosphates in urine.

Hyposecretion of the Parathyroid Hormone

The hyposecretion of the PTH hormone is called as hypoparathyroidism. It can be caused by some injury or surgical removal of the parathyroid gland or accidentally during thyroid surgery. Hypoparathyroidism is characterized by: Calcium being unable to enter into the bloodstream from bones, which leads to nerve and muscle weakness, spasm of muscles, which is called tetany.

Hypersecretion of the Parathyroid Hormone

The hypersecretion of the PTH is called as hyperparathyroidism. Usually, it is caused by the benign tumor of the parathyroid gland. Excessive secretion of the PTH hormone will cause:
- Calcium to leave the bones and to enter into the bloodstream, this condition is called hypercalcemia.
- Demineralization of bones making them highly prone to fracture or deformity. This condition is called osteitis fibrosa.
- Tendency to develop kidney stones due to hypercalcemia.

ADRENAL GLANDS

The adrenal glands are two small glands situated on top of each kidney. It is also called as suprarenal glands. Each gland consists of two parts, an outer portion called the adrenal cortex and inner portion called adrenal medulla. These two parts of each adrenal gland secretes different endocrine hormones. The adrenal cortex secretes hormones called steroids and medulla secretes hormones called catecholamine. The adrenal cortex secretes three types of steroid hormones, they are:

a. *Mineralocorticoids*: The most important mineralocorticoid hormone is called aldosterone. This hormone regulates the kidneys to conserve sodium and to excrete potassium. It also promotes water conservation and reduces urine output.

b. *Glucocorticoids*: The most important glucocorticoids is cortisol. It helps to regulate the metabolism of sugars, fats, and proteins within all body cells.

c. *Gonadocorticoids*: The most important gonadocorticoids are androgens, estrogens, and progesterone. These are male and female hormones, which maintain, secondary sex characteristics. These hormones are also produced in the ovaries and testes.

The adrenal medulla secretes two types of hormones epinephrine and norepinephrine (adrenaline and noradrenaline), which are closely related hormones. Both epinephrine and norepinephrine are called sympathomimetic agents, as they function on the sympathetic nervous system. They help the body to respond to crisis situations.

Addison's disease is characterized by the hyposecretion of cortical homones of adrenal cortex: which results, when the adrenal cortex is destroyed by atrophy of adrenals.

Cushing's disease: Hyperfunctioning of the adrenal cortex with increased glucocorticoid secretion. It is characterized by moon like fullness of the face, hypertension, high blood sugar, excess deposition of fat at the back of thoracic region, excess hair growth in unusual places (hirsutism) especially in females.

PANCREAS

The pancreas is located behind the stomach in the bed of duodenum. It functions as both endocrine and exocrine gland. The specialized cells in the pancreas, which produce hormones are called the islets of Langerhans. There are two kinds of main cells in the islets: α-cells (alpha cells) produce glucagons and constitute about 25 percent of the islets and β-cells (beta cells) produce insulin and constitute about 75 percent of the islets cells. Both the hormones, glucagon and insulin play an important role in the proper metabolism of sugars and starches in the body.

Hyposecretion of Insulin

The hyposecretion of the insulin is called as diabetes mellitus. It is the most common pancreatic disorder. It is recognized to exist in two forms: the insulin-dependent form caused by failure of the β-cells to produce insulin and non-insulin dependent form, caused by the insufficient insulin production to facilitate the oxidation of the glucose.

Hypersecretion of Insulin

This condition is known as hyperinsulinism. It may be caused by tumor in the pancreas. By excesive secretion of the insulin, excess glucose is drawn out of the bloodstream, resulting in hypoglycemia.

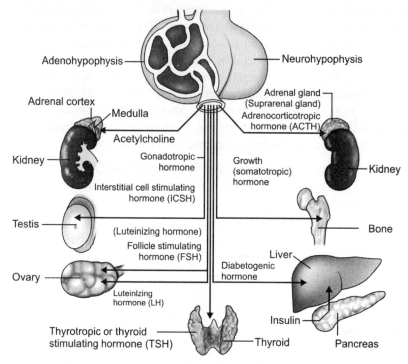

Fig. 7.2: Hormones of pituitary gland: direct and indirect effect on target organs

PITUITARY GLAND

The pituitary gland is a small, pea-sized gland located at the base of the brain. It is also known as master gland as it regulates many body activities and stimulates other glands to secrete their own specific hormones.

The pituitary gland consists of three distinct parts—an anterior lobe (adenohypophysis or pars distalis), middle lobe (pars intermedia) and a posterior lobe (neurohypophysis or pars nervosa). All these lobes secrete many hormones (Fig. 7.2), they are:

Anterior Lobe of Pituitary (Adenohypophysis)

See Table 7.1.

Middle Lobe of Pituitary (Pars Intermedia)

It secrets melanocyte stimulating hormone (MSH).

Posterior Lobe of Pituitary (Neurohypophysis)

See Table 7.2.

Table 7.1: Hormones secreted by anterior lobe of pituitary and its actions

S.No.	Hormone	Action
1.	Growth hormone (GH)	Acts on bone tissues to stimulate bone and body growth
2.	Thyroid stimulating hormones (TSH)	Controls the stimulation and secretion of thyroid hormones
3.	Prolactin	Promotes growth of breasts tissue during the puberty period of the female and stimulates milk production after the childbirth
4.	Adrenocorticotropic hormone (ACTH)	Stimulates the secretions by adrenal cortex especially corticoid
5.	Gonadotropic hormones	There are many gonadotrophic hormones, which influence the growth and hormone secretion of the ovaries in females and testes in males
6.	Follicle stimulating hormone (FSH)	Stimulates the growth of eggs in the ovaries, secretions of the estrogen in the females and stimulates the production of sperm cells in testes (in males)
7.	Luteinizing hormone (LH)	Induces the secretion of the progesterone for ovaries in females and promotes the secretion of sex hormones in both males and females

Diseases Related to Hypo- and Hypersecretions of Pituitary Glands

Anterior Pituitary Gland

1. *Gigantism*: Hyperfunctioning of the anterior pituitary gland before leading to abnormal overgrowth of body.
2. *Acromegaly*: Hyperfunctioning of the anterior pituitary gland, leads to abnormal enlargements of extremities. Hypersecretion of the growth hormone (GH) causes abnormally large growth of the bones in the hands, feet, face and jaw.

Table 7.2: Hormones secreted by posterior lobe of pituitary and its actions

S.No.	Hormone	Action
1.	Antidiuretic hormone (ADH)	This hormone is also known as vasopressin. It stimulates the reabsorption of water by the kidney and can also increase the blood pressure by constricting the arterioles
2.	Oxytocin	Stimulates the contraction of uterus during labor, and milk secretion after childbirth

3. *Dwarfism*: This is due to the hyposecretion of growth hormone. It is a congenital disorder characterized by bones remaining small and underdeveloped.
4. *Panhypopituitarism*: Hyposecretion of all hormones secreted by anterior pituitary gland. It largely affects the functions of the target glands such as adrenals, testes, ovaries and thyroid.

Posterior Pituitary Gland

1. *Inappropriate ADH (IADH)*: Hypersecretion of antidiuretic hormone (ADH). This condition is characterized by excessive retention of water in the body.
2. *Diabetes insipidus*: Hyposecretion of ADH. Clinical symptoms include polyuria and polydipsia.

Pineal Gland (Body)

The pineal gland is pinecone shaped gland attached to the posterior part of the third ventricle of the brain. The exact functioning of the gland is not found out so far. However, it is believed that it secretes melatonin hormone, which plays a vital role in inhibiting the activities of ovaries.

OVARIES

The ovaries are two small glands located in lower abdominal region of the female. The ovaries produce the female sex cells called ovum, as well as hormones, which are responsible for female sexual characteristics and regulation of the menstrual cycle.

The hormones secreted by the ovaries are estrogen and progesterone. Estrogen is responsible for the development and maintenance of secondary sex characteristics. Progesterone is responsible for the preparation and maintenance of the uterus during pregnancy.

TESTES

The testes are two small, ovoid gland suspended from the inguinal region of the male by the spermatic cord and surrounded by the scrotal sac. The testes produce the male sex cells spermatozoa, as well as the male hormone called testosterone. The testosterone hormone regulates the growth and maintenance of secondary sexual characteristics in the male.

ENDOCRINE AND METABOLIC DISORDERS

Origin of Terms

S.No.	Terms	Meanings	S.No.	Terms	Meanings
1.	Adren	Adrenal glands	20.	Pineal/o	Pineal gland
2.	Melano	Black	21.	-toxic	Poison
3.	Somat/o	Body	22.	Tophus	Porous stone
4.	Calc/o	Calcium			
5.	Metabole	Change	23.	Kal/I	Potassium
6.	Cortic/o	Cortex, outer region of an organ	24.	-phylaxis	Protection
			25.	Porphyr	Purple
7.	-phagia	Eating	26.	Gonad/o	Sex glands
8.	Acro	Extremity	27.	Thyro	Sheild
9.	Estr/o	Female	28.	Natr/o	Sodium
10.	-physis	Growth	29.	Ster/o	Solid structure
11.	Meli, Melit	Honey	30.	-tropin	Stimulate
12.	Keton	Ketone	31.	Gluc/o	Sugar
13.	-tocin	Labor, delivery	32.	Edema	Swelling
14.	Home/o	Likeness, resemblance	33.	-dipsia	Thirst
15.	Andro	Male	34.	Goiter	Throat
16.	Lact/o, Galact/o,	Milk	35.	Thym/o	Thymus
17.	Tropho, -trophy	Nourishment	36.	Thyr/o	Thyroid, shield
18.	Pancreat	Pancreas	37.	Hormone	To excite
19.	Parathyroid/o	Parathyroid glands	38.	-crine	To secrete

Symptomatic Diagnostic Terms

S.No.	Terms	Meanings
1.	Acromegaly	Disease characterized by enlarged features particularly of the face and hands as a result of over secretion of the pituitary growth hormone
2.	Adenoma	Benign glandular neoplasm
3.	Carcinoma	Malignant tumor with subsequent metastasis to cervical lymph node, lungs and the long bones
4.	Cushing's syndrome	Syndrome attributed to the hyperproduction of cortisone and hydrocortisone marked by obesity, weakness, and hypertension
5.	Diabetes insipidus	Metabolic disorders into hyposecretion of the antidiuretic hormone of the pituitary gland and clinically manifested by polyuria and polydipsia
6.	Diabetes mellitus	The most significant pancreatic disease in which pathogenic alterations of the islet cells cause a depletion in the insulin storage resulting in polyuria and polypepsia, hyperglycemia, glycosuria, ketoacidosis, etc.
7.	Diuresis	Increased excretion of urine. This occurs in diabetes mellitus. It can also be an early sign of chronic interstitial nephritis
8.	Dwarfism, pituitary	Congenital under development due to hyposecretion of growth hormone

Contd...

Contd...

S.No.	Terms	Meanings
9.	Exophthalmos	Abnormal protrusion of eyeballs, may be due to thyroid toxicosis, tumours of the orbit, orbital cellulitis, leukemia or aneurysm
10.	Gigantism	Abnormal growth particularly of long bones due to the over production of the growth hormone of pituitary gland
11.	Galactosemia	Inborn error of carbohydrate metabolism incapacity for metabolizing galactose characterized by hepato-megaly, cataract, mental retardation, weight gain, malnutrition in infancy and transmitted as an autosomal recessive trait
12.	Glycosuria	Presence of sugar in urine due to pancreatic insufficiency, excessive carbohydrate, disorders of the endocrine glands, etc.
13.	Goiter	Enlargement of the thyroid gland, which is classified as, follows: a. Nontoxic diffuse goiter c. Nontoxic nodular goiter b. Toxic diffuse goiter d. Toxic nodular goiter
14.	Gout, Gouty	Disorder of purine metabolism and recurrent form of arthritis manifested by an abnormal increase in purine in the blood with involvement of joint and renal failure.
15.	Hirsutism	Excessive growth of hair
16.	Homeostasis	State of equilibrium in the internal environment of the body
17.	Hypercalcemia	Abnormally high calcium level in the blood
18.	Hyperchloremia	Increasing chloride content in the blood
19.	Hypercholesterolemia	Presence of excess amount of cholesterol in the blood
20.	Hyperinsulinism	Hypoglycemic episode with blood sugar below 30 to 40 mg. Excessive secretion of insulin results in hypo-glycemia
21.	Hyperkalemia	Excessive amount of potassium in the blood, most often due to defective renal excretion
22.	Hyperkinesia	Hypermotility of increased movements
23.	Hyperparathyroidism	Over production and over activity of parathyroid hormone hypocalcemia and tissue calcification
24.	Hypertension paroxysmal	Sudden recurrents of high blood pressure which may be caused by the condition of adrenal glands
25.	Hyperthyroidism, Thyrotoxicosis Graves disease	Immunologic disorder, excessive hormone secretion, increased oxygen consumption with the result of high metabolic rate. Clinically manifested by goiter protrusion of the eye balls, tachycardia, emotional instability sweating and loss of water
26.	Hyponatremia	Abnormal condition of low sodium in the blood
27.	Hypoparathyroidism	Decreased production of parathyroid causing hypo-calcemia
28.	Hypothyroidism	Condition resulting from insufficiency of thyroid hormones in the blood

Contd...

Contd...

S.No.	Terms	Meanings
29.	Ketosis	Excess ketone bodies in the body fluid and tissues frequently associated with acidosis
30.	Melanosis	Unusual deposit of black pigment in different parts of the body
31.	Myxedema	Hypothyroidism causing lethargy, non-pitting edema weakness and slow speech
32.	Phenylketonuria	Phenyle pyruvic acid in the urine which is caused by the body failure to oxidise an amino acid to thyroxin because of the defective enzyme
33.	Polydipsia	Excessive thurst
34.	Polyphagia	Eating abnormally large amount of food
35.	Porphyria	Presence of porphyrin in the blood
36.	Proptosis	Forward displacement of globes in the orbit., same as exopthalmos or inflammatory condition of the orbit
37.	Remission	Decrease in severity
38.	Steatorrhea	Excess fat in stools
39.	Thymotoxicosis	Excessive secretion of thymin causing toxic effects
40.	Thyrotoxicosis	A morbid condition resulting from over activity of the thyroid gland also called as Graves' disease
41.	Thyroiditis	Inflammation of thyroid gland usually induced by drug
42.	Tophi	Deposit of sodium- bi-urate near a joint. Condition is peculiar to gout
43.	Virilism	Masculinisation in women or development of men's secondary characteristics in women
44.	Vitiligo	White patches on the skin may be seen in hyperthyroidism
45.	Panhypopituitarism	All pituitary hormones are deficient
46.	Calcium gluconate	Substance given to restore calcium levels in the blood
47.	Cushing's syndrome	A condition caused by over-secretion of cortisone and hydrocortisone
48.	Hormones	Secretions secreted by the endocrine glands
49.	Hypoglycemia	Lack of sugar in the blood
50.	Thyrotoxicosis	Over-activity of thyroid gland
51.	Uremia	Retention of urea in blood as a result of kidney failure

Operative Terms

S.No.	Terms	Meanings
1.	Adrenalectomy	Removal of adrenal gland
2.	Cryohypophysectomy	Removal of hypophysis by the application of cryoprobe
3.	Parathyroidectomy	Removal of parathyroid tissue to control hyperparathyroidism
4.	Thymectomy	Removal of thymus gland
5.	Thyroidectomy	Removal of subtotal or total thyroid in persistent hyperthyroidism
6.	Pinealectomy	Removal of the pineal body
7.	Hypophysectomy	Removal of pituitary gland
8.	Oophorectomy	Removal of ovary
9.	Orchidectomy	Removal of testicle
10.	Pancreatectomy	Removal of pancreas

COMMON ABBREVIATIONS

S.No.	Abbreviation	Term
1.	17-OH	17-Hydroxycorticosteroids
2.	ACE	Adrenocortical extraction
3.	ACH	Adrenal cortical hormone
4.	ACTH	Adrenocortico trophic hormone
5.	ADH	Antidiuretic hormone
6.	AP	Anterior pituitary
7.	ATP	Andenosine triphosphate
8.	BGTT	Borderline glucose tolerance test
9.	BMR	Basal metabolic rate
10.	CO_2	Carbondioxide
11.	CRH	Corticotrophin releasing hormone
12.	CZI	Crystalin zinc insulin
13.	DI	Diabetes insipidus
14.	DM	Diabetes mellitus
15.	DOC	Deoxy corticosterone
16.	FBS	Fasting blood sugar
17.	FFA	Free fatty acid
18.	FSH	Follicle stimulating hormone
19.	FTM	Fractional test meal
20.	GH	Growth hormone
21.	GTT	Glucose tolerance test
22.	HDL	High density lipoproteins
23.	ICF	Intracellular fluid
24.	ICSH	Intracellular or interstial cell stimulating hormone
25.	IF	Intertial fluid
26.	K	Potassium
27.	LDL	Low density lipoproteins
28.	LH	Leutinising hormone
29.	LTH	Prolactin
30.	MSH	Melonocyte stimulating hormone
31.	Na	Sodium
32.	NaCl	Sodium chloride
33.	NPH	Neutral protamine hagedorn (insulin)
34.	PBI	Protein bound iodin
35.	PGH	Pituitary growth hormone
36.	PP	Post parandial
37.	PPBS	Post parandial blood sugar
38.	PRL	Prolactin
39.	PTH	Parathyroid hormone
40.	PZI	Protamin zinc insulin
41.	RAI	Radioactive iodine
42.	RAIU	Radioactive iodine uptake
43.	RIA	Radioimmunoassay
44.	T_3	Tri-iodothyronine
45.	T_4	Thyroxine
46.	TSH	Thyroid stimulating hormone
47.	TTH	Thyrotropic hormone
48.	VLDL	Very low density lipoproteins
49.	XX	Female sex chromosomes
50.	XY	Male sex chromosomes

8

Respiratory System

INTRODUCTION

The essential features of respiratory system are the exchange of oxygen from atmosphere to the tissues and carbon dioxide from the tissue to the outer air. With the cooperation of the cardiovascular system, it supplies oxygen to the tissues of the body and takes away carbon dioxide. There are two phases in the respiration—external respiration and internal respiration.

External Respiration

Exchange of oxygen and carbon dioxide between the lungs and capillaries.

Internal Respiration

Exchange of gas (oxygen and carbon dioxide) between individual body cells and tiny capillaries.

During external respiration, the air inhaled contains 21 percent of oxygen, during exhalation the air contains 16 percent carbon dioxide.

PARTS OF THE RESPIRATORY SYSTEM (FIG. 8.1)

Nose

Air enters through the nose and passes through nasal cavities (turbinates) which are lined with mucous membranes and fine hairs, which help in filtering the dust as well as to warm and moisten the air. The nose is subdivided by a septum into two cavities. These are lined above by olfactory mucosa and below by the respiratory mucose and skin. The nose also acts as a sense organ to smell.

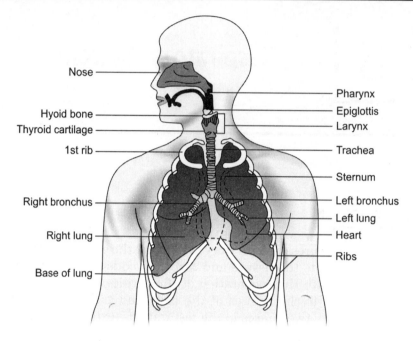

Fig. 8.1: Parts of the respiratory system

Paranasal Sinuses

Paranasal sinuses are hollow, air-containing cavities within the cranium which helps to produce the tunal quality of sound.

Pharynx

Pharynx is a muscular tube and it is about 5″ long. Pharynx is common for both respiratory and digestive systems. There are three sections:
1. Nasopharynx—Posterior to the nose
2. Oropharynx—Posterior to the mouth
3. Laryngopharynx—Above the larynx

The collection of lymphatic tissue known as adenoids or pharyngeal tonsil is located in the nasopharynx. Another type of lymphatic tissue known as tonsil is located in the oropharynx, which helps to filter and invade the bacteria present in the air and food.

Larynx

Larynx is located under the laryngopharynx in front of the neck. It is the prominent part of the windpipe and it is made up of sections of cartilage interspersed by membrane and ligaments. The largest cartilage is the thyroid cartilage (Adam's Apple) attached to the top of which is the epiglottis. The vocal cords are situated in larynx and are responsible for sound production (speech) or promotion. The cords are actually folds of tissues. Air passing through the glottis and across the cords produce vibrations which can be changed into sounds and varied by muscle actions.

Epiglottis

A leaf like structure present above the larynx and acts like a lid for the larynx, by closing and not allowing the food particles into the larynx while eating.

Trachea (Windpipe)

The trachea is a windpipe which is of 12 cm long and 2.5 cm in diameter, which extends from the larynx downwards in front of the esophagus and it divides to form the two main (principal) bronchi and crosses the arch of aorta. The trachea is composed of sixteen to twenty C-shaped rings of hyaline cartilage by fibrous tissue, which helps to keep the windpipe permanently open. The trachea is lined with ciliated epithelium.

Bronchi

The end of the trachea is divided into two small pipes called bronchi (left and right). The left and right bronchi passes to the corresponding sides of the lungs. The bronchi is divided into small branches called bronchioles, which ends with air sacs called alveoli which resemble a balloon like structure. The capillary structure (bed) lies close to the alveoli. The internal respiration (exchange of oxygen and carbon dioxide) is carried out between the alveoli and capillaries. The structure of bronchi is similar to the trachea and is lined with ciliated epithelium.

Lungs

The lungs are two roughly cone-shaped organs, situated in the right and left side of thoracic cavity protected by ribs, almost filling the thoracic cavity. The two lungs are separated by the heart and great vessels lying in the mediastinum. The base of the lungs lie on the diaphragm. Lungs are covered by pleural cavity containing pleural fluid, which helps to glide smoothly over the pleura during the respiration which helps in breathing. Mediastinum is the space between the two pleural sacs (lungs).

Each lung is divided into lobes. The right lung has three lobes and the left has two lobes. The lobes are further divided into lobules, which are bound together by loose connective tissue. Each lobules has bronchioles, which are divided and subdivided becoming finer until they end in small dilated air sacs or alveoli. The overall lung tissue is elastic and spongy in order to carry out its respiratory functions.

Diaphragm

A large muscular partition which lies between chest cavity and abdominal cavity. By contracting and relaxing the diaphragm produces the needed pressure differential for respiration (Flow chart 8.1).

MECHANISM OF EXTERNAL RESPIRATION

Inspiration

Inhaling oxygen into the lungs is called inspiration. During inspiration the diaphragm is forced down, the sternum and ribs move forward and outward respectively, thus increasing the space of thoracic cavity and the lungs enlarge. Being elastic, the lungs expand to fill up with oxygen 20 percent and carbon dioxide 0.04 percent and nitrogen 79 percent and water vapor depending on degree of humidity in the increased space.

In the alveoli, the basic part of the lung, the oxygen from the inspired air is able to pass through the thin alveolar-capillary membrane and is taken up by the hemoglobin in the red cells of the blood. This highly oxygenated blood is passed back to the heart through the pulmonary veins to be pumped around the body.

Expiration

Exhaling carbon dioxide from the lungs is called expiration. During expiration, the diaphragm regains its dome shape and sternum and ribs relax, thus the size of the thorax return to its normal size after the expansion during inspiration and the carbon dioxide (4%), oxygen (16%) and nitrogen (79%) present in the lungs are expelled.

The process of inspiration and expiration is called ventilation. Normal rate of ventilation in adults is 14 to 18 breaths per minute. In children this rate is more, up to 40 breaths per minute.

Process of Internal or Tissue Respiration (Fig. 8.2)

The well-oxygenated blood is circulated through the arteries and arterioles of the body. When it reaches the capillaries it moves very slowly, the tissue cells take oxygen from the hemoglobin and exchanges it with carbon dioxide, the waste product of metabolism (carbon dioxide) is returned through the venous system to the heart and back to the lungs.

Flow chart 8.1: Block diagram representing the mechanism of respiration

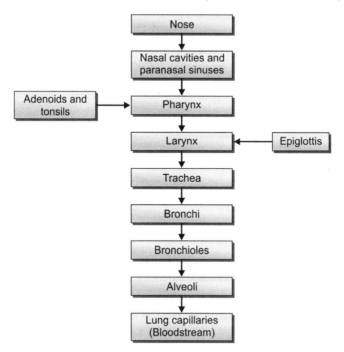

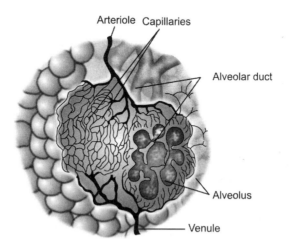

Fig. 8.2: Mechanism of internal or tissue respiration

VITAL CAPACITY

The volume of air that can be passed through the lungs is called as vital capacity. For men the normal vital capacity is 4–5 liters and for women 3–4 liters. The instrument used to measure the vital capacity is Spirometer.

FACTORS INFLUENCING THE RESPIRATORY SYSTEM

Normal rhythmic respiration continues even when a person is unconscious or asleep. This rhythm is maintained by a part of the brain referred to as the respiratory center, in the medulla oblongata. One part of the respiratory center facilitates inspiration and is called the inspiratory center. The other part which facilitates expiration is called expiratory center. The alternating activity of the inspiratory and expiratory centers brings about alternate inspiration and expiration. This alternate activity of the two centers is brought about by:
• A third part of the respiratory center known as pneumotoxic center
• Reflexes arising from the lung due to the stretching of the lungs during inspiration.

The factors which influence the respiration are the carbon dioxide content of the blood, if it is raised above the normal level it can stimulate respiration by acting on the respiratory center directly and through reflexes, producing an increase in both depth and rate. Hypoxia is a partial lack of oxygen in the blood and anoxia is a total lack of oxygen. Both stimulate respiration. The pH of blood is also another factor influencing respiration. Acidosis stimulates respiration and alkalosis inhibits it.

At high altitudes where the atmospheric pressure is low, less amount of oxygen is taken up by the blood resulting in hypoxia. Sudden transfer to high altitudes result in a condition called mountain sickness. Continued residence at high altitudes brings about certain compensatory changes in the mechanism of oxygen carriage referred to Acclimatization. The important changes are:
• The subjects begin to breath in a greater quantity of air by increasing both the rate and depth of respiration.
• The RBC count is increased by the red bone marrow producing more RBC so that the Hb content also increases and more oxygen can be carried.

RESPIRATORY SYSTEM

Origin of Terms

S.No.	Terms	Meaning	S.No.	Terms	Meaning	S.No.	Terms	Meaning
1.	Choane	Funnel	17.	Furca	Fork	33.	Trachea	Windpipe, rough
2.	Cricoid	Ringlike	18.	–ptysis	spitting	34.	Lob	Lobel lung
3.	Glottis	Aperture of larynx	19.	–phonia	Voice	35.	Adenoid	Adenoid
4.	Laryngo	Voice box, larynx	20.	Pyon	Pus	36.	Pleura	Pleura
5.	Naso	Nose	21.	Thorac	Chest	37.	Cyano	Blue
6.	Paries	Wall	22.	–osmia	Smell	38.	Tonsill	Tonsils
7.	Pector	Chest	23.	Phren	Diaphragm, mind	39.	Sinus	Sinus cavity
8.	Pneum, Pulmo	Lung	24.	Apex	Tip	40.	Segment	A portion
9.	Rhino	Nose	25.	Pnea	breathing	41.	Epiglott	Epiglottis
10.	Scope	To examine	26.	Alveolus	Little tub	42.	Pneumo	Air
11.	Septum	Partition	27.	Antrum	Cavity	43.	Maxilla	Jawbone
12.	Sinus	Hollow	28.	Ethmo	Sieve	44.	Chon-dros	Cartilage, gristle
13.	Steno	Narrow	29.	Bronchus	Windpipe	45.	Bron-chiolus	Air passage
14.	Viscus, vicer	Flesh, vital organ	30.	Thorax	Breast plate, chest			
15.	Meatus	Passage	31.	Rhin	Nose			
16.	Phono	Voice	32.	Vox	Voice			

Symptomatic and Diagnostic Terms

S.No.	Medical term	Description
1.	Anosmia	Absence of sense of smell and absence of the sense of taste
2.	Anoxemia	Deficient oxygen content of the blood below physiology level
3.	Anoxia	Deficiency of oxygen in tissues
4.	Aphonia	Loss of voice due to defect of vocal cord or injury to laryngeal nerve
5.	Asphyxia	Insufficient oxygen
6.	Asthma	Bronchial airway obstruction or difficulty in breathing due to allergy or related nervous tension or emotional problems
7.	Atelectasis	Imperfect expansion of the air sacs; functions, airless lung or portion of a lung
8.	Bronchial asthma	Distressing affliction, characterized by severe attacks of dyspnea and wheezing triggered by bronchospasm. It may be due to extrinsic factors; pollens, dusts, foods or intrinsic factors; infection, chilling or emotional upset or both.
9.	Bronchiectasis	Dilation of the bronchi

Contd...

Contd...

S.No.	Medical term	Description
10.	Bronchitis	Inflammation of the bronchial mucous membrane; endobronchial tuberculosis bronchitis due to tubercle bacillus
11.	Bronchogenic carcinoma	Cancerous tumor arising from a bronchus
12.	Bronchopneumonia	Inflammation of bronchi and air vesicles with scattered areas of consolidation
13.	Cor pulmonale	Heart and lung disease
14.	Coryza	Common cold
15.	Croup	Laryngeal spasm
16.	Cyanosis	Bluish color of skin due to deficient oxygenation
17.	Diphtheria	Acute infectious disease of the throat and upper respiratory tract caused by presence of diphtheria bacteria
18.	Dyspnea	Pain in breathing/painful breathing
19.	Deviated nasal septum (DNS)	Deviation in nasal septum bone causing interrupted breathing.
20.	Emphysema	Distention of alveoli with swelling and inflation of lung tissue
21.	Empyema	Pus in the lung tissue
22.	Epiglottitis	Inflammation of the epiglottis
23.	Epistaxis	Nasal bleeding
24.	Expectoration	Bringing out of sputum while coughing
25.	Hemoptysis	Spitting or of blood stained sputum
26.	Hemothorax	Blood in pleural cavity due to trauma or ruptured blood vessel
27.	Hydropneumothorax	Water effusion in the pleural cavity
28.	Hypercapnia	Excessive carbon dioxide in blood circulation
29.	Hyperpnea	Increased respiratory rate or abnormally rapid and deep breathing
30.	Hyperventilation	Excessive movement of air in and out of the lungs
31.	Hypoplasia of epiglottis	Defective development of epiglottis
32.	Hypoxia	Want of oxygen due to decreased amount of oxygen in organs and tissues
33.	Intercostal	Between the ribs
34.	Laryngitis	Inflammation of the larynx
35.	Laryngotracheobronchitis	Inflammation of larynx, trachea with bronchi
36.	Nasal polyp	Benign lesion which may cause considerable obstruction of the nasal airway
37.	Nasopharyngitis	Inflamed condition of the nasopharynx
38.	Pansinusitis	Inflammation of all paranasal sinuses

Contd...

Contd...

S.No	Medical term	Description
39.	Perichondritis	Inflammation of the perichondrium, a membrane of fibrous connective tissue which surrounds the cartilage
40.	Pertussis	Whooping cough; contagious bacterial infection of the UTI, characterized by painful cough.
41.	Pleurocentesis	Removal of fluid from lungs
42.	Pleural effusion	Excessive formation of serous fluid within the pleural cavity
43.	Pleurisy, pleuritis	Inflammation of the pleural membrane characterized by a stabbing pain that is intensified by coughing or deep breathing
44.	Pleurodynia	Pain in pleura
45.	Pneumonia	Acute inflammation and infection of the alveoli filled with fluid, blood cells or both
46.	Pneumonitis	Inflammation of the lung
47.	Pneumothorax	Air in the pleural cavity
48.	Pulmonary edema	Swelling and fluid in the air sacs and bronchioles
49.	Pulmonary embolism	Floating clot or other material blocking the blood vessels of the lung
50.	Pyopneumothorax	Accumulation of pus and air in the pleural cavity
51.	Quinsy	Peritonsillar abscess
52.	Rales	Abnormal rattling sounds heard on auscultation
53.	Rhinitis	Inflammation of the lining of the nose
54.	Rhinolith	Nasal concretion
55.	Rhinorrhea	Thin watery discharge from the nose
56.	Silicosis	Disease caused by inhalation of silica dust
57.	Sinusitis	Inflammation of the sinuses
58.	Sputum	Material expelled from the chest by coughing or clearing the throat
59.	Stridor	High-pitched, harsh sound heard during inspiration when the larynx is obstructed
60.	Tonsillitis	Inflammation of the tonsils
61.	Tuberculosis	Disease caused by acid-fast bacilli. It is acquired by inhaling viable tubercle bacilli into the lungs. It might affect any organ of the body
62.	Bronchiolitis	Inflammation of the bronchioles
63.	Adenotonsillitis	Inflammation of the tonsils and adenoids
64.	Chronic obstructive pulmonary disease	Prolonged airway obstruction causing disabling respiratory disease, frequently with irreversible functional deterioration and fatal prognosis
65.	Respiratory failure	Persistent condition of abnormally low arterial oxygen tension or abnormally high carbon dioxide tension

Operative Terms

S.No.	Medical term	Description
1.	Adenoidectomy	Removal of the adenoids
2.	Antrotomy	Opening of antral wall
3.	Bronchoscopy	Examination of the bronchi through a bronchoscope
4.	Bronchoplasty	Plastic operation for closing fistula
5.	Bronchotomy	Incision into a bronchus
6.	Deplectomy	Submucous resection of part of the nasal septum
7.	Dilatation of the larynx	Instrumental stretching of the larynx
8.	Ethmoidectomy	Excision of ethmoid cells or a portion of the ethmoid bone
9.	Laryngectomy	Removal of the larynx for carcinoma
10.	Laryngoplasty	Plastic repair of the larynx
11.	Laryngoscopy	Examination of interior larynx with a laryngoscope
12.	Laryngostomy	Establishing permanent opening through the neck in the larynx
13.	Lobectomy	Complete or partial excision of lobe or lobes of lung
14.	Mediastinoscopy	Examination of the mediastinal organs by a mediastinoscope under direct vision to aid in the diagnosis of disease and in assessing the severity of bronchogenic carcinoma
15.	Pleurectomy	Partial or complete removal of the pleura
16.	Pneumonectomy	Excision of lung or lobe of the lung
17.	Rhinoplasty	Plastic repair of the nose
18.	Septal dermoplasty	Excision of septal mucosa in telangiectatic area and its replacement with skin graft or oral mucous membrane to control bleeding
19.	Septectomy, submucous resection	Excision of the nasal septum or part of it
20.	Septoplasty	Plastic repair of the deviated nasal septum
21.	Therapeutic pneumothorax	Introduction of a measured amount of air into the pleural cavity through a needle in order to give the diseased lung temporary rest.
22.	Thoracocentesis	Puncture of pleural cavity to remove pleural effusion
23.	Thoracostomy	Excision of rib segment for drainage of empyema space
24.	Tonsillectomy	Removal of the tonsils
25.	Tracheoplasty	Plastic operation on trachea
26.	Tracheotomy	Incision of the trachea for exploration
27.	Tracheostomy	Formation of a more or less permanent opening into the trachea, usually for insertion of a tube. Tracheostomy (or laryngostomy) is absolutely imperative prior to total laryngectomy, to establish an open airway. It may be necessary after thyroidectomy, brain or lung surgery, to overcome a tracheal obstruction
28.	Tracheoscopy	Examination of interior of trachea by means of a reflected light
29.	Turbinectomy	Surgical removal of turbinate bone
30.	Turbinotomy	Incision of the turbinate bone

COMMON ABBREVIATIONS

S.No.	Abbreviation	Term
1.	A and P	Auscultation and percussion
2.	AB	Asthmatic bronchitis
3.	ABG	Arterial blood gases
4.	ABLB	Alternate biaural loudness balance
5.	AC	Air conduction
6.	AC and BC	Air and bone conduction
7.	AD	Auris dextra (right ear)
8.	AFB	Acid fast bacillus
9.	AFT	Acute follicular tonsillitis
10.	AHT	Augumented histamin test
11.	AP view	Anteroposterior view (radiology)
12.	ARD	Acute respiratory disease
13.	ARDS	Adult respiratory distress syndrome
14.	ARF	Acute respiratory failure
15.	ATD	Asphyxiating thoracic dystrophy
16.	BC	Bone conduction
17.	Br	Bronchitis
18.	Br Pn	Bronchopneumonia
19.	CB	Chronic bronchitis
20.	CBA	Chronic bronchitis with asthma
21.	CM	Cochlear microphonics
22.	CM	Costal margin
23.	CO2	Carbon dioxide
24.	COAD	Chronic obstructive airways disease
25.	COLD	Chronic obstructive lung disease
26.	COPD	Chronic obstructive pulmonary disease
27.	CPR	Cardiopulmonary resuscitation
28.	CXR	Chest X-ray; chest radiography
29.	ENG	Electronystagmogram
30.	ENT	Ear, nose and throat
31.	EP	Endochochlear potential
32.	ERA	Evoked response audiometry
33.	ETF	Eustachian tube function
34.	FBS	Fasting blood sugar
35.	FEF	Forced expiratory flow
36.	FVC	Forced vital capacity
37.	HD	Hearing distance
38.	ICM	Intercostal margin
39.	INH	Isoniazid
40.	IPPB	Intermittent positive-pressure breathing
41.	LCM	Left costal margin
42.	LL	Left lung
43.	LLL	Left lower lobe (lungs)
44.	LUL	Left upper lobe
45.	MACS	Mastoid air cell system
46.	O_2	Oxygen
47.	Oto	Otology
48.	PA View	Posteroanterior view (radiology)
49.	PAP	Primary atypical pneumonia
50.	PCO_2	Carbon dioxide pressure
51.	PND	Paroxysmal nocturnal dyspnea
52.	PO_2	Oxygen pressure
53.	PPD	Purified protein derivative

Contd...

Contd...

S.No.	Abbreviation	Term
54.	PS	Pulmonary stenosis
55.	PT	Pulmonary tuberculosis
56.	PVR	Pulmonary vascular resistance
57.	RCM	Right costal margin
58.	RD	Respiratory disease
59.	RDS	Respiratory distress syndrome
60.	RL	Right lobe
61.	RLE	Right lower extremity
62.	RLL	Right lower lobe
63.	RS	Respiratory system
64.	RUE	Right upper extremity
65.	RUL	Right upper lobe
66.	RURTI	Recurrent upper respiratory tract infection
67.	SAS	Sensorineural acuity level
68.	SEM	Scanning electromicroscopy
69.	SISI	Short increment sensitivity index
70.	SOB	Short (ness) of breath
71.	Stereo	Stereogram
72.	T and A	Tonsillectomy and adenoidectomy
73.	TB	Tuberculosis
74.	TPR	Temperature, pulse and respiration
75.	UL	Upper lobe
76.	URI	Upper respiratory infection
77.	URTI	Upper respiratory tract infection
78.	VASC	Visual auditary screening test for children
79.	VC	Vital capacity
80.	VRI	Viral respiratory infection
81.	WC	Whooping cough

9

Sense Organs

INTRODUCTION

The special senses of the body include the sense of sight, taste, hearing, smell and equilibrium. These senses allow us to detect changes in our environment, and each of them has structurally complex receptors organs. The sense organs are eye, ear, tongue, nose and skin.

EYE

Eye is one of the sense organs. We see the world around us through the eyes by sensing the light that gives off or reflects. Eyes look like two balls of jelly each about 2.5 cm apart, set in socket in the skull, on each side of the nose. There are six muscles to each eye, four straight and two sloping muscles. These muscles can move the eyes freely in all directions. The optic nerve joins the eyeball through the back of the eye, which transmits the reflexes to the brain.

The eye's functions are similar to that of a camera. Light rays pass through a small opening and are focussed by a lens upon a photoreceptive surface, retina. Then the image is transmitted from retina to the brain through the optic nerves.

The eye is a globe shaped organ that is composed of three distinct layers. They are:

1. *Sclera:* Outer most layer, which is a tough fibrous tissue, acting as a protective shield for the eye and maintains the shape of the eyeball. It also contains the cornea which is transparent.
2. *Choroid:* The middle layer which provides the blood supply for the entire eye. It also contains ciliary body and iris.
3. *Retina*: The innermost layer composed of nerve endings that are responsible for the reception and transmission of light impulses.

Anatomy of the Eye

Iris

A colored, contractile membrane, which functions as a sphincter.

Cornea

Cornea is the transparent layer situated in the external surface of the eyeball. It allows the light to enter into the eye. It is also called as the window of the eye.

Pupil

The perforated center for the iris, which regulates the entering of light by varying its size. As the environmental light increases, (bright) the pupil constricts, and as the light decreases (dark), the pupil dilates, which can be compared with the aperture of the camera.

Lens

The lens is a bi-convex transparent body attached to the ciliary body by the suspensory ligament. When the ligament is taut the lens is flattened and when it slackens the lens becomes thicker.

Ciliary Muscles

Muscle in which the lens are attached, used to alter the shape of the lens by relaxation and contraction depending upon the distance of the object and environmental light so as to get a clear view. This is like adjusting the camera lens. This process is called accommodation.

Aqueous Humor

One of the two major humors (fluids) of the eye. The fluid is filled in between the cornea and the lens. The iris divides the aqueous humor into two small chambers, the anterior chamber and the posterior chamber.

Vitreous Humor

Clear, jelly like fluid occupying the entire orbit of the eye behind the lens. The vitreous humor, lens and the aqueous humor are the refractive structures of the eye, which are responsible for the focussing of the rays sharply on the retina by bending the rays.

Retina

Delicate eye membrane, which is attached to the optic nerve. Retina has two types of light receptors on its surface, namely rods and cones. Rods function in dim light and provide black and white vision, whereas the cones functions in bright light and provide color vision.

Optic Nerve

The second cranial nerve is responsible for the sight and transmitting the nerve impulses caused by the chemical changes as the light strikes the retina (on rods and cones).

Accessory Organs of the Eye (Fig. 9.1)

Eyelids

It is in the anterior portion of the eye, which are movable folds, upper and lower. The upper part is large and more mobile than the lower. It protects the eyes from dust and injuries.

Eyelashes

Short thick hairs projecting from both the eyelids.

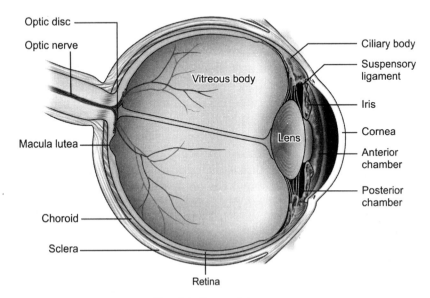

Fig. 9.1: Parts of the eye

Lacrimal Glands

Situated immediately above the lateral angle of the eye. A number of small canals connect it to the conjuctival sac in the opposite side. It produce tears during the emotional situations and when any foreign body enters. The tears produced by the lacrimal glands keep the eye moist, remove the dust and foreign bodies and acts as an antiseptic agent.

Lacrimal Duct

The lacrimal duct is a small tubule like structure which connect the orbit and lacrimal sac. The lacrimal glands produce tears, these tears when excess, passes down the lacrimal ducts and finally reaches nasal cavity.

Lacrimal Sac

The lacrimal sac is the continuation of the lacrimal duct which collects the tears produced by the lacrimal glands.

Nasolacrimal Duct

The duct which drains the lacrimal fluid from the lacrimal duct into the nose.

Physiology of Eye

Light enters the eye through the pupil, conjunctiva, lens, and cornea where the light rays are bent so as to focus properly on the sensitive receptor cells. The iris regulates the amount of light passing through the conjunctiva by constricting or relaxing the iris muscles. Then the light ray reaches the retina, where 6 million cones and 120 million rods act as receptors of the light. Light when focused on the retina, causes a chemical change in the rods and cones, initiating nerve impulses which travel from the eye to the brain through optic nerves. The rods and cones in the retina communicate with neurons, connecting to the optic nerve fibers. The optic chiasma is the point where the nerve fibers of the right and left eye meet. Nerve fibers from the right half of each retina now form an optic tract meeting in the thalamus of the brain and ending in the right visual region of the cerebral cortex. Similarly, nerve fibers from the left half of each retina merge to form the optic tract and pass from the thalamus to the left region of the cerebral cortex. The images are fused by a single visual sensation with a three-dimensional effect in the visual area of the cerebral cortex. This is called binocular vision.

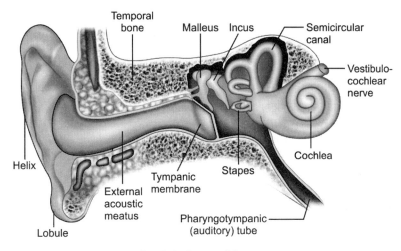

Fig. 9.2: Parts of the ear

EAR

Ear is the sense organ for hearing and for maintaining equilibrium of the body. It is divided into 3 sections namely, external ear, middle ear, and inner ear (Fig. 9.2).

Parts of External Ear

1. Pinna
2. External auditory meatus
3. Tympanic membrane or ear drum.

Pinna

Pinna is the external structure attached to the side of the head. It has a deep shell like cavity to collect the sound waves travelling through air.

External Auditory Meatus

It is like a tubule (canal) 2.5 cm long. It leads from the pinna to the tympanic membrane or ear drum (middle ear). The canal is lined with glands that produce a waxy secretion called cerumen. These waxy substances prevent dust and foreign particles from entering into the ear.

Tympanic Membrane

Tympanic membrane is a thin membrane covering the end of the external auditory canal. Sound waves that enter the ear canal, strike against the tympanum.

Eustachian Tube

It is the canal which connects the middle ear to the nasopharynx. Its functions are to regulate the pressure in the middle ear to that of environment and clear the fluid secretion from the middle ear to the nasopharynx.

Parts of Middle Ear

The middle ear or tympanic cavity is a small chamber containing air to equalize the pressure on both sides of the tympanic membrane. It has a narrow and bony membranous wall which communicates with the nasopharynx through the eustachian tube. The tympanic cavity contains three small bones or ossicles namely malleus, incus and stapes which are responsible for transmission of sound waves from the external ear (tympanic membrane) to the inner ear cochlea by conduction. Malleus the external bone which is shaped like a hammer with its handle attached to the tympanic membrane and its head in the tympanic cavity, articulating with the incus and the inner most bone the stapes, which is attached to the oval base of the fenestra vestibuli, transmit the sound vibration to the inner ear.

Parts of Inner Ear

1. Cochlea
2. Semicircular canals
3. Vestibule.

Cochlea

Cochlea is like a snail, which contains cochlear fluid and its inner surface is lined with nerve endings called corti. Disturbance of the fluid stimulates the hairs of corti, causing them to generate a series of nerve impulses. These impulses are transmitted to the brain by the auditory nerves which are interpreted as sound.

Semicircular Canals

It is situated to the posterior of the vestibule. Its main function is to maintain the balance and equilibrium.

Vestibule

It lies in the central part of the bony labyrinth. It is in the shape of oval. It connects the cochlea and semicircular canals.

Functioning of Ear

Sound is due to the vibrations of atmosphere. Sound waves vary by the rate and volume. The unit to measure the sound waves are frequency and intensity which are measured in hertz (speed) and decibels (dB). The human ear is able to hear the frequency of 20 to 20000 hertz and is sensitive to the intensity of 10 to 140 dB.

Sound waves pass along the external auditory canal and makes the eardrum vibrate. This causes the malleus to pass vibrations to the incus and stapes. The three bones moving against one another cause the vibrations to be magnified and thus they are passed through the vestibular membrane to the perilymph. Vibrations in the perilymph are transmitted to the endolymph in the canal of the cochlea and the stimuli reach the nerve endings to be passed to the brain by the auditory nerve.

SKIN

The outer surface of the body is covered by the skin. The skin and its accessory organs (hairs, nails and glands) are known as the integumentary system of the body. The skin consists of 2 layers, epidermis and dermis (corium). Integument means covering, and the skin is the outer covering of the body, hence, it is called integumentary system. The skin has specialized tissues, contains glands which secrete several types of fluids, nerves which carry impulses, and regulates the body temperature.

The important functions of the skin are:
1. Provides protection against injuries and invasion of the bacteria
2. Regulates the body temperature and the prevention of dehydration.
3. Works as a sensory receptor and is responsible for synthesis of vitamin D.

Structure of the Skin

The structure of the skin consists of two layers (Fig. 9.3) embedding one above the other. The two layers are:

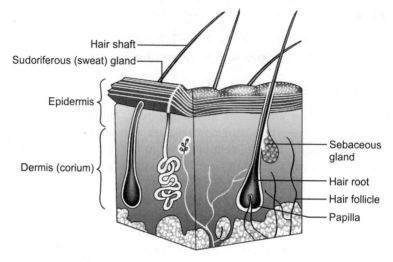

Fig. 9.3: Cross-section of structure of skin

Epidermis

It is the outermost cellular membrane layer of the skin. It has no blood supply. The cells of the epidermis will shed continuously. The mature cell of the dermis are pushed above which are finally sloughed off and replaced by new cells. The deepest layer of the epidermis is called basal layer. The cells in the basal layer are constantly growing and multiplying and give rise to all the other cells in the epidermis. As the basal layer cells divide, they are pushed upward and away from the blood supply of the corium layer by a steady stream of younger cells and finally these cells sheds from our body. This process of dividing, pushing upward and shedding of these cells takes 3 to 4 weeks. Thus, it is constantly renewing itself, cells dying at the same rate at which they are born. The basal layer of the epidermis contains special cells called melanocytes. Melanocytes form and contain a black pigment called melanin. The amount of black pigments accounts for the color variations. The presence of melanin in the epidermis protects against the harmful effects of ultraviolet radiation which can cause skin cancer.

Dermis

This layer of skin lies under the epidermis. It is a dense, fibrous, connective tissue layer. It has nerve endings, and numerous capillaries for blood supply. Apart from these, hair follicles, sebaceous glands, and sweat glands are also present in the dermis. This layer is also called as corium.

Subcutaneous

The subcutaneous layer of the skin is another connective tissue layer where the formation of fat is more. Lipocytes (fat cells) are predominant in the subcutaneous layer and they manufacture and store large quantities of fat. Functionally, this layer of the skin protects the deeper tissues of the body and serves as a heat insulator.

Hair

The hair has 3 parts namely, hair shaft, hair root, and hair follicle. The hair shaft is visible in the epidermis, the hair root and hair follicle are lying under the dermis. The hair follicle is a collection of capillaries enclosed in a covering called the papilla. Deep lying cells in the hair root produce horny cells which move upward through the follicles for the formation of the hair shaft. As long as these cells remain alive, hair will regenerate even though it is cut or plucked or otherwise removed. Baldness (alopecia) is evident when the hairs of the scalp are not replaced. Men rather than women are more susceptible to this condition, which is due to hereditary factors. Presence of the melanin pigment makes the hair look black and the pigment is supported by the melanocytes which are located at the root of the hair follicle. Hair turns gray when the melanocytes stop producing melanin.

Glands

There are two types of glands present under the skin, they are sebaceous and sweat glands. The sebaceous gland produce an oily secretion called sebum, while the sweat glands produce a watery secretion called sweat.

Sebaceous Glands

Sebaceous glands are filled with fatty substances, when these cells disintegrate, they yield an oily secretion called sebum. The acidic nature of sebum helps to destroy harmful organisms on the surface of the skin, and thus, prevents infections. Sebaceous glands are present over the entire body except the soles of the feet and palms of the hands.

Sweat Glands

Sweat glands are small structures that open as pores on the surface of the skin. They are found on the palms, soles, forehead, and armpits. On the palms of the hands, there are approximately 3000 sweat glands per square inch of skin. Sweat is a clear watery fluid containing 0.5 percent of solids such as sodium chloride, small amount of other mineral salts and urea. Sweating is one of the mechanisms by which the human body regulates its body temperature. Secretion of sweat is controlled by hypothalamus through the sympathetic nervous system. Sweating may also be induced by the emotional stress, anxiety, and fear. The main functions of the sudoriferous glands are to cool the body by evaporation, to excrete waste products through the pores of the skin and to moisturize surface cells. The **ceruminous glands** are modified sweat glands located in the skin that lines the external auditory canal. Instead of sweat, they secrete wax (cerumen).

These secretions are carried out to the outer edges of the skin by ducts and excreted from the skin through opening or pores.

Nails

Nails are solid plates present at dorsal end of fingers, which protect fingers and toes. The nail plate or body is firmly attached to the underlying nail bed which consists of modified epidermal cells. The nail body is pink because of the underlying vascular tissue. The half-moon shaped white area near the root of the nail bed is the lunula. The lunula is the area where the new growth occurs. The average growth rate is approximately 1 mm per week for finger nails, and slower for the toenails. The main function of the nails is to protect the tips of the fingers and toes from bruises and other kinds of injuries.

TONGUE

The tongue is a highly mobile organ composed of voluntary muscles. It is essential for speech, taste (bitter, sweet, sour and salt), mastication and swallowing. The root of the tongue is attached to the hyoid bone in the neck. On the dorsum of the tongue are numerous minute elevations of the mucous membrane called papillae (Fig. 9.4). Embedded in the papillae are the taste buds, which are situated more densely at the tip, sides and base of the tongue (up to 9000 tiny papillae). There are three types of papillae, namely fungiform, filiform and circumvallate papillae. The tongue is governed by facial and glossopharyngeal nerves.

NOSE

Nose is the organ for smell. Sensory nerve ends of the olfactory nerves are situated (Fig. 9.5) in the olfactory mucosa which forms the upper one-third of the nasal mucosa. Olfactory nerves transmit these signals to olfactory bulbs then through olfactory tracts to the smell center in the temporal lobes of the cerebral cortex. Nose smell the substances whose molecules are breathed into the roof of each nasal cavity and dissolved on a patch of olfactory membrane along with 100 million smell receptor cells equipped with tiny sensitive hairs. Smell molecule reacts with these to stimulate nerve impulses in the receptor cells. Some people can identify 10000 odors all evidently based on combinations of just seven.

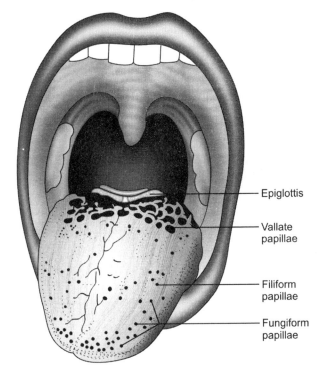

Fig. 9.4: Parts of the tongue

Epiglottis

Vallate papillae

Filiform papillae

Fungiform papillae

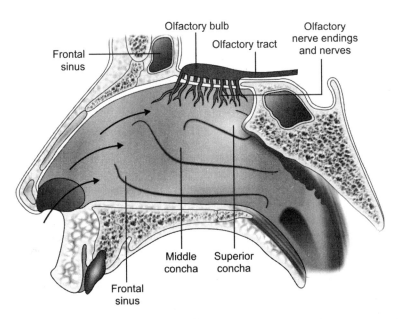

Fig. 9.5: The olfactory structures

Olfactory bulb

Olfactory tract

Olfactory nerve endings and nerves

Frontal sinus

Middle concha

Superior concha

Frontal sinus

EYE

Origin of Terms

S.No.	Terms	Meanings	S.No.	Terms	Meanings
1.	Ambly/o	Dull, dim	16.	Mi/o	Smaller, less
2.	Aque/o	Water	17.	Myc/o	Fungus
3.	Blephar/o	Eyelid	18.	Mydri/o	Wide
4.	chalasis	Relaxation	19.	Ocul/o, Ophthalm/o, Opt/o	Eye, vision
5.	Choroid/o	Choroids layer	20.	-Opia/opsia	Vision
6.	Conjunctiv/o	Conjunctiva	21.	Phac/o	Crystalline lens
7.	Core/o, Pupil/o	Pupil	22.	Phak/o	Lens
8.	Corne/o, Kerat/o	Cornea	23.	Phot/o	Light
9.	Cycl/o	Ciliary body of the eye	24.	Presby/o	Old age, elderly
10.	Dacry/o, Lacrim/o	Tear, tear duct, nasolacrimal duct	25.	Retin/o	Retina
11.	Dacryocyst/o	Lacrimal sac, tear sac	26.	Sclera/o	Sclera
12.	Emmert/o	Correct measure	27.	-tropia	Turning
13.	Gluac/o	Gray	28.	Uve/o	Vascular layer of the eye
14.	Ir/o, Irid/o	Iris	29.	Vitre/o	Glassy
15.	Is/o	Equal	30.	Xer/o	Dry

Symptomatic and Diagnostic Terms

S.No.	Terms	Meanings
1.	Aphakia	Absence of the crystalline lens of the eye. It may occur congenitally or from trauma, but is more commonly caused by extraction of a cataract
2.	Astigmatism	Unequal curvature of the refractive surfaces of the eye as a result of which a ray of light is not sharply focused on the retina
3.	Blepharitis	Inflammation of the eyelids
4.	Blepharoptosis	Drooping of the eyelids
5.	Cataract	Clouding of the lens, causing decreased vision
6.	Chalazion	Small, hard mass on the eyelid; formed from a sebaceous gland enlargement
7.	Color blindness	Reduced ability to distinguish between colors
8.	Conjunctivitis	Inflammation of the conjunctiva caused by bacteria, virus, allergy, or chemical or physical factors. When caused by virus or bacteria, it becomes highly contagious
9.	Corneal ulcer	A form of keratitis due to pathogenic organism entering the corneal epithelium, stroma may also breakdown
10.	Dactocystitis	Inflammation of the tear duct
11.	Diabetic retinopathy	Appearance of small aneurysms on retinal capillaries due to diabetes
12.	Diplopia	Double vision

Contd...

Contd...

S.No.	Terms	Meanings
13.	Ectopia lentis	Displacement of the crystalline lens of the eye
14.	Ectropion	Eversion of the edge of the eyelid
15.	Entropion	Inversion of the edge of the eyelid
16.	Exophthalmos, Exophthalmus	Abnormal protrusion of the eyeball
17.	Glaucoma	Increased intraocular pressure results in atrophy of the retina and optic nerve
18.	Hemianopia	Loss of one-half of the visual field
19.	Hordeolum	Stye; a localized purulent, inflammatory staphylococcal infection of a sebaceous gland in the eyelid
20.	Hypermetropia	Long-sightedness
21.	Iritis	Inflammation of the iris
22.	Iridocyclitis	Inflammation of the iris and ciliary body
23.	Keratitis	Inflammation of the cornea
24.	Myopia	Short-sightedness
25.	Nyctalopia	The individual cannot see well in faint light or at night
26.	Nystagmus	Involuntary rapid eye movement that appears jerky
27.	Optic neuritis	Inflammation of the optic nerve
28.	Papilledema, choked disc	Edema and hyperemia of the optic disc
29.	Presbyopia	Gradual decrease of visual acuity clarity due to old age
30.	Retinitis pigmentosa	Progressive retinal sclerosis, pigmentation, and atrophy
31.	Scotoma	Area of depressed vision surrounded by an area of normal vision (a blind spot in the vision)
32.	Strabismus	Abnormal deviation of the eye/squint
33.	Stye	Bacterial infection of the sebaceous gland of the eyelid.
34.	Trachoma	A chronic infectious disease of the conjunctive and cornea
35.	Diabetic retinopathy	Condition characterized by pinpoint aneurysm caused by dilation of the retinal capillaries, in uncontrolled diabetes mellitus
36.	Nyctalopia	Night blindness may be caused by vitamin A deficiency in children

Operative Terms

S.No.	Terms	Meanings
1.	Blepharectomy	Excision of a lesion of the eyelid
2.	Blepharorrhaphy	Suturing of an eyelid
3.	Cyclodialysis	Formation of an opening between the anterior chamber and the suprachoroidal space for the draining of aqueous humor on glaucoma
4.	Dacryocystotomy	Incision of lacrimal sac to provide drainage
5.	Dacryocystostomy	Creation of an opening into the nose for drainage of tears

Contd...

Contd...

S.No.	Terms	Meanings
6.	Extracapsular extraction	Removal of the lens material, separate from its capsule
7.	Enucleation	Removal of an organ or other mass intact from its supporting tissues. Removal of the eyeball from the orbit
8.	Enucleation of eye	Removal of eyeball
9.	Epilation	Removal of hair by its roots
10.	Evisceration	Removal of the contents of the eyeball leaving the sclera and cornea
11.	Intracapsular lens	Removal of the lens complete with its capsule
12.	Irisectomy	Surgical removal of part of the iris
13.	Keratocentesis	Surgical puncture of the cornea
14.	Keratoplasty	Replacement of a section of an opaque cornea
15.	Labyrinthectomy	Excision of the labyrinth of the ear
16.	Laminectomy	Excision of posterior arch of a vertebra
17.	Phakoemulsification	A method of treating cataracts by using ultrasonic waves to disintegrate the cataract, which is then aspirated and removed
18.	Scleral buckling	Surgical procedure to reduce the size of the globe
19.	Sclerostomy	Surgical formation of an opening in the sclera
20.	Stapedectomy	Excision of stapes
21.	Sympathectomy	Transections, cutting or division in resection of sympathetic nerve
22.	Vitrectomy	Diseased vitreous humor is removed and replaced with a clear solution

EAR

Origin of Terms

S.No.	Terms	Meanings	S.No.	Terms	Meanings
1.	Vestibule	Anterior chamber	10.	Audito, acoustic, acous/o, audi/o	Hearing
2.	Auditus	Approach, entrance	11.	-cusis	Hearing
3.	Cerumin/o	Cerumen (wax in the outer ear)	12.	Ossicle	Little bone
4.	-pyorrhea	Discharge of pus, purulent discharge	13.	Mastoid/o	Mastoid process
5.	Aur/o, aur/i	Ear	14.	Labyrinth	Maze/internal ear
6.	Ot,Oto	Ear	15.	Cochlea	Snail
7.	Myring/o, Tympan/o	Eardrum	16.	-phonia	Sound
8.	Auricle	External ear	17.	Staped/o	Stapes
9.	-mycosis	Fungal infection	18.	Salping/o	Tube, trumpet

Symptomatic and Diagnostic Terms

S.No.	Terms	Meanings
1.	Acoustic neuroma	Benign tumor of the eighth cranial nerve affecting more the vestibular branch than the cochlear branch of the nerve and causing vertigo and hearing impairment
2.	Aerotitis media, Barotitis media	Painful condition caused by atmosphere chiefly during air travel
3.	Anakusis	Sound perception as such complete loss
4.	Antral lavage	Washing out of sinuses
5.	Auditory agnosia	Sound perception at end organ intact but sound loss certainly (inability to recognize the sound correctly)
6.	Aural discharge	Drainage from ear
7.	Auriscope	Instrument for examining the ear
8.	Cholesteatoma	A pearly mass covered with a thin cell or epidermic and connective tissue. It usually forms following middle ear infections
9.	Congenital ossicular malformations	Abnormalities of ossicles which causes impaired hearing of connective type and may respond to surgical corrections
10.	Chronic Suppurative Otitis Media	Characterized by continuation of middle ear infection resulting in protracted suppuration
11.	Hearing Loss	Deafness
12.	Impacted cerumen	Dried ear wax
13.	Labyrinthitis	Inflammation of the labyrinth usually secondary to acute or chronic suppurative otitis media
14.	Mastoiditis	Infection of the middle ear which has extended to the antrum and mastoid cell, mastoiditis may be acute, subacute chronic and recurrent
15.	Middle ear effusion	Acute or chronic presence of fluid in the middle ear generally without infection
16.	Myringitis, tympanitis	Inflammation of the eardrum, otitis media
17.	Otalgia	Pain in ear
18.	Otitic meningitis	Inflammation of meninges following ear infection.
19.	Otitis externa	Inflammation of the outer ear
20.	Otitis media	Inflammation of the middle ear
21.	Otomycosis	Fungus infection of the ear
22.	Otorrhagia	Bleeding from the ear
23.	Otorrhea	Purulent discharge from the ear
24.	Otosclerosis	Hardening of the ear
25.	Paracusis of Willis	Ability of person with conductive hearing loss to hear better in the presence of noise
26.	Petrositis	Inflammation of petrose of the temporal bone
27.	Presbycusis	Impaired hearing which is part of the aging process
28.	Tinnitus	Ringing sound in the ear
29.	Tympanosclerosis	Involvement of mucous membrane of middle ear or drum sclerosis of exudate with fixation of the ossicles and drum

Contd...

Contd...

S.No.	Terms	Meanings
30.	Vertigo	Illusion of movement of individual in relation to his environment. The patient feels that he himself is spinning
31.	Vestibular neuronitis	Sudden vestibular failure in one ear without hearing impairment or tinnitus apparently due to viral infection
32.	Microtia	Abnormally small pinnae
33.	Macrotia	Abnormally large pinnae

Operative Terms

S.No.	Terms	Meanings
1.	Audiometry	Measurement of hearing for the purpose of accurately evaluating the extent and nature of hearing impairment
2.	Labyrinthectomy	Total destruction of labyrinth with or without removal of scar ganglion for interactive vertigo
3.	Mastoid antrotomy	Surgical opening of mastoid antrum, usually done for children with middle ear infection
4.	Mastoidectomy (Radical)	Removal of all diseased tissue in mastoid antrum and tympanic cavity and conversion of both into one dry cavity, which communicates with external ear. An operating microscope is used
5.	Myringoplasty	Surgical repair of tympanic membrane by tissue graft
6.	Otoplasty	Correction of deformed pinna
7.	Otoscopy with magnification	Inspection of auditory canal and eardrum for diagnosis or for removal of polyp or granulation tissue followed by microscopic study
8.	Pneumatic otoscopy	Inspection of the ear using an otoscope with an attachment for stimulating variation in pressure that put in the eardrum in motion. It provides a valuable aid in differential diagnosis of fluid ear, labyrinth fistula and other ear conditions
9.	Tympanoplasty	Reconstruction surgery of the sound conducting parts of the middle ear using skin graft
10.	Tympanotomy	Exploration of middle ear through tymponomeatal approach
11.	Stapedectomy	Removal of stapes, reestablishing connection between incus and oval window, by interposition of prosthesis and tissue or inert cover over oval window

NOSE AND TONGUE

Origin of Terms

S.No.	Terms	Meanings
1.	Naso, rhin	Nose
2.	Gloss, lingu	Tongue
3.	-centesis	Puncture
4.	Lingually	Towards the tongue
5.	Ala (vomer alar)	Winglike structure of bone forming septum of the nose

Symptomatic and Diagnostic Terms

S.No.	Terms	Meanings
1.	Anosmia	Absence of the sense of smell
2.	Choana	The paired openings between the nasal cavity and nasopharynx
3.	Coryza, acute nasopharyngitis	Common cold
4.	Dacryocystorhinostenosis	Narrowing of the duct leading from the lacrimal sac to the nasal cavity
5.	Ozena	Atrophic rhinitis
6.	Rhinitis	Inflammation of the nose
7.	Rhinophyma	A form of rosacea marked by redness, nodular swelling and congestion of the skin of the nose.
8.	Rosacea	Chronic disease affecting skin of nose
9.	Sinusitis	Inflammation of the sinuses
10.	Valsalva's maneuver	Forcible exhalation against closed nostrils and mouth causing increased pressure in eustachian tubes and middle ear
11.	Rhinitis	Inflammation of the nose

Operative Terms

S.No.	Terms	Meanings
1.	SMA operation	Submucous resection nose operation done in cases of chronic nasal congestion and rhinitis
2.	Nasal polypectomy	Removal of the nasal polyp usually caused by nasal obstruction but are not malignant
3.	Rhinoplasty	Plastic surgery to the nose
4.	SMD (Submucous diathermy)	Diathermy to the mucous membrane of the nasal passages
5.	SMR (Submucous resection)	Surgical procedure to relieve obstruction, irritation and infection in the nose and sinuses
6.	Intranasal antrostomy	A procedure to drain the sinus of a patient who suffers repeated attacks of acute maxillary sinusitis or who fails to respond to antibiotics and antral washouts
7.	Septoplasty (Septorhinoplasty)	Surgical repair of the deviated nasal septum
8.	Adenoidectomy	Removal of adenoids

DISORDERS OF THE SKIN

Origin of Terms

S.No.	Terms	Meanings	S.No.	Terms	Meanings
1.	Acanth/o	Thorny, spiny	17.	Onych/o	Nail
2.	Aden	Gland	18.	Onyx	Nail
3.	Adip/o, lip/o, steat/o	Fat	19.	Pachy/o	Thick, heavy
4.	Crypt/o	Hidden	20.	Papula	Pimple
5.	Derma, cutane/o, cutis	Skin	21.	Pemphix, vesic	Blister
6.	Diaphor/o	Profuse sweating	22.	-phyte	Plant
7.	Erythema	Red	23.	Pigmentum	Paint
8.	-gram	Record	24.	Pil/o, trich/o	Hair
9.	-graphy	Instrument used for recording	25.	Psora	Itch
10.	Hidr/o, sudor	Sweat	26.	Sclera/o	Hard
11.	Hist/o	Tissue	27.	Seb/o	Sebum
12.	Hyper	Excessive	28.	Sebum	Wax
13.	Itchy/o	Dry, scaly	29.	Sqam/o	Scale
14.	Kerat/o	Horny substance	30.	-therapy	Treatment
15.	Melan/o	Black	31.	Ungu/o	Nail
16.	Myc/o	Fungus			

Diagnostic Terms

S.No.	Terms	Meanings
1.	Acne	Any inflammatory condition of the sebaceous gland
2.	Adipose	Fat tissue
3.	Albinism	Defect of the melanin, due to which there will lack of normal skin pigments
4.	Allergy	Altered body tissue reaction to particular substance
5.	Alopecia	Loss of hair or baldness
6.	Cellulitis	Inflammation of skin and subcutaneous tissue with or without formation of pus
7.	Chloasma	An abnormal brown pigmentation of skin
8.	Comedo	Blackhead; discolored dry sebum plugging an excretory duct of skin
9.	Depigmentation	Partial or complete loss of pigment, occurs in albinism atrophic skin or scars
10.	Derm	Skin
11.	Dermatitis	Inflammation of the skin
12.	Discoid	Shape like a disc
13.	Eczema	Cutaneous inflammatory condition producing red papular and vesicular lesion, crust and scales
14.	Edema	Swelling

Contd...

Contd...

S.No.	Terms	Meanings
15.	Gangrene	Necrosis or putrefaction of tissue usually results from loss of blood supply to any organ
16.	Hirsutism	A condition characterized by the excessive growth of hair or the presence of hair in unusual places, especially in female
17.	Keratotic	Pertaining to a horny thickening
18.	Leukoderma	White patches of skin due to local absence of pigment
19.	Macule	Discolored patch or spot on the skin
20.	Melanoderma	Abnormal brown or black pigmentation of the skin
21.	Melanoma	A tumor made up of melanin-pigmented cells. When used alone, the term refers to malignant melanoma
22.	Onychia	Inflammation of the nail-bed
23.	Papule (pimple)	A small circumscribed, superficial, solid, elevation of the skin usually occurs on the face
24.	Paraonychia	Infected skin around the nail
25.	Pediculosis	Infestation with lice
26.	Proliferation	Process of rapid reproduction of similar cells
27.	Psoriasis	Chronic inflammatory skin disease with appearance of eruption in circular patches of various sizes and showing a definite line of demarcation
28.	Scabies	Skin lesions due to animal parasite associated with formation of vesicular eruption between the fingers, folds of axillae, buttocks, under the breasts and other areas
29.	Steatoma	Itching and its highly communicable smooth shiny globular cutaneous or subcutaneous tumor arising from the sebaceous gland
30.	Tinea	A fungal skin disease frequently caused by ringworms
31.	Urticaria	Skin eruption of pale or reddish patches usually associated with itching may occur as an acute cell. It is usually caused by food allergy, drug reaction of emotional stress
32.	Impetigo	Infectious condition of the skin
33.	Pustule	Raised spot in skin containing pus
34.	Seborrhea	A disease of the sebaceous glands, marked by an excessive secretion of sebum which collects on the skin in oily scales
35.	Tinea pedis	Athletes foot, fungal infection
36.	Urticaria	Allergic reaction
37.	Verruca	Plantar wart
38.	Pilonidal cyst	An epidermal inclusion cyst of the sacral area, usually a tatratomatous (hair containing) cyst which may become infected and undergo suppuration

Operative Terms

S.No.	Terms	Meanings
1.	Autograft	Surgical transplantation of any tissue from one part of the body to another location in the same individual. Autografts are commonly used to replace skin lost in severe burns
2.	Dermabrasion	Surgical removal of scars using sand paper or other abrasives
3.	Electrodesiccation	The use of short high frequency electric sparks for drying cells and tissue
4.	Electrolysis	The decomposition of a substance by passage of an electrical current through it. Hair follicles may be destroyed by use of this method
5.	Fulguration	Destruction of tissue by means of long, high-frequency electric sparks
6.	Lumpectomy	Excision of a small primary breast tumor with the remainder of the breast left intact

COMMON ABBREVIATIONS

Ophthalmology

S.No.	Abbreviation	Term
1.	Clgl	Correction with glasses
2.	ERG	Electroretino gram
3.	LE	Left eye
4.	OD, RE	Right eye (ocular dexter)
5.	OMD	Ocular media
6.	OS, LE	Left eye (oculus sinister)
7.	OU	Each eye (oculi uterque)
8.	VA	Visual acuity
9.	VE	Visual efficiency

Ear

S.No.	Abbreviation	Term
1.	AM	Auditory meatus
2.	AOM	Acute otitis media
3.	BOM	Bilateral otitis media
4.	BSOM	Bilateral suppurative otitis media
5.	CSOM	Chronic suppurative otitis media
6.	DNS	Deflected/deviated nasal septum
7.	EAM	External auditory meatus
8.	ENT	Ear, nose and throat
9.	OM	Otitis media
10.	AC	Air conduction
11.	AC and BC	Air and bone conduction
12.	AD	Auris dextra (right ear)
13.	AP view	Anteroposterior view (radiology)
14.	BC	Bone conduction
15.	CM	Cochlear microphonics
16.	ENG	Electronystagmogram
17.	ENT	Ear, nose and throat
18.	EP	Endochochlear potential
19.	ERA	Evoked response audiometry
20.	HD	Hearing distance
21.	MACS	Mastoid air cell system
22.	Oto	Otology
23.	PA view	Posteroanterior view (radiology)
24.	SAS	Sensoryneural acuity level
25.	SEM	Scanning electromicroscopy
26.	VASC	Visual auditory screening test for children

Dermatology

S.No.	Abbreviation	Term
1.	bx	biopsy
2.	Derm	Dermatology
3.	DLE	Discoid Lupus Erythematosus
4.	FS	Frozen Section
5.	H	Hypodermic
6.	I and D	Incision and Drainage
7.	ID	Intradermal
8.	SLE	Systemic Lupus Erythematosus
9.	SSG	Split Skin Graft
10.	STD	Skin Test Dose
		Sexually Transmitted Disease
11.	Subcu	Subcutaneous
12.	ung	Ointment

10 Excretory System

INTRODUCTION

The urinary system is one of the important systems, which excretes the waste (end) products of metabolism that tend to change the normal internal and external environment of the cell. This is also called as excretory system (Fig. 10.1). The wastes produced by the body such as carbon dioxide and water in the form of vapor are removed from the body by the exhalation through the lungs. Whereas the nitrous waste, produced when proteins combine with oxygen is more difficult to excrete from the body by exhalation. Hence, the body excretes it in the form of a water-soluble substance called urea. The major function of the urinary system is to remove urea from the bloodstream so that it does not accumulate in the body and become toxic. Besides removing the urea, the urinary system maintains the proper balance of water, salts and acids in the body fluids, salts such as sodium, potassium and some acids known as electrolytes. Nephrology is the study of the urinary system or kidney and a specialist in this field is called a nephrologist.

PARTS OF URINARY SYSTEM

The urinary system is composed of:
1. Two kidneys
2. Two ureters
3. Urinary bladder
4. Urethra.

Kidneys

There are two kidneys, which are bean-shaped organs situated behind the abdominal cavity on either side of the vertebral column in the lumbar region of the spine. They lie behind the peritoneum and are embedded in renal fat for protection. They are dark reddish brown in color measuring the size of a fist and about half a pound each. The left kidney is situated at higher level on the posterior abdominal wall than the right kidney (Fig. 10.2).

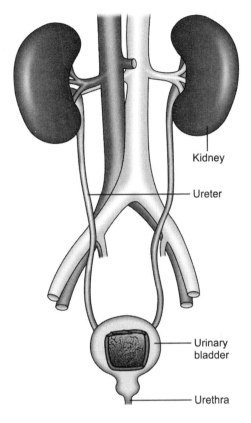

Fig. 10.1: Excretory system

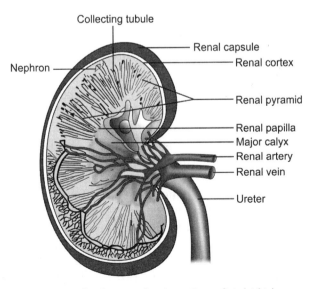

Fig. 10.2: The longitudinal section of right kidney

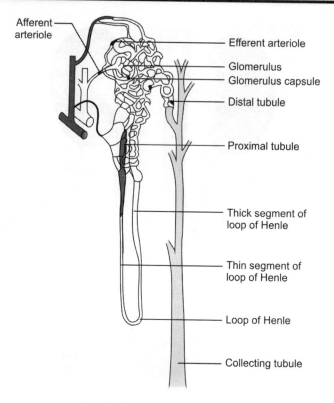

Afferent arteriole

Efferent arteriole

Glomerulus

Glomerulus capsule

Distal tubule

Proximal tubule

Thick segment of loop of Henle

Thin segment of loop of Henle

Loop of Henle

Collecting tubule

Fig. 10.3: Diagram of nephron

The kidney can be divided into three parts namely:

1. The cortex (or) outer part
2. The medulla (or) inner part
3. The hilum depression at the medial part of the kidney.

The cortex (outer) part of the kidney contains tiny glomeruli, together with the renal tubules, which lie partly in the medulla also. These two are commonly called as nephrons, (Fig. 10.3) the functional units of the kidney. There are about 1 million nephrons.

Each nephron has a renal corpuscle and a renal tubule. The renal corpuscle is composed of a tuft of capillaries, the glomerulus and a modified funnel shaped end of the renal tubule called the Bowman's capsule, which encases the glomerulus. An afferent arteriole conveys blood to the glomerulus and an efferent arteriole carries the blood away from the glomerulus. The renal tubule has four sections, the proximal convoluted tubule, loop of Henle, distal convoluted tubule, and collecting tubule, where the excretion process for removing the waste products from the blood takes place. After this process, blood leaves the kidney by way of the renal vein. The waste material is carried out to the hollow chamber, the renal pelvis, that is situated in the hilus. The adrenal gland lies on top of each kidney.

The concave central part of the kidney is called hilum, where the renal artery enters the kidney and renal vein leaves the kidney. The inner area is called medulla. Calices are the ducts, which join the renal pelvis. Pelvis is the collection point of urine as it is formed. The main function of the urinary system is to filter and remove waste products from the blood.

Ureters

There are two ureters which start from the pelvis of each kidney and opens into the urinary bladder. Each ureter is 25 cm long and they are fine, muscular tubes lined with mucous membrane. They convey urine in peristaltic waves from the kidney to the urinary bladder.

Urinary Bladder

The urinary bladder is a triangle-shaped muscular bag, situated in the pelvic cavity. It acts as a temporary reservoir for the urine. The neck of the bladder has a sphincter muscle to stop the back flow of the urine from the bladder. The voluntary action controls the external muscle sphincter, which opens only when the desire to void arises. The trigone is a triangular space at the base of the bladder where the ureters enter and the urethra leads out.

Urethra

It is a canal leading from the bladder to discharge urine from the urinary bladder. The external opening of the urethra is called the urethral or urinary meatus. Urethra is a common passage for urine and seminal fluid in the male while in the female it is the passage for urine only. The length of the male urethra is longer than the female. It measures about 20 cm in male and 8 cm in female. The male urethra has three parts, prostatic part is surrounded by the prostate gland; the ejaculatory ducts and the ducts of the prostate gland open into it, the membranous part and penile part is surrounded by the corpus spongiosum of the penis.

Adrenal Glands (Suprarenal Glands)

There are two glands, which are endocrine glands located above each kidney. The functioning of the adrenal glands are explained in the endocrine system.

EXCRETION PROCESS OF URINE (FLOW CHART 10.1)

Blood enters each kidney through the renal artery. These arteries, divides into small arteries called arterioles and these are located throughout the cortex of the kidney. The blood from the arteriole leads to the tiny smaller blood vessels called capillaries, which are collectively called as glomeruli, and here the process of formation of urine begins. The three steps involved in this process are filtration, reabsorption, and secretion.

The filtration process starts at the glomeruli, where the water, salts, sugar and nitrogenous waste such as urea, creatinine, and uric acid are filtered out through the thin walls of the glomeruli. These filtered products are collected by the Bowman's capsule, a cup like structure

Flow chart 10.1: Excretion process of urine

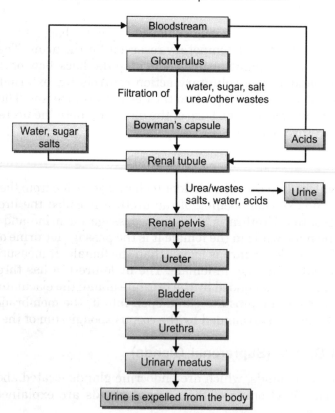

holding the glomeruli. The fluid formed is called filtrate. During filtration, some of the essential chemicals for healthy living such as water, sugar, salts are also filtered out with the wastes.

When this filtrate passes through the four sections of the renal tubule, certain amount of these filtered products such as water, some of the electrolytes and amino acids are absorbed by the peritubular capillaries, thus re-entering the circulating blood. In the convoluted tubules much of the water, salts, etc. are returned to the blood supply while the remainder is passed into the collecting tubules and then into the kidney pelvis via the pyramids and calyces as urine. The final stage of urine production occurs when specialized cells of the collecting tubules secrete ammonia, uric acid and other substances directly into the lumen of the tubule. Here thousands of renal tubule deposit urine into the central renal pelvis, a space that fills most of the medulla of the kidney. Blood leaves the kidney via the renal vein. The urine is then passed via the ureters into the urinary bladder, where it is temporarily stored. The exit area of the bladder to the urethra is closed by sphincters, which do not permit urine to leave the bladder. As the bladder fills up, however, there is a point at which muscular contractions of the walls of the bladder begin and pressure is placed on the base of the urethra, which causes the desire to urinate. This process of muscular contractions so as to pass urine is called *micturition*.

Blood flow should be maintained constantly through the kidneys. When the flow of blood is reduced, a substance called renin is released by the kidney, which ultimately increases the blood pressure and blood flow in the kidneys is restored to normal.

EXCRETORY SYSTEM

Origin of Terms

S.No.	Terms	Meanings	S.No.	Terms	Meanings
1.	Calyx	Cup	10.	Pyelo	Pelvis
2.	Cortex	Ring, outer portion	11.	Pyo	Pus
3.	-genesis	Origin, beginning process	12.	Trigone	Triangle
4.	Glomerul/o	Glomerulus	13.	Urethra	Urethra
5.	Glomerulus	Little skin	14.	-uria	Urine
6.	Glyc/o	Sugar	15.	-lith	Calculus, stone
7.	Junction	Joining	16.	-lithiasis	Presence, condition
8.	Medulla	Marrow			or formation of
9.	Nephron, Ren	Kidney			calculi

Symptomatic and Diagnostic Terms

S.No.	Terms	Meanings
1.	Agenesis	Absence of an organ
2.	Albuminuria, proteinuria	Albumin or protein in urine
3.	Anuria	Complete failure of secretion of urine due to renal failure or blockage of urinary tract
4.	Azotemia	Presence of nitrogen bodies in increased amount especially urea in the blood
5.	Cystitis	Inflammation of bladder due to infection
6.	Dysplasia	Abnormal tissue development
7.	Dysuria	Difficult or painful urination
8.	Ectopy kidney	Displaced kidney usually low in position
9.	Enuresis	Bedwetting, involuntary discharge of urine
10.	Exstrophy of bladder	Congenital absence of the lower abdominal and anterior vesicle walls with *eversion* of the bladder; absence of closure or formation of the anterior one half of the bladder. It is often associated with epispadiasis
11.	Glomerulonephritis	Inflammation of kidney due to injury to the glomeruli due to antigen-antibody reaction
12.	Glycosuria	Sugar in urine
13.	Hematuria	Blood in urine
14.	Hesitancy	Dysuria due to nervous inhibition or due to obstruction of vesical outlet
15.	Hydronephrosis	Accumulation of fluid in renal pelvis resulting in enlargement of kidney
16.	Hydroureter	Ureter overdistended with urine due to obstruction
17.	Hypertrophy of kidney	Increased in size of kidney
18.	Hyperuricemia	Disorder resulting from a sudden high increase of serum uric acid level in blood prone to occur in patients receiving massive antineoplastic therapy
19.	Interstitial nephritis	Renal disease in which the interstitial connective tissue is involved
20.	Megalocystis, megabladder	Enormous dilation of urinary bladder
21.	Micturition	Act of passing urine
22.	Nephritis	Inflammation of kidney
23.	Nephrolithiasis	Stone in the Kidney generally in the pelvis.
24.	Nephroptosis	A movable, floating kidney which is displaced downward
25.	Nocturia	Passing urine during the night
26.	Oliguria	Scanty urinary output due to acute tubular necrosis, advanced fluid and electrolyte imbalance, organic kidney lesions, obstructive uropathy and other causes.
27.	Polyuria\	Excessive urinary output
28.	Pyelitis	Inflammation of the renal pelvis
29.	Pyoureter	Infection in the ureter, generally secondary to infection of the bladder or kidney with pus formation

Contd...

Contd...

S.No.	Terms	Meaning
30.	Pyuria	Pus in the urine
31.	Renal calculus	Stones in kidney
32.	Renal colic	Spasm in kidney
33.	Renal insufficiency	Severe disturbance of excretory kidney function in renal disease or following surgery or trauma. Anuria may develop from blood transfusions
34.	Trigonitis	Inflammation of the trigone, the triangular base of the bladder
35.	Urinary retention	Inability to expel urine. This may be acute or chronic, complete or incomplete
36.	Uremia	Excess of nitrogenous end products of protein and amino acid metabolism in the blood
37.	Ureteritis	Inflammation of the ureter
38.	Urethritis	Inflammation of urethra which may be due to gonococcic infection
39.	Urethroplasty	Repair of the urethra
40.	Urgency	Intense need to urinate at once

Operative Terms

S.No.	Terms	Meaning
1.	Cystectomy	Excision of bladder
2.	Cystolithotomy	Incision into bladder for removal of stones
3.	Cystoplasty	Surgical repair of the bladder
4.	Cystorrhaphy	Suture of ruptured or lacerated bladder
5.	Cystoscopy	Endoscopic examination of the bladder
6.	Cystostomy	Surgical creation of a cutaneous bladder fistula for urinary drainage
7.	Meatotomy	Incision of urinary meatus to increase its caliber
8.	Nephrectomy	Excision of kidney primarily for advanced calculus, pyonephrosis, hydronephrosis or malignant tumor
9.	Nephrolithotomy	Incision into kidney for removal of stones
10.	Nephrolysis	Surgical destruction of renal adhesions
11.	Nephropexy	Surgical fixation of a displaced kidney
12.	Nephrorrhaphy	Suture of an injured kidney
13.	Nephrostomy	Surgical creation of renal fistula for drainage
14.	Nephrotomy	Incision into kidney
15.	Nephroureterectomy	Removal of ureter and kidney for tumor of the renal pelvis or for malignant tumor of the ureter
16.	Pyelolithotomy	Incision into renal pelvis for removal of calculi
17.	Pyeloplasty	Plastic repair of renal pelvis
18.	Pyelotomy	Incision into renal pelvis

Contd...

Contd...

S.No.	Terms	Meaning
19.	Ureterectomy	Partial or complete removal of ureter
20.	Ureterocystostomy	Re-implantation of ureter into bladder
21.	Ureterolithotomy	Incision into ureter for removal of calculi
22.	Ureterolysis	Freeing the ureter from adhesions to relieve secondary obstruction
23.	Ureteropelvioplasty	Plastic operation at the ureteropelvic junction
24.	Ureterostomy	Creation of new outlet for ureter
25.	Ureterovesicoplasty	Corrective surgery for persistent reflux by repair of the ureterovesical junctions
26.	Ureteropyelostomy	Anastomosis of ureter and renal pelvis
27.	Hemodialysis	Removal of waste chemical substances from the blood by passing it through tubes made of semipermeable membranes. The tubes are continually bathed by solutions that selectively remove harmful products in renal failure cases
28.	Urethropexy	Surgical fixation of the urethra
29.	Urethroplasty	Surgical correction of the urethra
30.	Ureteropyelostomy	Anastomosis of ureter and renal pelvis
31.	Ureterovesicostomy	Reimplantation of a ureter into the bladder

COMMON ABBREVIATIONS

S.No.	Abbreviation	Term
1.	A/G	Albumin/globulin ratio
2.	ADH	Antiuretic hormone
3.	AGN	Acute glomerulonephritis
4.	ATN	Acute tubular necrosis
5.	B/K	Bladder kidney (scan ratio)
6.	BPH	Benign prostatic hypertrophy
7.	BUN	Blood urea nitrogen
8.	Cl	Chloride; an electrolyte excreted by the kidney
9.	CPK	Creatinine phosphokinase
10.	CRF	Chronic renal failure
11.	CSU	Catheter specimen of urine
12.	cysto	Cystoscopic examination
13.	GFR	Glomerular filtration rate
14.	GU	Genitourinary
15.	HCO_3	Bicarbonate; an electrolyte conserved by the kidney
16.	IVP	Intravenous pyelogram
17.	IVU	Intravenous urography
18.	K	Potassium; an electrolyte
19.	KUB	Kidney, ureter, bladder
20.	LK	Left kidney
21.	MSSU	Midstream specimen of urine
22.	Na	Sodium; an electrolyte
23.	NPU	Not passer urine

Contd...

Contd...

S.No.	Abbreviation	Term
24.	pH	Hydrogen ion concentration
25.	pH	Test of acidity or alkalinity
26.	PKU	Phenylketonuria
27.	RFT	Renal function test
28.	RK	Right kidney
29.	RP	Retrograde pyelogram
30.	RU	Retrograde urogram
31.	SEP	Senile enlarge prostate
32.	SPP	Suprapubic prostatectomy
33.	TPUR	Transperineal urethral resection
34.	TUR; TURP	Transuretheral resection (for prostatectomy)
35.	U/A	Urinalysis
36.	UD	Urethral discharge
37.	UDT	Undescended testicle
38.	UTI	Urinary tract infection
39.	VCC	Voiding cystouretherogram
40.	VD	Veneral disease

11

Reproductive System

INTRODUCTION

The reproductive system plays a vital role in the reproduction of an individual. The organs and functions of the reproductive system differ in male and female. Reproduction is the union of the female sex cell (ovum) and male sex cell (sperm), which contains the genetic material called chromosomes. Each sex cell (male and female) has exactly 23 chromosomes. Male has 21 chromosomes and 2 autosomes (X and Y) which decides the sex of the newborn, where as female has 23 chromosomes, when the ovum and sperm cell unite, the cell produced receives half of its genetic material complement of hereditary material. These sex cells are produced in special organs called gonads in the male and female. The female gonads are the ovaries and male gonads are the testes.

MALE REPRODUCTIVE SYSTEM

The male reproductive system performs two important functions, viz production of the male sex cells (sperm), storage and transportation of the sperm.

The organs of the male reproductive system (Fig. 11.1) are:
1. Testes (singular: testis)
2. Scrotum
3. Seminiferous tubules
4. Epididymis
5. Vas deferens
6. Seminal vesicles
7. Ejaculatory duct
8. Prostate gland
9. Penis
10. Urethra.

Testes

The primary organ of male reproductive system is testis. The male gonad consists of pair of testes. The testes develop in the kidney region

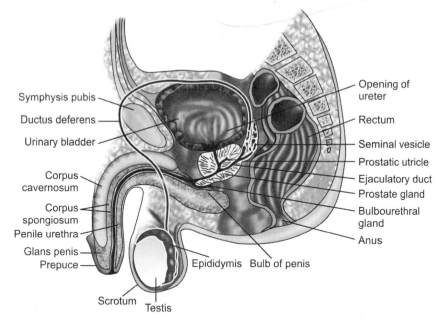

Fig. 11.1: Parts of the male reproductive system

of the body and descends into the scrotum during embryonic development. They produce an important male hormone called testosterone,
which is responsible for the secondary sexual character such as beard,
pubic hair, voice deepening and proper development of male gonads
and accessory organs which secretes fluid to insure the lubrication
and viability of the sperm.

Scrotum

The scrotum is a muscular sac enclosing the testes on the outside of
the body. It lies between the thighs, and maintains the testes at lower
temperature than that of the body, facilitating adequate maturation
and development of sperm, which requires quite low temperature.

Seminiferous Tubule

Seminiferous tubules are small-coiled tubules in the testis and they
produce sperm.

Epididymis

The epididymis is the tightly coiled tubule lying over the surface of
the testis. The seminiferous tubule collectively meets at the epididymis.
The spermatozoa become motile and are temporarily stored in
epididymis.

Vas Deferens

The vas deferens is a narrow tubule, which starts from the epididymis runs down through the length of the testes then turns upward again to reach the seminal vesicle. The vas deferens is about 2 feet long and carries the sperm up into the pelvic region, around the urinary bladder and down toward the urethra.

Seminal Vesicle

The seminal vesicles are glands located at the base of the urinary bladder and open into the vas deferens as it joins the urethra. It secretes a thick yellowish substance that nourishes the sperm cells and forms much of the volume of ejaculated semen.

Ejaculatory Duct

The ejaculatory duct is a tubule like structure where the vas deferens and seminal vesicle meet together.

Prostate Gland

The prostate gland is triple lobed cone-shaped organ, situated below the urinary bladder and surrounding the upper part of the urethra near the bladder neck. The prostate gland secretes a thin, alkaline substance that accounts for about 30 percent of seminal fluid and helps to protect the sperms from the acidic environment and aids the motility of the sperms.

Two pea-shaped glands Cowper's gland or bulbourethral glands are located below the prostate and they also secrete fluid into the urethra.

Penis

The penis is the organ for copulation. It is cylindrical in shape composed of erectile tissue made up of three cylindrical bodies viz. a pair of corpus cavernosum and one corpus spongiosum. It is enclosed by the urethra. The tip of the penis is soft and sensitive region called glans penis. A fold of skin known as the prepuce, which is freely movable, protects the glans penis.

Urethra

The urethra expels both semen and urine from the body. During ejaculation, the sphincter at the base of the bladder is closed. This not only stops the urine from being expelled with the semen, but also prevents the sperm from entering the bladder.

SEMEN

Semen is a combination of fluid and spermatozoa, which is ejected from the body through the urethra. In the male, as opposed to the female, the genital orifice combines with the urinary opening.

The male sex cell, the spermatozoon (sperm) is microscopic-in volume, only one-third of the size of an erythrocyte and less than 1/100000th size of female ovum. It is relatively uncomplicated cell, composed of a head region, which contains nuclear hereditary material and a tail region, consisting of flagellum (hairlike process), which makes the sperm motile, somewhat resembling a tadpole.

Only one spermatozoon of approximately 100 million sperm cells, which may be, released during a single ejaculation can penetrate a single ovum and produce fertilization of the ovum. If more than one egg is passing down the fallopian tube when sperms are present, multiple fertilization are possible and twins, triplets, quadruplets and so fifth may occur. Twins resulting from the fertilization of separate ova by a separate sperm called fraternal twins. These twins develop in separate placentae. Identical twins are formed from the fertilization of a single egg cell by a single sperm, where both the embryos share the same placenta.

FEMALE REPRODUCTIVE SYSTEM

The female reproductive system consists of organs, which produce ova and provide space for the growth of embryo. The female reproductive organs (Figs. 11.2 and 11.3) also secrete hormones such as estrogen and progesterone that contribute the secondary female sexual characteristics such as body hair, breast development, structural changes in bones and fat. The period when the secondary female sexual characteristics develop is called puberty. Ova are produced during the onset of the puberty period. When the ova is not fertilized the hormonal changes result in the shedding of the uterine lining, and bleeding. This is called menstruation. When ova is fertilized in uterus, that condition is called pregnancy, the normal gestation period is approximately 9 calendar months. The cessation of the fertility and diminishing of the hormone production is called menopause. The period between the puberty and menopause is called the reproductive period or child bearing age, it is normally between age of 15 to 44 years of a woman's age.

The major organs of female reproductive system can be divided into two: they are internal genitalia and external genitalia. The organs of the internal and external genitalia are as follows:

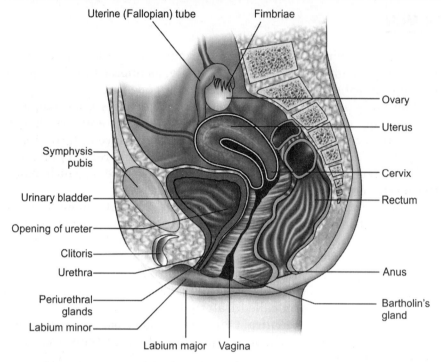

Fig. 11.2: Organs of the female reproductive system—lateral view

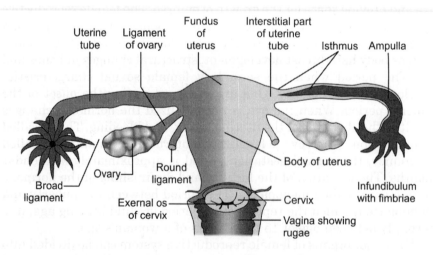

Fig. 11.3: Organs of the female reproductive system—anterior view

Internal genitalia	External genitalia
a. Ovaries	a. Vulva:
b. Fallopian tubes	i. Labia majora
c. Uterus	ii. Labia minora
d. Vagina	iii. Hymen

The accessory organ of the female reproductive system is breasts.

Ovaries

The ovaries are the bean-shaped glands located in the pelvic cavity on either side of the uterus to which they are attached by the ovarian ligament. They produce ovum, which is the female reproductive cell and hormones such as progesterone and estrogen. These hormones are responsible for the menstrual cycle and prepare the uterus for pregnancy when the fertilization takes place and also plays a vital role in development of secondary sexual characteristics.

Fallopian Tubes

The fallopian tubes are the muscular tube like structure measuring five and half inches which extends from ovaries to either side of the uterus. It transport ovum by a wavelike movement (peristalsis) from the ovary to the uterus. It takes for an ovum about five days to pass through the fallopian tube. It also acts as a passage for the ovum to pass from the uterus towards the ovaries.

Uterus

Uterus is a muscular pear-shaped organ. It lies in the pelvic cavity behind the urinary bladder and infront of the rectum. It is supported in position by ligaments and covered by three layers of tissue:
1. Endometrium   inner lining of the uterus
2. Myometrium   middle muscular lining of the uterus
3. Perimetrium   outer covering of the uterus.

It is the organ, which stores and nourishes the embryo from the time of fertilization until the fetus is born. It has three parts namely: the fundus, which is the upper round part; the corpus, which is the central part and the cervix the external part, which extends to vagina.

Vagina

The vagina is a muscular tube of 7.5 cm long, extending from the uterus to the exterior of the body. It is lined by mucous membranous fold, which provides elastic quality. It serves as an organ for sexual intercourse and receptor of semen and passageway for the delivery of the fetus. Besides these, it discharges the menstrual flow.

There are two glands situated on either side of the vaginal orifice, they are called Bartholin's gland. The clitoris is an organ of sensitive erectile tissue located anterior to the vaginal orifice and in front of the urethral meatus. The clitoris is similar in structure to the penis in the male.

External Genitalia

The organs of the external genitalia are collectively called vulva. The vulva consists of labia majora the outer lips of the vagina and labia minora are the small and inner lips. The hymen is a mucous membrane, partially covering the entrance to the vagina. It is normally perforated, which permits the exit of menstrual discharge. The clitoris and Bartholin's gland are also parts of the vulva.

The Breast

The breasts (Fig. 11.4) are two mammary (milk-producing) organs, located in the upper anterior region of the chest. The breasts also contain fatty tissue, special lactiferous ducts and sinuses which carry milk to the opening of nipple. The breast nipple is called the mammary papilla and the dark-pigmented area around the mammary papilla is called the areola. They are in rudimentary stage during the birth and they develop during the puberty period and the size of the breast increases during the pregnancy and when lactation takes place.

Menstrual Cycle

The menstrual cycle, which last long for 28 days is divided into 4 phases. They are:

Menstrual phase (1–5 days): These are the days during which bloody fluid containing disintegrated endometrial cells, glandular secretion and blood cells passing from the uterus are discharged through vagina.

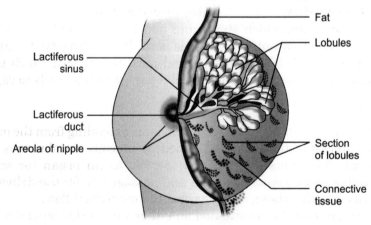

Fig. 11.4: Cross-section of the breast and its parts

Pre-ovulatory phase (6–13 days): Estrogen is released by the ovarian follicles to repair the endometrium (uterus lining). During this phase, one of the secondary follicles matures into a graafian follicle, which is ready for ovulation.

Ovulatory phase (13–14 days): On about the 14th day of the cycle, the graafian follicle ruptures (ovulation) and the egg leaves the ovary to travel slowly down to the fallopian tube. This phase (14th day) is said to be the best period of copulation for the fertilization of ovum.

Menstrual phase (15–28 days): This represents the time between ovulation and the onset of next menses.

Following ovulation, the graafian follicle collapses and forms a clot which is absorbed by the remaining follicular cells. These follicular cells enlarge, change character and form the corpus luteum, or yellow body. The corpus luteum then secretes increasing quantities of estrogen and progesterone.

If fertilization and implantation do not occur, the decreased secretion of progesterone and estrogen then initiates the next menstrual cycle.

PREGNANCY

Pregnancy is the condition in which a zygote (the union of male gonad and female ovum) develops in the uterus. The placenta, which is the organ of communication between the mother and embryo, now forms within the uterine wall. The placenta is filled with a fluid called amniotic fluid, which breaks during the onset of labor. The hormone oxitocin instigate the vigorous contraction of the uterus to effect the delivery of the fetus. The normal gestation period is about 40 weeks. Immediately after delivery a hormone called prolactin promotes the milk secretion to feed the newborn.

The product of conception up to the 3rd month is called as embryo and later it is referred as fetus. During pregnancy, there will be a change in uterus, vagina and breasts.

Labor and Birth

The labor and birth can be classified into three stages: they are:
1. *Dilation stage:* During this stage the uterus contracts and the complete dilation of the cervix occurs.
2. *Expulsion stage:* This stage starts from complete dilation of the cervix to the birth of baby.
3. *Placental stage:* After the childbirth, when the uterine contractions discharge the placenta from the uterus.

REPRODUCTIVE SYSTEM

MALE

Origin of Terms

S.No.	Terms	Meanings	S.No.	Terms	Meanings
1.	Andr	Male	8.	Epdidym/o	Epididymis
2.	Balano	Glans penis	9.	Zo/o	Animal life
3.	Test/o, orchid	Testis, testicle	10.	Cry/o	Cold
4.	Prostat	Prostate gland	11.	-chrome	Color
5.	Sperm	Spermatozoa	12.	-genesis	Origin, beginning, process
6.	Vas	Vessel duct	13.	-uria	Urine
7.	Vesiculo	Seminal vesicles			

Symptomatic and Diagnostic Terms

S.No.	Medical terms	Description
1.	Actinomycosis	Fungal disease affecting genital organ
2.	Anorchism	Absence of testis
3.	Aspermia	Lack of or failure to ejaculate semen
4.	Benign prostatic hypertrophy	Overgrowth of the glandular tissue of the prostate
5.	Balanitis	Inflammation of the glans penis
6.	Cryptorchism	Undescended testicles
7.	Epispadias; epispadia	Congenital opening of the male urethra on the upper surface of the penis
8.	Glans penis	Sensitive tip of the penis
9.	Gonorrhea	Venereal disease, characterized by inflammation of the genital tract mucous membranes; caused by infection with gonococcus
10.	Hydrocele	Hernia (sac) of fluid in the testes or in the tubes leading from the testes
11.	Hypospadias; hypospadia	Congenital opening of male urethra on the undersurface of the penis
12.	Impotence	Condition characterized by the inability to achieve an erection
13.	Orchitis	Inflammation of the testis
14.	Perineum	Area between the anus and scrotum
15.	Phimosis	Narrowing of the opening of the foreskin over the glans penis
16.	Prepuce	Foreskin
17.	Semen	Thick, white secretion of the reproductive organ of the male. This fluid is composed of spermatozoa and the mixed product of various glands, including the prostate and bulbourethral glands
18.	Sterilization	Procedure rendering an individual incapable of reproduction; vasectomy in males and salpingectomy in females are common procedures

Contd...

Contd...

S.No.	Medical terms	Description
19.	Syphilis	Venereal disease caused by *Treponema pallidum* leading to structural and cutaneous lesions.
20.	Testicular carcinoma	Malignant tumor of the testes
21.	Testis	Male gonad which produces spermatozoa and the hormone testosterone
22.	Testosterone	Hormone secreted by the interstitial tissue of the testes; responsible for male sex characteristics
23.	Trichomoniasis	Infection of the genitourinary tract of either sex; caused by *Trichomonas*.
24.	Varicocele	Enlarged, herniated, swollen veins near the testicle
25.	Vas deferens	Narrow tube which carries sperm from the epididymis to the urethra
26.	Azoospermia	Semen without living spermatozoa causing infertility in the male

Operative Terms

S.No.	Medical Terms	Description
1.	Circumcision	Surgical removal of the end of the prepuce of the glands penis
2.	Epididymectomy	Excision of the epididymis
3.	Orchidoplasty Orchiopexy	Surgical transfer of an undescended testicle to the scrotum
4.	Orchiectomy orchidectomy orchectomy	Removal of testis
5.	Prostatomy	Incision into the prostate
6.	Vasectomy	Removal of all or a segment of the vas deferens
7.	Varicocelectomy	Excision of varicocele
8.	Orchotomy	Incision of a testis
9.	Prostatectomy	Removal of the prostate gland
10.	Transurethral resection of prostate (TURP)	Resection of the hypertrophy of the prostate

FEMALE

Origin of Terms

S.No.	Terms	Meanings	S.No.	Terms	Meanings
1.	Albus	White	17.	Isthmus	Narrow passage
2.	Ampulla	Little jar	18.	Labi /o	Lip
3.	-arche	Beginning	19.	Luteum	Yellow
4.	Cervic/o	Neck, cervix	20.	Mamm/o, mast/o	Breast
5.	Colp/o, vigin/o	Vagina	21.	Men/o	Menses, menstruation
6.	Episi/o vulv/o	Vulva	22.	Nat/a	Birth
7.	Fimbria	Fringe	23.	Oopher, ovari/o	Ovary
8.	Fistula	Pipe, tube	24.	Ostium	Small opening
9.	Folliculus	Little bag	25.	Ovarium, ova	Egg holder
10.	Fundus	Base	26.	-para	To bear
11.	Galact/o, lact/o	Milk	27.	Perine/o	Perineum
12.	-gravida	Pregnancy	28.	Salpingo	Tube
13.	Gyne	Female	29.	Salpinx	Fallopian tubes
14.	Hymen	Membrane	30.	-tocia	Childbirth, labor
15.	Hyster, metra	Uterus, womb	31.	Vestibule	Antechamber
16.	Infundibulum	Funnel	32.	Vulva	Covering

Symptomatic and Diagnostic Terms

S.No.	Medical terms	Description
1.	Abortion	Deliberate termination of pregnancy before the fetus is capable of surviving outside the uterus
2.	Abrupitio-placenta	Premature separation of a normally situated placenta
3.	Adnexa	Accessory parts of a structure
4.	Amenorrhea	Absence of menstruation
5.	Amnion	The innermost membrane enclosing the developing fetus and the fluid in which the fetus is bathed
6.	Atresia	Congenital absence or closure of a normal body opening
7.	Cervicitis	Inflammation of the cervix
8.	Choriocarcinoma	A malignant neoplasm of the uterus
9.	Corpus luteum	Scar tissue of the ovary that results from the rupturing of a follicle during ovulation
10.	Cystocele	Herniation of the bladder into the vagina
11.	Down's syndrome	Preferred terms for mongolism
12.	Dyspareunia	Painful sexual intercourse
13.	Eclampsia toxemia	Major disorder of pregnancy that may be manifested by high blood pressure, edema, convulsions, renal dysfunction, proteinuria, and in severe cases, coma
14.	Ectopic pregnancy	A pregnancy in which the fertilized ovum developed outside the uterine cavity
15.	Endocervicitis	A fairly common problem that results when organisms gain access to the cervical glands after delivery, abortion, or intrauterine manipulation
16.	Endometriosis	Condition of endometrium

Contd...

Contd...

S.No.	Medical terms	Description
17.	Fibroids, fibromyoma uteri	Benign uterine tumors that are composed of muscle and fibrous tissue
18.	Hematocolpos	Blood in vagina
19.	Hematometra	Collection of blood in uterus
20.	Hematosalpinx	Infection to fallopian tubes
21.	Hydrosalpinx	Collection of watery fluid in a uterine tube, occurring as the end stage of pyosalpinx
22.	Hydrocephalus	Increased accumulation of cerebrospinal fluid within the ventricles of the brain
23.	IUD (intrauterine device)	A small coil is placed inside the uterus to prevent implantation of the fertilized egg in the uterine lining
24.	Lactation	Period when infant is nourished from breast
25.	Leukorrhea	White vaginal discharge
26.	Leukoplakia vulva	Condition of white patches on vulva
27.	Mastitis	Inflammation of the breast
28.	Menarche	Establishment or beginning of the menstrual function
29.	Menorrhagia	Excessive bleeding
30.	Metrorrhagia	Bleeding between periods
31.	Miscarriage, spontaneous abortion	A natural, spontaneous termination of pregnancy before the fetus is able to survive outside the uterus
32.	Multigravida	A woman who has been pregnant two or more times
33.	Oophritis	Inflammation of ovary
34.	Multipara	A woman who has borne more than one viable fetus, whether or not the offspring were alive at birth
35.	Parametrium	Loose connective tissue around the uterus
36.	Primipara	A woman during her first pregnancy
37.	Procidentia	Prolapse of uterus
38.	Pruritus vulvae	Disorders marked by severe itching of external female genitalia
39.	Puberty	The period during which the secondary sex characteristics begin to develop and capability for sexual reproduction is attained
40.	Puerperium	The period of 42 days following childbirth and expulsion of the placenta and membranes.
41.	Pyosalpinx	Pus in the fallopian tubes
42.	Salpingitis	Inflammation of fallopian tubes
43.	Salpingo-oophoritis	Inflammation of the fallopian tubes and ovaries
44.	Trichomonas vaginitis	Infection of vagina by a parasite called flagellate protozoa
45.	Uretheral carbuncle	Small red swelling of the urethra
46.	Vaginismus	Painful spasm of the vagina from contraction of the muscles surrounding the vagina
47.	Vaginitis	Inflammation of vagina
48.	Vulvovaginitis	Inflammation of vulva and vagina
49.	Dysfunctional uterine bleeding (DUB)	Functional bleeding not due to any local disease may result from irregular production of estrogen or progesterone

Operative Terms

S.No.	Medical terms	Description
1.	Amniocentesis	Transabdominal puncture of the amniotic sac, using a needle and syringe, in order to remove amniotic fluid
2.	Chorion villus biopsy	Guided by an ultrasound display, the doctor inserts an aspirator into the uterus to obtain a sample of the chorionic villi
3.	Colpectomy	Excision of vagina
4.	Colpectomy, vaginectomy	Excision of the vagina
5.	Colpocleisis	Closure of the vaginal canal
6.	Colpoperineoplasty colpoperineorrhaphy	Plastic surgery on vagina and perineum
7.	Colporrhaphy	Suture of vagina
8.	Conization	Excision of a cone of tissue as of the mucous membrane to promote healing of the cervix
9.	Colposcopy	Examination of vagina
10.	Cryosurgery, cryocautery	The process of freezing tissue for the purpose of destroying cells
11.	Dilatation and curettage (D and C)	Therapeutic measure for incomplete abortion
12.	Episiorrhaphy	Suturing of a lacerated perineum
13.	Episiotomy	Incision of perineum from the vaginal orifice, usually done to facilitate childbirth
14.	Hymenotomy	Incision of the hymen
15.	Hysterectomy	Excision of uterus
16.	Myomectomy	Excision of myomatous tumor in uterus
17.	Panhysterectomy	Removal of the entire uterus, including the cervix
18.	Perineorrhaphy	Repair of lacerated perineum
19.	Salpingectomy	Removal of a fallopian tube
20.	Salpingo-oophorectomy	Removal of a fallopian tube and ovary
21.	Tubal ligation	Ligation of the uterine tubes to prevent pregnancy; sterilization surgery
22.	Episioplasty	Plastic repair of vulva and perineum due to injury during deliveries
23.	Vulvectomy	Partial removal of vulva
24.	Oophorectomy	Partial and complete removal of ovary
25.	Oophoropexy	Fixation of displaced ovary
26.	Oophoroplasty	Plastic repair of an ovary
27.	Tuboplasty	Reconstructive tubal surgery for the correction of infertility
28.	Salphingolysis	Breaking up or releasing of peritubal adhesions which damage the fimbriated end of the tube

MATERNAL, ANTENATAL AND NEONATAL CONDITIONS

Origin of Terms

1.	Gravida	(L)	=	Pregnancy	5.	Pelvis	(L)	=	Basin
2.	Multi	(L)	=	Many	6.	Placenta	(L)	=	Cake
3.	Nulli	(L)	=	None	7.	Primi	(L)	=	First
4.	Pario	(L)	=	To bear					

General Terms

S.No.	Terms	Meanings
1.	Blighted ovum	Impregnanted ovum that has ceased to grow within the first trimester (Three months)
2.	Contraception	Voluntary prevention of pregnancy
3.	Gestation	Period of pregnancy. Intrauterine development of fetus a) *Embryonic period:* Approximately in a first trimester b) *Fetal period:* Approximately in a second and third trimester
4.	Gravida	Pregnant women
5.	High-risk gravida	Being too young or too old, under or over weight, having any one of the conditions such as diabetes, hypertension, urinary infection, hepatitis, Rh incompatibility, etc. during the current pregnancy
6.	High-risk neonate	Newborn in need of resuscitation due to abnormally brief or prolonged gestation, too low or high birth weight, defective apgar score, fetal diseases and congenital anomalies
7.	Multipara	A woman who is bearing more than one child
8.	Natural childbirth	Childbirth in a normal physiologic manner without anesthetic or instruments. The women participate actively and consciously in her delivery. This is also called as normal or spontaneous vaginal delivery
9.	Parturient	A women in labor
10.	Perinatology	The study of infant before, during and after birth
11.	Primipara	A women who has delivered her first child
12.	Teratogens	Noxious agents, capable of disrupting normal gestation, with subsequent antenatal death
13.	Teratology	Branch of science dealing with the study of congenital deformed fetus

Diagnostic Terms

S.No.	Terms	Meanings
1.	Abortion	The termination of fetus, before the stage of viability. Sometime between the 20th and 28th week of gestation. The fetus measuring less than 14 inches and weight less than 500 gm

Contd...

Contd...

S.No.	Terms	Meanings
2.	Ectopic pregnancy	Implantation of the fertilized ovum outside of the uterine cavity, in tube, ovary or free in abdomen attached to viscus
3.	Hyperemesis gravidum	Severe nausea and vomiting during the first month of pregnancy, which may cause dehydration and serious metabolic disturbances in mother and fetus
	Habitual abortion	Spontaneous abortion occurring in three or more pregnancy with no other cause
	Imminent threatened	Threatened abortion characterized by vaginal bleeding by with or without pain and cervical dilation usually terminating the product of conception by expulsion of uterus
	Incomplete	Abortion in which part of product of consumption has been retained in the uterus and subsequent bleeding occur
	Induced	Abortion may be induced by use of drugs and instruments
	Inevitable	Rupture of membrane associated with cervical dilation and followed by fetal expulsion
	Missed	Fetal dead but retained in uterus for at least eight weeks.
	Septic	Condition in which there is a serious infection of the uterus leading
4.	Hypertensive disorders	High blood pressure of 140/90 and above during pregnancy. Proteinuria, edema, convulsion of coma may also occur
5.	Eclampsia	Major disorders of pregnancy manifested by high blood pressure, convulsion, renal dysfunction, headache, edema and severe causes of coma
6.	Pre-eclampsia	Usually a disorder of first pregnancy but also may occur in multiparas who are severely hypertensive or diabetic characterized by high blood pressure sudden and excessive weight gain and kidney dysfunction
7.	Involution of uterus	After delivery return of uterus to its normal shape and size
8.	Oligohydramnios	Deficient amount of aminotic fluid
9.	Phlegmasia alba dolens	Inflammation of the femoral vein. Inflammation with pain may occur after delivery
10.	Placenta abruptio	Premature detachment of placenta from the uterus due to severe hemorrhage
11.	Placenta accreta	Adherent placenta remains attached to uterus after delivery
12.	Placenta previa	Displaced placenta implanted in lower segment of uterine wall.
13.	Polyhydramnios	Excessive amount of aminotic fluid
14.	Hysterorrhexis	Laceration of uterus
15.	Subinvolution	Failure of the uterus to reduce to the normal size after delivery

Operative Terms

S.No.	Terms	Meanings
1.	Cesarean section	Removal of the fetus through an insertion into uterus
2.	Classical	Incision into corpus uteri
3.	Lower uterine segment	Incision into lower segment of the uterus
4.	Cesarean hysterectomy	Delivery of the child by section followed by supravaginal or supracervical hysterectomy
5.	Vaginal hysterectomy	Removal of the uterus through the vagina
6.	Breech extraction	Method of delivery when the presenting parts are the buttock or feet of the fetus is pulled out
7.	Episiotomy	Incision of perineum to facilitate delivery and prevent perineal laceration
8.	Forceps operation	Instrumental delivery of child
	Low forceps	Application of forceps when head is on perineum
	High forceps	Application of forceps before head has passed though the pelvic inlet
	Mid forceps	Application of forceps when head is at level of ischial spine (hip bone)
9.	Saline abortion	Intra-amniotic insertion of hypertonic salt solution after 14 weeks of gestation to induce abortion
10.	Vacuum extraction	Application of vacuum extracted to assist delivery indicated in fetal
11.	Fetal distress	Life-threatening condition due to fetal anoxia, hemolytic disease or other causes

Symptomatic Terms

S.No.	Terms	Meanings
1.	Dilation of cervix	Gradual opening of the cervix to permit passage of fetus
2.	Dystocia	Difficult of birth
3.	Effacement	Complete closure of the cervix. The process of thinning and shortening of uterine cervix
4.	Engagement	Entrance of the fetal head through the pelvic inlet
5.	Engorgement	Excessive veins and lymph stasis of lactating breast usually refer to as caked breast
6.	Gestation	Pregnancy
7.	Hemorrhage	Excessive blood loss
8.	Antepartum	Before birth
9.	Intrapartum	During birth
10.	Postpartum	After birth
11.	Labor	Normal uterine contraction that results in the delivery of fetus
	Missed	A few contractions at full term then cessation of labor, and fetal retention
	Preterm	Before full term that is before 37 completed weeks of gestation

Contd...

Contd...

S.No.	Terms	Meanings
	Premature	Labor coming on between the seventh month of gestation and full term
	Protracted	(Prolonged labor) unduly prolonged labor
12.	Lochia	Discharge from the birth canal following delivery
13.	Pica	Peculiar craving of the pregnant women for strange food of non-edible nature
14.	Presentation or lie	Placing before
15.	Breech presentation	Presentation of the fetal buttocks
	complete breech	thigh flexed on abdomen and leg flexed on thigh
	footling	foot presents
	frankbreech	legs extended over ventral body surface
16.	Face presentation	Presentation of the fetal head
	brow	face or the forehead present
	sinciput	the large frontalial presence
	vertex	top of the head—the upper and back part of the head present
17.	Quickening	The pregnant women's first perception of fetal life
18.	Sterility	Infertility— reproductive failure

ANTENATAL

Origin of Terms

1. Amnion (G) = Membrane around fetus
2. Chorion (G) = Membrane around fetus
3. Teras (G) = Monster
4. Antigen (G/L) = Against begetting
5. Fetus (L) = Offspring
6. Toxico (G) = Poison

Anatomic Terms

S.No.	Terms	Meanings
1.	Amnion	The inner of the fetal membrane, a thin transparent sac which holds the fetus
2.	Amniotic fluid	Fluid in the amniotic sac
3.	Embryo	The product of conception, especially during the first three months of life
4.	Fetus	The unborn child after the first three months of development
5.	Chorion	An extraembryonic membrane which in early development form the outer wall of the blastocyst

Diagnostic Terms

S.No.	Terms	Meanings
1.	Abortus	Fetus that weight about 500 gm or less when expelled from the uterus and thus unable to survive
2.	Fetal anomaly	Malformed fetus caused by the mother taking teratogenic drug during pregnancy
3.	Fetal anoxia	Oxygen wants of the fetus that may result from prolapse of the cord, placenta abruptio, compression of the umblical vein or other causes. Death is inevitable if fetus is not delivered promptly
4.	Fetal hemolytic disease	Blood disorder caused by antibody antigen reaction in ABO, Rh or other blood group incompatibility
5.	Fetotoxicity	Toxic effects of the maternal medication on fetus and neonatal
6.	Prolapse of cord	Premature descent of the umblical cord because of fetal death

Terms Related to Special Procedure

S.No.	Terms	Meanings
1.	Amniocentesis	Puncture of the amniotic cavity
2.	Anti-D antibody injection	Preparation for passive or non active immunization Rh - negative mothers of Rh-positive babies administered intramuscularly
3.	Fetal electrocardiography	A method of detecting and recording electrical impulses of the fetal heart
4.	Fetal monitoring	Continuous recording of fetal heart rate
5.	Fetal phonocardiography	The findout of fetal heart sound by means of phonograph
6.	Fetal telemetry	A wireless radio transmission which provide remote records of the fetal electrocardiography or other data

NEONATAL PERIOD

Origin of Terms

1. Natus (L) = Birth
2. Neo (G) = New, recent
3. Neonate (L) = Newborn
4. Umblicus (L) = Naval

Diagnostic Terms

S.No.	Terms	Meanings
1.	Asphyxia neonatorum	Lack of oxygen in the blood of the newborn
2.	Atelectasis neonatorum	Failure of lungs to expand at brith
3.	Cerebral hemorrhage	Brain hemorrhage due to birth injury resulting in anoxia, cyanosis and convulsion

Contd...

Contd...

S.No.	Terms	Meanings
4.	Congenital stridors	Breathing disorder associated with a high pitched sound during first 3 weeks of life caused by malformation or abnormal position or functioning of trachea or vocal cord
5.	Cord hemorrhage	Bleeding from umbilical cord
6.	Down's syndrome	Chromosome abnormalities characterized by mental retardation and many physical features such as slanting eye, flat facial profile, thick fisher's tongue, protruding from open mouth, and broad neck
7.	Erythroblastosis fetalis	Hemolytic disease of the newborn
8.	Hydrocephalus	Abnormal fluid collection in the ventricle of the brain resulting in an enlargement of the head
9.	Hyperbilirubinemia	Abnormal high bilirubin content of the circulating blood of the newborn, it is also called as neonatal jaundice
10.	Meningocele	Meninges protruding through a defect in the spine or skull
11.	Ankyloglossia	Short frenulum linguae preventing neonate from taking feeding. It is also called as tongue tie
12.	Apgar score	Assessing a neonate's physical condition by evaluating his heart rate, respiratory effort, reflex irritability and skin color according to a scoring system
13.	Congenital	Born with a certain condition
14.	Meconium	Black stools of the newborn

COMMON ABBREVIATIONS

S.No.	Abbreviation	Term
1.	AB	Abortion
2.	ABD HYST	Abdominal hysterectomy
3.	AFP	Alphafetoprotein
4.	AGA	Appropriate for gestational age
5.	AN	Antenatal
6.	ANC	Antenatal clinic
7.	APH	Antepartum hemorrhage
8.	ARM	Artificial rupture of the membranes
9.	BBA	Born before arrival
10.	BBT	Basal body temperature
11.	BPD	Bipartial diamete
12.	BSO	Bilateral salpingo-oophorectomy
13.	BW	Birth weight
14.	C and D	Cystoscopy and dilatation
15.	CAV	Congenital absence of vagina
16.	CDC	Calculated day of confinement
17.	CPD	Cephalopelvic disproportion
18.	CS	Cesarian section
19.	CWP	Childbirth without pain

Contd...

Contd...

S.No.	Abbreviation	Term
20.	D and C	Dilation and curettage
21.	DES	Diethylstillbestrol
22.	DOB	Date of birth
23.	DOC	Date of confinement
24.	DUB	Dysfunctional uterine bleeding
25.	EDC	Estimated days of confinement
26.	EDC	Expected date of delivery
27.	FD	Forceps delivery
28.	FDIU	Fetal death *in utero*
29.	FECG	Fetal electrocardiogram
30.	FHR	Fetal heart rate
31.	FHT	Fetal heart tone
32.	FHT	Fetal heart tones
33.	FSH	Follicel stimulating hormone
34.	FTND	Full term normal delivery
35.	GC	Gonorrhea
36.	Gyn	Gynecology
37.	HBW	High birth weight
38.	HCG	Human chronic gonadotrophin
39.	HDN	Hemolytic disease of newborn
40.	HPL	Human placental lactogen
41.	HSG	Hystero salpingography
42.	IU	Intrauterine
43.	IUD	Intrauterine device
44.	IUFB	Intrauterine foreign body
45.	IUP	Intrauterine pressure
46.	LB	Live birth
47.	LBW	Low birth weight
48.	LH	Luteinizing hormone
49.	LMP	Last menstrual period
50.	LSCS	Lower segment cesarean section
51.	MFD	Mid forceps delivery
52.	MH	Marital history
53.	NB	Newborn
54.	NBW	Normal birth weight
55.	ND	Normal delivery
56.	NFTD	Normal full term delivery
57.	OB	Obstetric
58.	OBG	Obstetrics and gynecology
59.	OGN	Obstetric, gynecology and neonatal
60.	OH	Obstetric history
61.	Path	Pathology
62.	PET	Pre-eclamptic toxemia
63.	PID	Pelvic inflammatory disease
64.	PMB	Postmenopausal bleeding
65.	PMP	Previous menstrual period
66.	PN	Postnatal
67.	PPA Pos	Phenyl pyruvic acid positive
68.	PU	Pregnancy urine
69.	PV	Per vaginum (through the vaginum)
70.	ROM	Rupture of membrane
71.	Rh Neg	Rhesus factor negative
72.	Rh Pos	Rhesus factor positive

Contd...

Contd...

S.No.	Abbreviation	Term
73.	RM	Radical mastectomy
74.	RML	Right mediolateral
75.	SB	Stillbirth
76.	SD	Spontaneous delivery
77.	STOP	Suction termination of pregnancy
78.	SVD	Spontaneous vertex delivery
79.	TAH	Total abdominal hysterectomy
80.	TVH	Total vaginal hysterectomy
81.	TVP	Trans vesical prostatectomy
82.	UC	Uterine contraction
83.		Vertex presentation
a	LOA	Left occipitoanterior
b	LOP	Left occipitoposterior
c	LOT	Left occipitotransverse
d	ROA	Right occipitoanterior
e	ROP	Right occipitoposterior
f	ROT	Right occipitotransverse
84.		Face presentation
a	LMA	Left mentoanterior
b	LMP	Left mentoposterior
c	LMT	Left mentotransverse
d	RMA	Right mentoanterior
e	RMP	Right mentoposterior
f	RMT	Right mentotransverse
85.		Breech presentation
a	LSA	Left sacroanterior
b	LSP	Left sacroposterior
c	RSA	Right sacroanterior
d	RSP	Right sacroposterior
86.		Transverse presentation
a	LScA	Left scapula anterior
b	LSCcP	Left scapula posterior
c	RScA	Right scapula anterior
d	RScP	Right scapula posterior

12

Oncology

INTRODUCTION

Oncology is the study of tumors. Unrestrained and excessive multiplication of body cells producing lump or swelling, known as tumor or neoplasm. The neoplasm may be either benign or malignant. Malignant tumors or neoplasm accumulate as growth, which penetrate, compress and ultimately destroy the surrounding normal tissue. The malignant cells from the primary tumor site find their way into lymph channels or blood vessels and are carried to remote body structures by which secondary malignant neoplasm develop. This is called metastasis. Benign neoplasms are new growths that develop in body tissues. They are composed of the same type of cells as the tissue in which they are growing. When they grow bigger in size, then they harm the place by exerting pressure on surrounding structures. In general, benign tumors are not life-threatening, once they are removed they usually do not reoccur.

DIFFERENCES BETWEEN THE MALIGNANT AND BENIGN NEOPLASM

See Table 12.1.

CARCINOMAS

Carcinomas, the largest group, are solid tumors, which are derived from epithelial tissue. Epithelial tissue is found on external and internal body surfaces, including skin, glands, digestive, urinary and reproductive organs. Almost all-malignant neoplasm are carcinomas.

Table 12.1: Differences between the malignant and benign neoplasm

S.No.	Malignant	Benign
1.	Rapid growth could be seen	Grows slowly
2.	Invasive and infiltrative	Encapsulated
3.	Composed of tissue that does not resemble the tissue in which the neoplasm arises	Composed of highly organized and specialized tissue, that closely resembles the tissue in which the neoplasm arises
4.	If left untreated, establish a new tumor site by infiltrating through blood and lymphatic vessels in the remote regions of the body	Does not spread to remote areas to form a secondary tumor
5.	If left untreated, poses a risk to the patient	Generally poses little risk, if any, to the patient

SARCOMAS

Sarcomas are a rare type of cancer when compared to carcinomas and are derived from supportive and connective tissue, such as bone, fat, muscle, cartilage, bone marrow, and lymphatic tissue, or from blood cells. Sarcomas account approximately 10 percent of all malignant neoplasm.

MIXED TISSUE TUMORS

Mixed tissue tumors are derived from tissue, which is capable of differentiating into epithelial as well as connective tissue. The tumors are thus composed of several different types of cells. Examples are: mixed tissue tumors can be found in kidney, ovaries and testes.

STAGING

Staging is an attempt to define the extent of cancer by classifying it into three categories: T, N, and M. T represents the primary tumor site or place of origin; N represents local or regional node involvement; and M indicates whether metastasis is there or not. When the primary site contains classifications of T_1, T_2, T_3 or T_4, the higher number indicate progressive increases in tumor size and involvement. Similarly N_0, N_1, N_2, or N_3, represent progressively advancing nodular involvement. Finally, M_0, or M+ defines absence or presence of metastasis, respectively (Table 12.2).

Table 12.2: Staging

	T	Primary tumor
	N	Regional lymph nodes
	M	Distant metastasis
Tumor		
	T_0	No evidence of primary tumor
	TIS	Carcinoma *in situ*
	T_1, T_2, T_3, T_4	Progressive increase in tumor size and involvement
	T_X	Tumor cannot be assessed
Nodes		
	N_0	Regional lymph nodes not demonstrably abnormal
	N_1, N_2, N_3, etc.	Increasing degrees of demonstrable abnormality of regional lymph nodes
	N_X	Regional lymph nodes cannot be assessed clinically
Metastasis		
	M_0	No evidence of distant metastasis
	M_1, M_2, M_3	Ascending degrees of distant metastasis, including metastasis to distant lymph nodes
		TNM assignments may be grouped into small number of stages

GRADING

Grading is concerned with the microscopic appearance of the tumor cells, in other words, the degree of anaplasia. Generally, four grades are employed, which are numbered from 1 through 4. Neoplasms that are composed of cells that closely resemble the tissue from which they arise are given a grade 1 rating. The tissue demonstrates a minimum amount of anaplasia. Patients with grade 1 tumors have high survival rate, while patients with grades 2, 3, and 4 tumors, have a poorer survival rate. At the other extreme is grade 4, in which there is a great deal of anaplasia within the tumor. Such tumors are more serious and the prognosis is very poor. Grades 2 and 3 are intermediate grades between these two extremes.

CANCER TREATMENT

Cancer is treated by three major approaches namely, surgery, radiation therapy and chemotherapy.

SURGERY

The surgery is performed when the tumor is localized, and gets the effective means of cure. Some common cancers in which surgery may be curative are, those of the stomach, large bowel, breasts and endometrium, especially the accessory organs of the system.

RADIATION THERAPY

The goal of the radiation therapy is to deliver a maximal dose of ionizing radiation to the tumor tissue and a minimal dose to the surrounding normal tissue. In reality, this goal is difficult to obtain and usually one accepts a degree of residual normal cell damage as a sequel to the destruction of the tumor. The effect of high-dose radiation to cells is to produce damage to DNA and thus inhibit cell replication and growth.

CHEMOTHERAPY

Chemotherapy is the treatment of cancer using drugs. It is probably the most important factor responsible for long-term survival in several types of cancer. Chemotherapy may be used alone or in combination with surgery and radiation.

ONCOLOGY

Origin of Terms

S.No.	Terms	Meanings	S.No.	Terms	Meanings
1.	Ana-	Backward, up	20.	Mut/a	Genetic change
2.	Astro	Start	21.	Ne/o	New, recent
3.	Benign	Mild	22.	Onco	Mass
4.	Blasto	Embryonic	23.	Papil/o	Elevation
5.	Carcin/o, oma	Tumor	24.	Plakia	Plate
6.	Cauter/o	Heat, burn	25.	-plasia, -plasm	Formation, growth, development
7.	Chem/o Pharmacy/o	Chemical, drug	26.	-plasm	Formation
8.	Cirrh/o	Hard	27.	Ple/o	Many, more
9.	Cry/o	Cold	28.	Polyp/o	Polyps; small growths
10.	Cyst/o	Bladder, sac of fluid	29.	proliferate	To bear offspring
11.	Ependyma	Wrap	30.	Radi/o	Rays, X-rays
12.	Epi-	Upon	31.	Rhabdomy/o	Striated muscle
13.	Follicul/o	Small sac	32.	Sarco	Flesh
14.	Glia	Glue	33.	-stasis	Control, stop, stand still
15.	Kerato	Horny	34.	Terat/o	Monster, malformed fetus
16.	Leiomy/o	Smooth muscle	35.	-therapy	Treatment
17.	Malignant	of bad kind	36.	Therm/o	Heat
18.	Medulla	Marrow	37.	Tox/o	Poison
19.	Meta-	Beyond, change	38.	Tumor	Swelling

Symptomatic and Diagnostic Terms

S.No.	Terms	Meanings
1.	Adenocarcinoma	Malignancy arising from glandular structure
2.	Adenomyosis	A benign condition characterized by growth of the endometrium
3.	Angiokeratoma	Warty growth in groups
4.	Angiolipoma	Benign blood vessel tumor containing fatty tissue
5.	Angioscotoma	A defect in the visual field caused by the shadow of the retinal blood vessels
6.	Astrocytoma	Tumor of the brain or spinal cord composed of astrocytes
7.	Basal cell carcinoma	Skin cancer, malignant tumor arising from skin cells
8.	Carcinoma	Malignant new growth from epithelial cells
9.	Cementoma	Mass of cementum lying free at apex of tooth, probably a reaction to injury
10.	Cholesteatoma	Cyst-like mass commonly occurring in the middle ear and mastoid region
11.	Chondrosarcoma	Sarcoma of the cartilage tissue
12.	Fibrosarcoma	Sarcoma containing connective tissue
13.	Fungating	Mushrooming pattern of growth in which tumor cells pile on top of another and project from a tissue surface
14.	Dermatofibroma	A fibrous tumor-like nodule of the skin
15.	Glioblastoma	Tumor usually of cerebral hemispheres composed of spongioblasts, astroblasts and astrocytes
16.	Glioma	Sarcoma of neurological origin
17.	Hemangioma	Tumor composed of dilated blood vessels usually birth marks
18.	Hematoma	Localized internal collection of blood that sometimes occurs after injury or operation
19.	Hepatoma	Tumor of the liver
20.	Hodgkin's disease	Solid tumor of the lymphatic system
21.	Kaposi's sarcoma	Malignant disease chiefly involved in the skin seen in some patients with AIDS
22.	Keratocanthoma	Benign popular lesion usually on the face
23.	Lymphangioma	Tumor composed of new lymph spaces and channels
24.	Lymphoma	Any neoplastic disorder of the lymphoid tissue
25.	Leukemia	Malignant disease of blood forming organs (spleen, lymphatic system and bone marrow) marked by abnormal increase of WBC
26.	Leukoplakia	Formation of white patches on the mucous membranes of the cheek and tongue
27.	Malignant melanoma	Malignant, dark pigmented tumor or mole of the skin
28.	Mastocytoma	A benign aggregation of mast cells forming a nodular tumor
29.	Metastasis	Spreading of cancer cells from one part of the body to another. The plural is metastasis

Contd...

Contd...

S.No.	Terms	Meanings
30.	Melanoma	Dark mole like tumor
31.	Mycetoma	Chronic disease caused by one of a variety of fungi affecting usually hands, neck and feet
32.	Myeloma	Tumor formed of cells found in the bone marrow
33.	Mucinous	Filled with mucus, thick sticky fluid
34.	Non-Hodgkin's lymphoma	Malignant, solid tumors of the lymphatic tissue
35.	Neuroma	Tumor of nerve cells and fibers
36.	Papilloma	Benign tumor derived from epithelium
37.	Pilomatrixoma	A benign calcifying epithelial neoplasm derived from hair and matrix cells
38.	Retinoblastoma	Malignant tumor arising from retinal cells
39.	Scotoma	An area of depressed vision with the visual field surrounded by an area of normal or less depressed vision
40.	Syringocystadenoma	Adenoma of the sweat glands
41.	Xanthoma	A papule, nodule or plaque in the skin due to lipid deposit
42.	Diffuse	Spreading evenly throughout the affected tissue
43.	Dysplastic	Pertaining to abnormal formation of cell
44.	Epidermoid	Resembling squamous epithelial cells (respiratory tract)
45.	Follicular	Forming small microscopic gland type sacs (thyroid gland)
46.	Necrotic	Containing dead tissue
47.	Nodular	A small node or mass, which is solid and can be detected by touch
48.	Papillary	Forming small finger-like/nipple-like projection of cells
49.	Polypoid	Growths that are like projections extending outward from the base
50.	Scirrhous	Densely packed tumors overgrown with fibrous tissues
51.	Serous	Filled with thin water/fluid
52.	Sessile	Polypoid tumors extend from a broad base
53.	Trachoma	Chronic infectious disease of the congestive and cornea
54.	Ulcerating	Characterized by open, exposed surface resulting from death of overlying tissue
55.	Undifferentiated	Lacking microscopic structures typical of normal mature cells
56.	Verrucous	Resembling a wart like growth (cheeks)

13 | Psychiatry

INTRODUCTION

The branch of medicine, which deals with study, treatment and prevention of mental illness. Madness is different from psychiatry. A psychiatric condition, if untreated, may develop into insane condition, which may become madness.

Psychotherapy is the treatment of emotional problems by psychological techniques. There are different techniques involved in psychotherapy, they are:

S.No.	Types	Explanation
1.	Behavior therapy	Conditioning the primary feelings of the patients
2.	Group therapy	Patients are educated through group discussions in front of invited audience
3.	Sex therapy	Mainly deals with solving psychosexual disorders such as frigidity, impotence, and premature ejaculation
4.	Family therapy	This deals with the common problems of a family
5.	Psychoanalysis	This is a long-term form of psychotherapy, to resolve internal conflicts, by allowing the patients, to bring their unconscious emotions, such as free association, and transference (recollecting the early past incidence)
6.	Hypnosis	Therapy by recovery of deeply repressed memories
7.	Play therapy	Therapy given to children through toys, and plays to express conflicts, and feelings, which he or she is unable to communicate directly
8.	Electroshock therapy	Treatment applied to the brain by producing convulsions, through electric current, chiefly for severe depressions
9.	Drug therapy	Treatment by drugs such as antianxiety agents (diazepam), antipsychotic tranquilizers (chlorpromazine), lithium, anti-depressants, etc.

PSYCHIATRY DISORDERS

Affective Disorders

Disorder of mood, e.g. manic depressive illness, major depressions, etc. Manic depressive illness is characterized by alternating moods of mania such as excitement, activity, exalted feelings and decreased in need for sleep. Major depression, involves, severe, dysphoric mood like sadness, hopelessness, irritability and worry, etc.

Anxiety Disorders

These disorders are characterized by the experience of unpleasant tension, distress, and troubled feelings, like phobias and anxiety states.

Somatoform Disorders

These disorders in which the patient's mental conflicts, are expressed as physical symptoms, like abdominal pain, nausea, vomiting, chest pain, loss of functions in parts of body (difficulty in swallowing), loss of voice, deafness, etc. In conversion disorders (hysterical neurosis), the patient usually has a feared but unconscious conflict, which threatens to escape from repression. Hypochondriosis, is a somatoform disorders, in which the patient has preoccupation, with body pains, and discomforts.

Disassociate Disorders (Hysterical Neurosis)

The symptoms of this disorder are psychogenic amnesia and multiple personality. This disorder is characterized by inability to remember important personal information, unexpected travel away from home or work (with amnesia).

Psychosexual Disorders

These disorders includes sexual perversion, in which the patient's psychological sexual identity from his or her gender identity.

Transvestism

Dressing in the clothes of opposite sex.

Exhibitionism

Compulsive need to expose one's genitals.

Sexual Masochism

Achievement of sexual pleasure from suffering.

Transsexualism

Desire to change anatomic sexual characteristics, stemming from the fixed conviction that one is a member of the opposite sex. Such a person often seeks medical and surgical treatment to bring their anatomy into conformity with their belief.

Fetishism

Achieving sexual gratification by substituting an inanimate object for a human love object.

Voyeurism

An abnormal desire, to look at sexual organs or acts.

Sexual Sadism

Achievement of sexual pleasure, by inflicting physical or psychological pain.

Personality Disorders

These are behavioral disorders acceptable to the individuals, but produce, conflict with others who interact with the same individuals.

Antisocial

No loyalty or concern for others and without moral standards.

Passive Aggression

Showing aggressive feelings in passive ways, such as stubbornness, helplessness, etc.

Histrionic

Emotional immaturity, and dependent having general dissatisfaction with themselves and angry feelings about the world.

Narcissistic

Pompous sense of self-importance, and preoccupation, with the fantasy of success and power.

Paranoid

Pervasive, suspiciousness, and mistrust of people, jealous and quick to take offence.

Delirium

Mental disturbances associated with illness characterized by mental cloudiness, and visual hallucinations.

Dementia

Characterized by loss of memory and intelligence. The most common is Senile Dementia.

Schizophrenic Disorders

This is a major psychotic disorder characterized by withdrawal from reality into inner world of disorganized thinking and feeling. Symptoms are bizarre delusions, auditory hallucinations, hearing imaginary voices, and incoherent speech.

Paranoic Disorders

In this disorder, patient will have persistent delusions or persecution and jealousy.

Chronic Alcoholism

Addition to alcohol consumption, may present psychological symptoms such as hallucinations, amnesia, with physical ailments, such as cirrhosis of liver, and brain damage. Patient will be unable to remember and resorts to confabulation (lying).

Drug Dependence (Substance Induced Disorders)

Diseases due to addiction to drugs like opioids (heroin, morphine, etc.), sedatives (barbiturates, diazepam, etc.), cocaine and hallucinogen-type drugs.

PSYCHIATRIC DISORDERS

Origin of Terms

S.No.	Terms	Meanings	S.No.	Terms	Meanings
1.	Dement	Unsound mind	2.	Catatonia	Stupor
3.	Hallucinate	To wander in mind	4.	Dynamo	Power
5.	Ment	Mind	6.	Mania	Madness
7.	Psyche	Soul, mind	8.	Phren	Mind
9.	Schizo	Split	10.	Psychedelic	Mind manifesting
11.	Soma	Body			

General Terms

S.No.	Terms	Meanings
1.	Commitment	Legal consignment of a mentally unsound patient to an institution for treatment
2.	Descriptive psychiatry	Psychiatry based on clinical patterns, symptoms and classification (branch of treatment and thinking and emotions)
3.	Dynamic psychiatry	Study of emotional process their origin and mental mechanisms under lying them. Study of behavior, activeness, motivation, etc. Dynamic principles convey concept of change of evaluation and progression or regression (act of moving)
4.	Ego	Acting of reality, principles, ethics, morality consciousness
5.	Mental health	Activity to get along with proper satisfaction of living, achievement and level of maturity attained and flexibility
6.	Orthopsychiatry	Deals with mental and emotional development of child psychiatry and mental hygiene "preventive aspects of psychiatry"
7.	Psychiatry	Study, treatment and prevention of mental illness
8.	Psychodynamics	The science of mental process in the prediction and recognition of unconsciousness in human behavior
9.	Psychometry	The testing and measuring of mental and psychologic ability, efficiency and potentials

Diagnostic Terms

S.No.	Terms	Meanings
1.	Mental retardation, Mental deficiency	Abnormal low intellectual functioning from birth of childhood with impairment of maturation and social adjustment
2.	Neurosis (Pl: neuroses)	Mental disorders based on basic sense of reality and changed condition of fear after any cause
3.	Anxiety neurosis	Condition of fear without any cause
4.	Hysterical neurosis	Physical symptoms instrumental basis caused by emotional factor

Contd...

Contd...

S.No.	Terms	Meanings
5.	Traumatic neurosis	Functional nervous emotions following accidents
6.	Personality disorder	Mental disorder associated with physical cause and nonpsychotic alcohol addiction
7.	Alcohol addiction	Unconditional desire for alcoholic beverages
8.	Psychophysiologic disorder	A mental disorder in which physical symptoms are presumed to be of psychogenic origin. Examples irritable colon, mucous conditions, heart burn, peptic ulcer, blood pressure, etc.
9.	Psychosis (Pl: psychoses)	Major mental disorder of organic or emotional origin
10.	Presenile dementia	Dementia of unknown origin. Cortical brain syndrome, at the beginning of middle-age and below
11.	Senile dementia	Mental deterioration in old age also with organic brain changes due to brain atrophying
12.	Schizophrenia	Severe mental disorder of psychotic depth marked by disturbances in behavior, mood and ability to think. Altered concept formation may lead to a distortion or reality, delusions, and hallucinations, which tend to be self protective. Emotional disharmony and bizarre regressive behavior are frequently present

Symptomatic Terms

S.No.	Terms	Meanings
1.	Agitation	Exceeding restlessness, associate mental distress
2.	Ambivalence	A simultaneous existence of conflicting attitude
3.	Amnesia	Loss of memory, inability to remember
4.	Anaclitic	Depending on some thing
5.	Autism	Form of thinking that seeks to satisfy unfulfilled desires but completely disregards reality factors
6.	Blocking	A mental condition in which the patient expresses himself with difficulty (seen in schizophrenia)
7.	Body image	The conscious and unconscious picture of the person of his own body at any movement variation from person to person
8.	Catalepsy	Diminished responsiveness usually characterized by trancelike states. May occur in organic or psychologic disorders or under hypnosis
9.	Catharsis	Expression and discharge of repressed emotions and ideas
10.	Circumstantially	The mental symptom marked by the inclusion of details in conversation either related or unrelated to the main subject
11.	Confabulation	Fabrication of stories in response to questions about situations or events that are not recalled
12.	Cyclothymic	The temperament caused by cyclic alternatives between elevations and depressions

Contd...

Contd...

S.No.	Terms	Meanings
13.	Delirium	The mental interbalance marked by illusions hallucinations and unsystematized delusion excitement restlessness, etc. usually reflects toxic state
14.	Dementia	Organic loss of intellectual function
15.	Depersonalization	Loss of sense of personal identity
16.	Delusions	False beliefs which cannot be corrected by reasonism
17.	Empathy	Sharing with others feelings not because of sympathy but because of emotions
18.	Hallucinations	False sensory perceptions without actual external stimulation
19.	Illusions	False interpretation of real sensory image
20.	Incoherence in speech	Talking without proper sequence
21.	Libido	A psychoanalytic term denoting the psychic drive that energizes living
22.	Malingering	Pretending only having illness or symptoms to avoid unpleasant situation or perusal gains
23.	Mental mechanism	An unconscious and indirect manner of gratifying a repressed desire
24.	Phobia	Morbid fear
25.	Sensory deprivation	Loss of sensory powers because of loneliness. Traveling space which leads to depression, panic delusions, hallucination, etc.
26.	Hysteria	A psychoneurosis condition characterized by lack of control over acts and emotions
27.	Conversion reaction	The conversion type of hysterical neurosis
28.	Schizophrenia	Severe emotional disorder, usually of psychotic proportions, characterized by misinterpretation and retreat from reality, delusions, hallucinations, bizarre or regressive behavior
29.	Depression	A psychiatric syndrome consisting of dejected mood, psychomotor retardation, guilty feelings, weight loss, etc.
30.	Anxiety	A feeling of apprehension, uncertainty and fear associated with physiological changes like increased heart beats, sweating, tremor, etc.
31.	Personality disorder	Mental disorder which stems from the personality of the individual and in which there is minimal feeling of subjective anxiety or no feeling of distress
32.	Psychosomatic disorder	Group of disorders characterized by physical symptoms and demonstrable physiological changes in which emotional factors are believed to play a major etiologic or pathogenic role
33.	Perversion	Sexual deviation, turning aside from the normal course
34.	Mental retardation	Subnormal general intellectual development, originating during the developmental period, and associated with impairment of either learning and social adjustment or maturation or both

14

Medical (History and Physical) Examination and Diagnostic Technique

INTRODUCTION

The term diagnosis (from Greek diagignosko "to judge, discriminate") has several closely related meanings in medicine, which few of us take the trouble to distinguish in practice. Diagnosis means, first, the intellectual process of analyzing, identifying, or explaining a disease. Diagnosis forms the subject matter of the branch of medicine called physical diagnosis. Secondly, in a somewhat more concrete sense, diagnosis means the explanation proposed for a given patient's problems. Thus, we speak of "arriving at a diagnosis" or of "making a tentative diagnosis of pancreatitis". Thirdly diagnosis is often used synonymously with disease or the name of a particular disease: " The diagnosis is multiple sclerosis." "Patients with this diagnosis often progress to renal failure."

Most of the errors in classification and naming arise from peculiarities in the phenomena of disease, which is due to gaps in our knowledge, limitations of language itself and the difficulty of altering a system of terminology that is classified in thousands of books and used daily by hundreds of thousands of professionals. With all their shortcomings, our current systems of classifying and naming diseases at least have the pragmatic justification that they "work"-in medical field, in the compilation of records and statistics, and in clinical practice.

Few physicians are logicians, much less philosophers. The "logic" of physical diagnosis is a rough-and-ready deductive process learned largely through imitation and experience. It's goal is the formulation of a diagnosis, which will enable the physician to get on with the business of instituting rational treatment.

The method of the medical diagnostics is an empirical one based upon a few elementary techniques and a "memory bank" of diseases and symptoms. A medical student learns not only the characteristic features of hundreds of diseases but also possible causes for each of the hundreds of diseases and causes for each of the hundreds of symptoms. By combining these two bodies of information into one, so to speak, vertical and the other horizontal—he learns to determine the most likely cause or causes for a given set of complaints or abnormalities. Starting with a specific problem like chest pain/fever/loss of appetite/ inability to urinate, the physician considers the full range of diagnostic possibilities (called, in professional jargon, the "different diagnosis") raised by the problem.

In the first place, the physician must distinguish normal and abnormal, often a Herculean task. He must also establish an accurate chronology of symptoms and events prior to the time when he became involved in the case, work out cause-and-effect relationships, and exclude irrelevant data (red herrings) from consideration.

The ability to recognize and identify patterns and complex assemblages of historical and observed facts-in what seems to be a single, intuitive act of the mind. Such mental shortcuts can greatly simplify diagnosis but unfortunately they often yield wrong answers.

The techniques used by the physician to groups data for a diagnosis are embodied in the two procedures known as history and physical examination. The history is the patient's own account of his experiences and observations of his illness—his symptoms—elicited by careful, methodical questioning. Physical examination is the process whereby the physician seeks and observes objective changes and abnormalities— the signs of illness. It is not generally appreciated by laypersons that in a typical case, a skillfully obtained history supplies both a larger number of diagnostic clues and more useful and specific ones that of the physical examination.

By convention, the term physical examination includes only those procedures performed directly by the physician relying on his own senses, with the aid of few simple, hand-held instruments. Although X-ray and laboratory studies, electrocardiography and electromyo- graphy, various kinds of scans, or other elaborate techniques may be absolutely essential to a precise and accurate diagnosis, they are not considered as a part of the physical examination.

The scope and nature of the history and physical examination depend on several variables. The patient's complaints give direction and focus to both history taking and examination. The physician's field of specia- lization often determines the type and extent of diagnostic maneuvers he employs. The setting of the examination spot-doctor's office or clinic, hospital emergency room, intensive care unit, or the patient's home- will have a bearing on what is done and not done. The patient's condition-whether alert, confused, belligerent, or unconscious-will influence the type of history that can be obtained and the degree of co- operation that can be enlisted during examination. Much may depend on formally established, quasi-legal requirements—forms to be filled out for a prospective employer or insurer, or hospital staff bylaws to be complied with.

The standard outline of history and physical examination is as follows:

History
- Chief complaint
- History of present illness
- Family history
- Social history
- Habits/addictions.

Past medical history
- General
- Review of systems
  - Head, eyes, ears, nose, throat, mouth, teeth
  - Cardiovascular
  - Respiratory
  - Gastrointestinal
  - Genitourinary
  - Neuromuscular
  - Psychiatric
  - Skin
- Physical examination
  - General appearance
  - Skin
  - Head, face, neck
  - Eyes
  - Ears
  - Nose, mouth, throat, teeth
  - Thorax, breasts, axillae
  - Heart
  - Lungs
  - Abdomen, groins, rectum, anus, genitalia
  - Back and extremities
  - Neurologic
  - Formal mental status (psychiatric).

GENERAL REMARKS ON THE HISTORY

As a rule, the physician compiles the medical history by questioning the patient himself. A physician should not invite specific answers.

The volume and validity of information obtained through history taking are limited by the informant's memory, intelligence, and ability and willingness to communicate. The answer to a dozen questions may be consolidated into a single telling phrase. The physician often translates the patient's statements into medical jargon, e.g. " I vomited five times" becomes, " he experienced emesis five times". As mentioned earlier, the physician often translates the patient statements into medical jargon. The physician explores its impact, intensity, onset, duration, intermittency, location and radiation, as well as any aggravating or alleviating factors, prior episodes of similar pain, and associated symptoms. The way in which this information presented is assembled can be seen in the following fictitious interview between a physician at a neighborhood clinic:

Location of pain	Physician: Mr. Salim, can you show me where your pain is right now? Patient: It is right here (He points to the left side of his chest, just above the nipple) Physician: Does it cover a pretty wide area or is it always right at the spot ? Patient: Always right here. Physician: Does not ever bother you anywhere else in your chest?
Radiation	Physician: Or seem to move or spread out from there, into your neck, shoulder, or arm; on either side ? Patient: Has not so far Physician: Never seems to bore through to your back ? Patient: No.
Duration	Physician: And when did this pain start ? Patient: I noticed it a little bit on sunday night before I went to bed.
Onset	Physician: Did come on little slowly or all of a sudden ? Patient: Just built up slowly sunday night Physician: What were you doing when you first noticed it ? Patient: Reading the paper, I guess. I watched TV a little, too. Physician: Anyway you were sitting down, not exerting yourself ? Patient: No.
Intermittency	Physician: Now, has the pain been there ever since it started or does it come and go ? Patient: It stays pretty steady. Of course, I do not notice it when I'm asleep.
Intensity	Physician: It has not kept you awake ? Patient: No Physician: Has it been really severe at any time ? Patient: I would not say real severe. I notice it pretty much all the time during the day, but I worked yesterday and today without any trouble.
Quality	Physician: How would you describe the pain? Is it sharp, like a knife stuck in your chest, or dull ? Patient: It is not sharp. Just like a pressure, maybe. Physician: Not burning ? Patient: No, not really.
Aggravating	Physician: Does it get worse when you take a deep breath, or cough, or move that left arm, or get in certain positions ? Patient: No, it stays pretty much the same. Physician: Does eating have any effect on it ? Patient: Not that I have noticed. Been eating well.

Contd...

Alleviating factors	Physician: Is there anything that makes it better lying down, or holding your breath? Patient: Seems like if I can burp it feels better for a few minutes. Physician: Did you take anything for it? Patient: No. My wife wanted me to take some of her ulcer medicine but I thought I better have you to check it out first.
Associated symptoms	Physician: Have you had anything else along with this pain-any shortness of breath, coughing, sweating? Patient: No. Physician: And you say your appetite is okay? Patient: My appetite's fine. Too good. Physician: Bowels moving okay? Patient: Okay for me. Physician: Do you take any medicine regularly ? Laxatives, vitamins, and prescription medicine? Patient: No Physician: You mentioned burping. Have you had a lot of burping or gas release lately? Patient: Yes, just since Sunday.
Prior episodes	Physician: Did you ever have anything like this before ? Patient: I had a pain like this about seven or eight years ago when we used to go to Dr Johnson. He said it was indigestion. Physician: This seems exactly the same ? Patient: Pretty much.
Inciting factors	Physician: Did you eat anything unusual on Saturday or Sunday ? Patient: We went to a steak house Saturday night and I had one of those things with all the mushrooms and onions on top. Physician: Has the particular kind of food bothered you before? Patient: Onions always do.

Chief Complaint and History of Present Illness

Some physicians prefer to state the chief complaint exactly in the patient's words ("I cannot sleep", "My left arm is numb"), while others strive for maximum conciseness and precision ("insomnia", "hyperesthesia of the dorsum of the left forearm"). Often the statement of the chief complaint includes an indication of its duration or other features: "Intermittent pain and pressure in the epigastrium for one week". Sometimes several apparently related complaints are mentioned together: "Fever, vomiting, diarrhea, and severe headache." Even when the patient himself cannot give any history, the heading "chief complaint" is still used: "Sudden loss of consciousness at home and deepening coma."

The history of the present illness is the heart of the medical history, for it contains all historical details leading up to and in any way pertaining to the patient's current status. If, for example, a patient is hospitalized for pneumonia, the history of present illness might include mention of his smoking habits, current medicines, previous treatments or hospitalizations for respiratory disease, and all negative and positive answers to questions.

By convention, the physician starts with a brief description of the patient, including age and sex and often race and social status. He then records the date (or time) and nature of onset of the first symptoms and traces the progress of the illness—the appearance of additional symptoms, their effect on the patient's lifestyle and well-being, and the results of treatment, physician-prescribed or otherwise-finally reporting the events that prompted the present consultation or hospitalization.

Family History

The importance of the family history lies in the fact that many developmental abnormalities, disease and tendencies to disease are not only hereditary (genetically transmitted from parent to child) but familial (occurring in some or all members of family).

The complete family history includes the age and state of health of each member of the patient's immediate family (parents, siblings, and children), selected data about other blood relatives, and a general statement regarding family history of certain conditions. Irrelevant, and sometimes it is omitted altogether.

Social History

This part of the history includes any personal information about the patient's past or present life, which, though non-medical, may have a bearing on his health. The ideal social history would include data on the patient's birth, upbringing, academic career, marital history and present status, spouse's health history, military service, occupational past and present, avocations and hobbies, social and cultural pursuits, political and religious activities, foreign travel or residence, financial status, police record, and current family structure, living arrangements, and personal responsibilities.

Hence the social history is often omitted, a brief note of the patient's age, marital status, and occupation having been inserted in the history of present illness. Other elements of the social history may also appear in the history of present illness.

Habits

Under this heading comes information about the patient's lifestyle, specifically his regular or customary practices with respect to eating, sleeping, exercise, recreation, and the use of prescribed or non-prescribed, medicines, caffeine, nicotine, alcohol, and other substances of abuse.

Dietary habits need to be investigated if the patient has a weight problem or digestive tract symptoms. A full dietary history covers the number of meals taken daily; regularity of mealtimes; circumstances of eating; composition and balance of meals as to fats, carbohydrates, and proteins; any self-imposed dietary restrictions (fat or weight-reduction diets, religious, abstinence, vegetarianism); snacking and fasting practices; weight history; use of dietary supplements, health foods, and vitamins; and an estimation of average daily caloric intake.

The sleep habits includes hours of sleep each night, ease of falling, asleep, tendency to awaken during the night, deepness of sleep, use of sleep inducing medicines, daytime napping, nightmares, and sleep-walking.

It is desirable to compile, as a part of every patient's history, a complete list of all medicines presently being taken, including ointments, eye or nasal drops, and popular or over the counter (OTC) medicines and medicines taken irregularly for specific indications. Patients are often unable to tell the names or purposes of medicines prescribed for them by physicians. A satisfactory record of medicine used should include the name-preferably the generic name of each medicine, the dosage form, strength, frequency and duration of use, and the purpose for which it was prescribed.

PAST MEDICAL HISTORY: GENERAL

The past medical history provides a concluding survey of all medical information not covered in any previous section of the history. The inclusion of material here implies that it is considered irrelevant to the history of present illness. Hence, the past medical history may be run through, or at least recorded, in perfunctory fashion, and may consist largely of negatives.

History reports past episodes or attacks of clearly defined, named diseases. When asked to recall all prior illnesses, most of us perform poorly. The physician's customary strategy is to listen ten to twenty common, serious diseases (diabetes, tuberculosis, asthma, pneumonia, high blood pressure, heart attack or heart disease, stroke, epilepsy, ulcer, cancer, anemia, arthritis, kidney disease, nervous or mental disease) and ask the patient if he has ever had any of them. An affirmative answer prompts inquiries about dates, severity, treatment, complications, or sequel. Physicians sometimes ask about the hospitalizations rather than about illnesses, and it yields a better return. Often the patient's recollections must be supplemented or corrected by reference to written records. The frequency with which "old" hospital charts and medical files, when they can be obtained, supply crucial historical data shall give all health professionals continued motivation to keep full and accurate records.

Injuries

To the physician, the terms injury and trauma suggest a broader range of probabilities than they do to the average lay person. For the purposes of this part of the history, the term is limited to serious injuries—fractures, dislocations, severe sprains and strains, open wounds or burns leading to scarring or deformity, loss of a body part, significant damage to internal organs, or impairment of function-resulting from falls, road traffic accidents, industrial injuries, military operations and criminal violence.

Surgical Operations

Even the most minor surgical procedure can result in changes of structure or function or both that are later mistaken for signs of disease. They also tend to forget childhood procedures (tonsillectomy, herniorrhaphy) or very minor ones (laparoscopy, arthroscopy, vasectomy) when asked point blank about any surgical operations.

Chronic Diseases and Disabilities

Chronic disabilities such as diabetes, hypertension, rheumatoid arthritis, coronary artery disease, and schizophrenia are more likely to receive attention here than acute illnesses which may well prove to be related to or part of the history or present illness. Significant functional impairments such as blindness, paralysis, absence of a limb, confinement to bed or wheelchair should also be recorded.

Allergies

Any prior history of allergy or sensitivity, especially to medicines, should be a part of the patient's written records. Usually such information is prominently displayed on the front of a hospital chart or medical record to prevent inadvertent administration or prescription of a medicine to which the patient has had an untoward response.

Immunizations

Routine childhood immunizations must usually be taken for granted unless written records are available.

Review of Systems

Head, eyes, ears, nose, throat, mouth, teeth.

Head

The head is not a system but an anatomic region. In this part of the history the physician records any diseases or injuries of the scalp, skull, and brain and any significant history of headaches. Alternatively, conditions, affecting the brain may be taken up in the neurologic history, and disorders of the hair and scalp recorded as skin conditions. The organs of special sense (eyes and ears, including balance centers), the upper respiratory tract (nose, sinuses, pharynx), and the mouth and teeth are treated as separate.

Full details of any significant head injury such as concussion, skull fracture, should be included in the past medical history irrespective of how the old injuries had happened.

Eyes

A thorough review of ocular history elicits information about past or present symptoms such as blurring of vision, double vision, partial or complete loss of vision, difficult of near adaptation, seeing spots or flashes, seeing halos or rings around lights, undue visual impairment with reduced illumination, pain in, on or behind the eyeball, redness, discharge, watering, abnormal sensitivity to light, swelling, drooping, itching, or crusting of lids, as well as full details about the use of glasses or contact lenses and the date of the most recent eye examination. Eye symptoms can indicate neurologic or systemic condition rather than purely local disease.

Ears

The examiner inquires about the duration, degree and pitch range of hearing loss in one or both ears; ringing, popping, or other abnormal sounds heard by the patient; pain, pressure, itching, swelling, bleeding, or discharge; history of occupational, vocational, or military exposure to loud noises; history of injury to the ear, particularly perforation of the tympanic membrane; recent air travel or diving; any previous operations on the ear; and use of hearing aid.

Vertigo and dysequilibrium, suggesting disease of the inner ear, are usually dealt with ear also. The distinction between these two symptoms are sometimes difficult to make; lay persons refer to both as "dizziness". Vertigo is a constant or intermittent feeling that one is spinning ("like I just got off a merry-go-round"). In contrast, disequilibrium means difficulty maintaining one's balance when standing or walking.

Nose

The nasal history includes mention of any acute or chronic pain, swelling, obstruction, or discharge affecting the nose; sneezing, nosebleeds, or frequent colds; seasonal or occasional allergies; sinus infections; disturbance of the sense of smell; history of fracture or other injuries;

submucous resection of deviated septum, removal of polyps; cautery for nosebleeds, or other surgical procedures. The common cold is an universal human experience. Hence, careful and detailed questioning may be needed to elicit clues to nasal allergy, chronic irritation from dust or smoke, or obstruction due to a tumor. The lay meaning of congestion usually diverges from the correct technical sense "swelling due to engorgement of blood vessels".

Throat

It includes the pharynx, the common channel shared by the respiratory and digestive tracts, but also the larynx. Important clinical symptoms include sore throat (the most common presenting symptom in many outpatient practices), postnasal drip, choking and difficulty swallowing; atypical pain, which may be due to foreign body, abscess, tumor, or neurologic disease; hoarseness or other change in the voice; and history of tonsillectomy or other throat operation. Pain, swelling or mass in the neck is included here for assessment.

Mouth and Teeth

The oral and dental history can have important health implications. Chronic, painful conditions of the mouth, gums, or teeth can severely impair nutrition. Many systemic diseases are reflected in oral and dental symptoms. The complete oral and dental history includes soreness, swelling, or ulceration of the lips, gums, or tongue; excessive salivation or excessive dryness of the mouth; abnormal taste or absence of taste; bleeding gums; frequent toothache or sensitivity of teeth to sweet, hot, or cold food or drinks; dental caries and loose, damaged, or missing teeth; regularity of dental care; and wearing of orthodontic braces, dentures, or other appliances.

Cardiovascular

The cardiovascular system includes the heart with its covering membrane, the pericardium, and all the blood vessels of the body-arteries, arterioles, capillaries, venules and veins.

Patients' complaints with respect to the cardiovascular system can be divided into three groups: those rightly perceived as related to the heart or blood vessels, such as angina pectoris, an irregular pulse, or varicose veins; those due to heart or blood vessel disease but not so perceived by the patient, such as anorexia, orthopnea and ankle edema due to congestive heart failure; and those wrongly assumed by the patient as cardiovascular disorders, such as chest pain due to indigestion or tingling in the extremities falsely blamed on "poor circulation".

The cardiovascular history begins with a review of past diagnoses of congenital or acquired heart murmurs, rheumatic fever, enlarged heart, coronary artery disease, heart attack, high blood pressure, varicose veins, thrombophlebitis, and treatments of the past and present, prescribed for any of these conditions. Note is made of the results of past diagnostic studies such as electrocardiograms, echocardiograms, stress testing, cardiac catheterization, or angiography, and of any surgical procedures, such as pacemaker implantation, valve repair or replacement, and coronary artery bypass graft.

The physician tends to bracket cardiovascular symptoms according to six or seven well-defined diagnostic categories: coronary arteriosclerosis, valvular heart disease, and hypertension, any of which can lead to the group of syndromes called congestive heart failure; pericardial disease, local or generalized arteriosclerosis, and venous disease (varicose veins, phlebitis, thromboembolism).

Respiratory

The respiratory system includes all bodily structure concerned with the handling of air: the nose and paranasal sinuses; the mouth and pharynx; the larynx and trachea; the lungs with their bronchi, bronchioles, alveoli, and terminal air sacs; the pleura; and the chest wall and diaphragm with their nerve supplies. The respiratory history begins with a survey of past or current diagnoses or respiratory problems such as asthma, bronchitis, pneumonia, emphysema, pleurisy, pneumothorax, tuberculosis, and lung cancer, with treatments prescribed for any of these.

Gastrointestinal

The gastrointestinal history is concerned mainly with two types of symptoms: abdominal pain of any type or degree (though abdominal pain often results from nondigestive causes) and any disturbances of digestive function, including anorexia, nausea, vomiting and diarrhea. Symptoms due to disorders of the liver or biliary tract, the pancreas, or the rectum or anus are also included here.

In reviewing the past digestive tract history, the examiner inquires about previous diagnoses of hiatal hernia, ulcer, gallstones or gallbladder disease, pancreatitis, colitis, any tumors of the alimentary canal or associated structures; results of gastrointestinal X-rays or other diagnostic studies; operations on the digestive organs, including appendectomy and hemorrhoid surgery; and use of antacids, laxatives, enemas, or prescription medicines for digestive symptoms. Lay persons often diagnose their own condition as gas, ulcers or indigestion, and the physician must exercise caution in accepting such diagram.

Abdominal pain may be described as burning, crampy, or dull. It may be constant, intermittent, or of varying intensity. It may remain in one place or radiate or migrate to another, perhaps in the back or chest. It may be brought on, aggravated, or relieved by eating, non-eating, drinking, defecation, or assuming certain positions. It may be provoked by eating certain foods; a record of any food intolerances is an important part of the digestive history.

Inguinal hernia may also be considered with the gastrointestinal history because most hernias contain loops of bowel and eventually affect digestive function. The groin or scrotum that is accentuated by coughing or straining and diminishes or disappears in the recumbent position.

Genitourinary

The kidneys and urinary tract (ureters, bladder and urethra) and the reproductive system are considered together because of their close anatomic association and the frequency with which one disease affects both the organs or systems. A thorough review of genitourinary history includes past diagnoses of congenital anomalies of the urinary or genital tract; urinary tract infections; stone in kidney, ureter, or bladder; sexually transmitted (venereal) diseases; genitourinary surgery; and menstrual and reproductive history.

The menstrual history includes age of onset of menses (menarche), regularity of cycles, interval between periods, duration of periods and the date of last normal menstrual period. The female reproductive history covers pregnancies, miscarriages, abortions, stillbirths, normal deliveries, and cesarean births; any complications of pregnancy such as hemorrhage or toxemia; use of diaphragm, oral contraceptives, or other contraceptive methods. Questions about pelvic pain, vaginal discharge, vulvar itching, sores, or rash, and any breast complaints (pain, swelling, masses, bleeding or discharge from the nipple).

Men will be questioned about urethral discharge or burning itching, rash, ulcers, or other lesions of the genitals; pain or swelling in the testicles; scrotal masses; and infertility.

Neuromuscular

The central and peripheral nervous system and injuries and diseases not only of skeletal muscle but also of bones, joints, ligaments, and associated structures. Treatment of seizures, brain concussion, brain tumor, stroke, paralysis, neuritis, any fractures or dislocations, severe sprains, bursitis, tendonitis, or arthritis.

Symptoms suggestive of central nervous system disease are severe. Unusual headache, unexplainable drowsiness or dysequilibrium; confusion; disorientation; sudden deterioration of memory, judgment, or emotional stability; tremors; in coordination; disorders of speech;

weakness, clumsiness, paralysis, or spasticity of the extremities; and seizures. Often, detailed information on these points must be obtained from the relatives of the patient.

Peripheral nerve disorders are suggested by numbness, tingling, weakness, or paralysis in an extremity. The pain of peripheral neuritis is often described as stinging or burning and often seems to shoot up along or just under the surface like electric shock.

Most of the painful, inflammatory conditions of the back and extremities are due to injury-either a single violent event or repeated strains or overuse. Hence, the interviewer will attempt to elicit a history of trauma or unusual activities (moving furniture, sudden excessive athletic activity, change of job). Less likely possibilities are local infection and systemic disorders such as rheumatoid arthritis and gout.

Psychiatric

The psychiatric history is even more intimate and sensitive, if possible, than the sexual history. Person with severe psychiatric impairment makes a most unreliable historian. A person with even mild neurotic problems frequently resists talking about them. Hence, a part or whole of the psychiatric history may have to be obtained from the patient's family or friends or from medical records.

Skin

The dermatologic history is usually omitted unless the patient has cutaneous complaints or a condition in which such complaints might be expected. The skin is subjected to numerous injuries and local diseases and often reflects systemic diseases as well.

The most common skin complaints are local or general eruptions or rashes, itching, dryness or scaling, pigment changes, and solid tumors of various kinds. Disorders of the hair (abnormal appearance of the hair, excessive hair, hair loss) and nails (deformity, discoloration) are also part of dermatologic history.

GENERAL REMARKS ON THE PHYSICAL EXAMINATION

Each physician performs a physical examination in the manner that seems most reasonable and convenient to him. Regardless of the sequence in which data are obtained, they are generally recorded in a format something like this:
• General appearance
• Skin
• Head and face
• Eyes

- Ears
- Nose, throat, mouth, teeth
- Neck
- Thorax, breasts, axillae
- Heart, peripheral vessels
- Lungs
- Abdomen, groins, anus, rectum, genitalia
- Back and extremities
- Neurologic
- Psychiatric.

Only simple portable instruments are used. The following is a fairly comprehensive list of equipments used in the performance of a physical examination:

- Flashlight, head mirror, or other light source
- Magnifying glass
- Measuring tape
- Ruler
- Tongue depressor
- Nasal speculum or rhinoscope
- Otoscope with various sizes of specula
- Ophthalmoscope
- Reflex hammer
- Pin or pinwheel
- Soft brush or cotton ball
- Diascope
- Clinical thermometer
- Watch with second hand
- Goniometer
- Skin-fold caliper
- Laryngeal mirror
- Tuning fork
- Stethoscope
- Sphygmomanometer
- Rubber gloves and lubricant
- Vaginal speculum
- Vision-testing chart.

Virtually all diagnostic maneuvers employed in the physical examination have variations on four basic classical techniques: inspection (looking), palpation (feeling), auscultation (listening), and percussion (tapping). Inspection in medicine implies far more than just looking. A diagnostic inspection is objective, systematic, and thorough, with removal of clothing as needed, adequate lighting, and sometimes use of instrument to expose, illuminate, or magnify. The examiner correlates what he sees with visual images stored in his memory, with other physical findings, and with relevant details of the history. Inspection thus includes not only search and discovery but also recognition and interpretation.

Auscultation of internal organs is performed with a stethoscope but the technique also embraces listening to sounds produced by or in any part of the body. Percussion, first developed in the eighteenth century to assess the state of internal organs, particularly in the thorax, is already becoming something of a lost art with the development of radiography, computed tomography, magnetic resonance imaging and various other types of noninvasive examinations.

The rationale of physical examination rest on three basic assumptions: that, there is such a thing as normality of bodily structure and function, corresponding to a state of health; that deviates from this norm of structural and functional integrity consistently result from or correlate with specific abnormal states or diseases; and that systematic examination can detect these abnormalities and appraise them in such a way as to yield grounds for an accurate diagnosis.

What is normal ? The term has two overlapping senses in medicine, which physicians rarely face trouble to distinguish. First, normal means "usual, ordinary, average, common unremarkable." In this sense, a condition or finding that is encountered in a majority of persons of a given sex and age would be considered normal. This type of normality can be established on a statistical basis, at least with respect to features or events that can be measured quantitatively, such as heart rate, ratio of height to weight, and age of onset of menstruation. The fact of biologic variation is acknowledged in such phrasing as "normal variant," "within normal limits," and "within the range of normal." From this perspective, abnormal means "anomalous, atypical, unusual, extra-ordinary," and at times "excessive" or "deficient."

Secondly, normal means "healthy, sound, intact, natural, un-impaired by disease or injury." It should be obvious that in most medical contexts, normal (or abnormal) applies equally in both senses. Moreover, physicians often use the term negative interchangeably with normal. Negative implies the lack of absence of something. Since, the diagnostician is searching for abnormalities, he is apt to use the term negative whenever a particular line of inquiry fails to turn up any: "The family history is negative for hypertension," "The left breast is entirely negative," "Rectal examination is negative," The expression, "The Romberg is negative," is shorthand for "The Romberg test yields negative (normal, expected) result." The Babinski is negative means, "The Babinski reflex (which would be abnormal if present) is absent." (Conversely, positive often implies abnormal: "positive Romberg", positive findings in the fundus."). The ubiquitous phrases essentially normal and essentially negative mean "sound, unimpaired, normal with allowance for expected and insignificant variations". A physical examination is a set of standard procedures designed to identify and assess any significant deviations from normal.

A visible palpable abnormality that represents more than a mere malformation or quantitative deviation from normal structure may be called a lesion (Lation laesio "injury"). Physicians apply this generic term not only to the results of injury but also to abnormal masses and inflammatory or degenerative processes, particularly when these are readily visible on skin or mucous membranes. They may even use it in an abstract as "the biochemical lesion of diabetes mellitus".

An abnormal mass can form in any part of the body, and can be a benign or malignant growth, a malformed or enlarged organ, a product of inflammation, or a foreign body, to name the most likely possibilities. Lymph nodes are fat layer under the skin, particularly in the neck, axillae, and groins, quite commonly enlarge and become palpable in response to various local and systemic processes, most often infectious or malignant condition.

The term inflammation refers to one of the cardinal concepts of pathology. Inflammation is a stereotyped pattern of biochemical, hematological, and mechanical events that occur in living tissue in response to injury of any kind, whether due to cutting, crushing, burning, freezing, electrical shock, chemical irritants, bacterial toxins, viral invasion, or antigen-antibody reactions.

Heart rate is recorded in beats per minute. Unless the cardiac rhythm is irregular the examiner usually counts beats for only fifteen seconds and multiplies by four. The heart rate may be counted as pulsations in a peripheral artery, most often the radial artery at the wrist (radial pulse) or beats heard with stethoscope placed on the chest near the cardiac apex (apical pulse). The respiratory rate, recorded as respirations per minute, is also usually determined by fifteen seconds actual observation. The examiner usually counts respirations while ostensible doing something else (e.g. still feeling the pulse at the wrist). This is because a person who knows that his breathing is being observed finds it almost impossible to breathe at a natural rate and depth.

Blood pressure is determined in the brachial artery above the elbow with the help of a stethoscope and sphygmomanometer. The latter consists of an inflatable cuff with a pressure gauge. The examiner wraps the cuff around the patients' arm and inflates it until no pulsations are transmitted from the heart to the artery below the cuff. While listening to this artery with a stethoscope, he then slowly deflates the cuff, noting the pressure at which pulsations can just be heard and the lower pressure at which they cease to be audible. The higher of these readings is taken as the maximum pressure attained by the blood in response to a contraction of the heart (systolic pressure); the lower, the pressure to which the blood drops between contractions (diastolic pressure), e.g. 120/80, 140/100.

The physician while performing physical examination strives to keep the patient relaxed and comfortable. Often these goals are incompatible. Some parts of the examination inevitably generate fear, embarrassment, or pain. The presence of a nurse or aide who can help the patient to remove clothing or assume certain positions while providing moral and physical support is essential.

While recording his findings, the physician makes note of factors that have limited the thoroughness or accuracy of his examination, such as the patient's inability to cooperate because of lethargy, pain, or fear.

General Appearance

The physical examination report usually begins with a description of the patient's general built up and appearance. The first glance at a patient conveys volumes of information. Before he has finished taking the history he would have observed many features of the patient's general state of mental and physical health. By performing the physical examination he gets the opportunities to make further observations and to confirm or correct his impressions before writing.

General appearance includes shape of the body (muscular development, proportions, skeletal deformities), nutritional status, apparent age and general state of health, skin color (pallor, cyanosis, jaundice), alertness and responsiveness, mood, posture, gait, mobility, grooming and personal hygiene, quality and clarity of voice and speech, evidence of distress (dyspnea, signs of pain or anxiety), abnormal odors of breath or body, and any other readily observable abnormalities (facial scars, absence of limb).

Examination of the Skin

The skin is the largest and most conspicuous organ of the body. Hence, the diagnostician is widely observing the skin for evidence of injury or disease, whatever region he is examining.

The physician requires adequate exposure of the body surface by removing clothing, dressings, bandages and ointments. He uses bright natural or artificial light and, if needed, a magnifying lens. Examination of the skin is not carried out by inspection alone. The examiner palpates any area of skin that appears abnormal and observes its temperature, texture, tenseness or laxness, moistness or dryness.

Evaluating skin color, the examiner considers the intensity of distribution of normal pigment (melanin) and any abnormal coloration (cynosis, erythema, jaundice, bronzing).

Cutaneous diagnosis depends on a consideration to many factors: the type, number, grouping and location of lesions; combinations of features occurring together; signs of evolutionary change, secondary infection, or the contradictions of treatment; and the presence of associated symptoms such as fever, headache, or pain in the joints or abdomen. Multiple problems arise of the skin may be the sign of systemic diseases.

Malignant tumors of the skin are common in older persons, particularly on sun-exposed parts of the body such as the face and neck. In addition, a very small percentage of pigmented lesions in younger persons tend to be highly malignant melanomas. For these reasons all skin tumors and pigmented lesions are subjected to critical scrutiny.

Oil and sweat glands, hair and nails are known as dermal appendages because they arise in or from skin tissue. Abnormal sweating may have neural or endocrine origins. Nail disorders are seldom of more than local significance but occasionally reflect systemic disease. Excessive hair growth, abnormal hair loss, and discoloration or deformation of hair shafts may also indicate either local or general disease. Abnormalities of the distribution of body hair can indicate chromosomal or gonadal disorders.

In most of the cases of trauma, the skin is affected in some way. Open injuries are described as abrasions (due to scraping away of the skin surface), incised wounds (due to sharp, blade-like objects), punctures, and lacerations (bursting of skin due to blunt trauma). Closed injuries are generally contusions, sometimes with hematoma formation. Burns may be described as partial or full thickness burns, or graded: first degree, erythema; second degree, blistering; third degree, charring.

Infections of the skin and adjacent soft tissues are common, as a result of penetrating injury but occasionally from invasion of diseased tissue by opportunistic bacteria. The examiner notes the pattern of lesions, the degree of inflammation, and any pus or exudates present.

Examination of Head, Face and Neck

The physician usually begins his examination with the head and face, since they are normally uncovered by clothing and are the parts at which one naturally looks first in viewing or studying another person. The amount, distribution, texture and color of scalp hair are observed, as well as the pattern of any hair loss. The scalp is inspected for scaling dermatitis, signs of present or past trauma and other lesions. Any tremors or involuntary movement of the head are also noted.

Parkinsonism, myxedema, acromegaly, myasthenia gravis, allergic rhinitis, and Cushing's syndrome produce characteristic changes in facial features. Generalized changes in skin color (pallor, puffiness, cyanosis, jaundice, abnormal pigmentation) are pertinent to be noted first in the face. Facial configuration and symmetricity can be distorted by various congenital syndromes. Cutaneous eruptions may be largely confined to the face (acne vulgaris, acne rosacea, the rash of systemic lupus erythematosus). Masses or cutaneous nodules are carefully evaluated for signs of malignancy. The examiner notes the presence and nature of any facial hair. Pain in the lower jaw, difficulty in chewing or speaking will prompt an assessment of the mandible, the temporomandibular joints, and the muscles of mastication for mobility, spasm, swelling, crepitus, or tenderness. The neck is not simply a column for supporting the head. Through it pass all nerve connections between brain and body, all inspired oxygen and exhaled carbon dioxide, all swallowed food and drink, and all blood supply to the brain, which consumes 25 percent of the body's oxygen intake. The neck is subject to many musculoskeletal injuries and disorders, some of which can affect its configuration and mobility in obvious ways. The examiner tests neck mobility by gently grasping the patient's head and putting it through a range of movements, noting any abnormalities due to joint stiffness, muscle spasm, or pain.

Any swelling or mass are palpated for size, shape, consistency, mobility, pulsatility, and tenderness. Additionally, the entire neck is examined for enlarged lymph nodes, which may appear in any of several locations. Each anatomic group of nodes "drains" (receives lymphatic channels from) through a specific region of the head, face, neck or thorax. The thyroid gland is felt and its size and consistency assessed. The larynx and the uppermost part of the trachea are also felt and any lesion or lateral deviation noted.

The carotid pulsations are gently palpated and compared. The physician applies a stethoscope over each carotid in turn to listen for bruits-harsh sounds synchronous with the pulse, caused by passage of blood through a vessel narrowed by arteriosclerosis.

The external jugular veins at the sides of the neck are normally not distended with blood when one is in an upright position, but can be seen to be filled with blood in the recumbent position.

Examination of the Eyes

The eyes are subject to many acute and chronic diseases, some of them can threaten vision loss. Moreover, the eyes register or reflect many systemic disorders such as jaundice, arteriosclerosis, diabetes, thyrotoxicosis, and the diseases of the nervous system. Hence, they deserve thorough examination. Unless some historical point has drawn specific attention relation to one or both eyes, the physician's evaluation will usually be limited to an inspection of the lids and lashes and the parts of the eye exposed between them, a test of the papillary light reflexes, a rough check of ocular movements and visual fields, and an inspection of the ocular fundus. A test of vision is often included. All of these procedures can be performed quickly and easily with standard equipment, but several of them require the cooperation of the patient.

The physician looks for opacities in the cornea and anterior chamber, abnormalities of the iris, and abnormalities in the shape of the pupil, incidentally observing whether the pupil constricts when light is focused directly into the eye. A check of the accommodation reflex may also be made by asking the patient to look at a distant object and notice whether the pupils constrict. Astigmatism, a warping of the cornea out of its natural spherical form, can sometimes be detected by noticing distortion in the reflection of some regularly shaped object on the cornea, but is usually determined by vision testing. Abnormalities of the white of the eye can be due to discoloration of disease of the sclera or of the overlying conjunctiva, usually the later. Mild or early jaundice is typically more evident in the sclera than in the skin. Conjunctival swelling and discharge or lacrimation are noted, as well as the degree and distribution of any redness. Very thin sclera, such as occur in some connective tissue disorders, appears blue.

The physician tests extraocular movements by having the examinee follow with the gaze the movements of a hand-held objects such as a lamp while holding his head immobile. Abnormalities of ocular movement can be due to disease or injury of the brain of the third, fourth, or sixth cranial nerve on either side, or due to orbital disease or injury affecting one or more of the six extraocular muscles that control the positioning of each eye.

The optic fundus is the portion of the interior of the eye that can be seen by an examiner looking through the pupil with an ophthalmoscope, a hand-held instrument with a light source and a set of magnifying lenses that can be quickly changed. The principal features of the fundus are the retina, the optic disk or nerve head, and branches of the central retinal artery and vein. Retinal and optic nerve disease as well as the effects of systemic conditions such as diabetes, arteriosclerosis, and hypertension, are readily observed in the fundus, provided that the examiner's view is not blocked by an opaque lens (cataract) or a hemorrhage or foreign body within the eye. Vision testing is usually performed with familiar snellen wall chart for distant vision and set of jaeger test types for a near vision. The subject reads the smallest letters he can see on the wall chart at a distance of 20 feet, and his performance is expressed as a fraction of normal. Thus 20/20 vision indicates normal far visual acuity, while 20/40 means that the subject can see no letters at 20 feet smaller than those that a normal person can see at 40 feet.

Examination of the Ears

The anatomist divides the human ear into three parts. The external ear, consisting of pinna, external auditory meatus or ear canal. The middle ear, or eardrum, is a hollow space within the temporal bone, lined with mucous membrane and communicating through the Eustachian or auditory tube with the nasopharynx. The middle ear is separated from the external ear by the tympanic membrane, and it contain three small bones connected in sequence that transmit sound waves from the tympanic membrane to the cochlea. The inner ear consists of cochlea, with receptors for the auditory division of the eighth cranial nerve; and the vestibular apparatus, with receptors for the vestibular division of the eighth cranial nerve, which is concerned with equilibrium.

The diagnostician has full access to the external ear, very limited access to the middle ear, and none at all to the inner ear except through testing of hearing and equilibrium. Examination of the ear begins with inspection of the pinna for deformity, inflammation, injury and abnormal masses. Malformation of the external ear occur as part of various genetic dysmorphic syndromes. They may also indicate congenital renal diseases. There is a high correlation between diagonal earlobe creases and coronary artery disease in middle-aged and elderly men. Hearing can be tested in various ways. Pure-tone audiometry (PTA) with sophisticated electronic equipment in a soundproof booth is the method used by otologists, and may also be a part of school and industrial health testing, but is not included in a standard physical examination. A rough notion of auditory acuity can be obtained by testing the examinee's ability to hear the spoken and whispered voice at various distances, with first one ear and then the other occluded.

Hearing loss can be of two types: conductive and neurosensory. Conductive hearing loss results from disease or injury of middle ear structures, neurosensory loss from deterioration of the acoustic nerve due to aging (presbycusis), noise exposure, or certain drugs and chemicals. Both conductive and neurosensory hearing loss can exist together in varying degrees. Two tests of value in distinguishing types of hearing impairment are the Rinne and the Weber test, both requiring the use of a tuning fork.

Examination of the Nose, Throat, Mouth and Teeth

It begins with the external inspection for developmental abnormalities, traumatic deformities, enlargement (rhinophyma), nodules, ulcers and other cutaneous lesions. The interior of each nostril is then viewed with a beam of light from a head mirror or other source. When a head mirror is used, the nostril is gently dilated with a bivalve nasal speculum. Alternatively, a cone-shaped speculum larger than those used for ear examination can be attached to an otoscope. The interior of the nose is inspected for septal deviation or perforation; mucosal edema, ingestion, ulcers, erosions, or polyps; discharge, hemorrhage, foreign bodies and tumors.

The paranasal sinuses are irregular cavities within certain bones of the skull. They are lined with mucous membrane and communicate with the nasal cavity by very small openings.

Examination of the Thorax, Breasts and Axillae

The thorax comprises roughly the upper half of the trunk, from the neck to the diaphragm, which at full inspiration lies just above the lower rib margins. Some examiners proceed directly from the head and neck to the thorax, while others prefer to interpose examinations of the extremities or part of the neurological examination that can be performed before the patient undresses.

The physician inspects all surfaces of the chest for cutaneous lesions, surgical or traumatic scars, swellings, or masses, noting pigment and hair distribution (including axillary hair) and palpating abnormal areas to assess their consistency and note any tenderness. The breasts are palpated in both sexes but in women the procedure is more elaborate. The female breasts are inspected for abnormalities of shape, lack of symmetry, deformity or retraction of nipples, cutaneous changes, surgical scars, and lack of mobility when arms are raised over the head. They are systematically palpated for masses or tenderness in both the erect and supine postures. Finally, the axillae are palpated to detect enlarged or tender lymph nodes or other lesions.

Examination of the Heart

Even a routine physical examination may include many of these procedures, and when cardiac disease is suspected or recognized, many more will be used. Because the circulatory system extends throughout the entire body, tests of its integrity and function are included in the examination of various regions and also so many be found recorded in various parts of the physical examination report. For example, inspection of retinal aviculture is performed as part of the eye examination, and so recorded. Peripheral pulses are felt at the neck, arms, and legs are being examined, and so on.

Very little information can be obtained about the structure of the heart through direct examination. Virtually, the entire cardiac examination consists of observation of the functions of the heart rate, regularity, and intensity of ventricular contractions, the resulting impulses imparted to the circulating blood and to the chest wall, and the sounds generated by cardiac contractions and the movement of blood. Congenital anomalies, vascular diseases, arrhythmias, pericardial effusions and adhesions, ventricular dilatation and hypertrophy, congestive heart failure-all must be detected or inferred by examination of cardiac function. X-rays, cardiograms, and other noninvasive and invasive diagnostic procedures can yield more precise data about structural alterations in the heart and great vessels, but even these depend largely on assessment of cardiac function.

Auscultation of the heart provides more information than any other procedures. Stethoscopes used for cardiac auscultation have two chest pieces, a narrow, cone-shaped "bell" for lower pitched sounds and a wide, flat diaphragm for higher pitched sounds. He applies the stethoscope to the chest in a number of areas, following a basic routine but varying it as circumstances dictate. Four areas of the anterior chest are designated according to the valves whose sounds are best heard there: the mitral area, pulmonic area, the aortic area, and the tricuspid area. The patient may need to change his position, such as by leaning forward or lying on his left side, to enable the examiner to evaluate heart sounds adequately.

Although an electrocardiogram is needed for precise diagnosis of abnormalities in cardiac rhythm, auscultation can yield much valuable information about the rhythm. A slight or even marked variation in heart rate with the breathing cycle (increase on inspiration, decrease on expiration) is normal and is known as sinus arrhythmia. Occasionally extrabeats (extrasystoles, premature ventricular contractions) can also be normal. Occurrence of a premature beat after each normal beat is more ominous.

Cardiac murmurs are produced by turbulence in the flow of blood passing forward through a stenotic valve, leaking back through an incompetent valve, or crossing from a place of higher to a place of lower pressure through an abnormal orifice, such as an interventricular septal defect. The diagnostician characterizes a murmur by recording its location (the point on the chest wall where it is heard best); its radiation or transmission (e.g. to the carotid arteries or left axilla); its character, intensity (graded on a scale of 1 to 6; less often, 1 to 4), and duration; and its timing within the cardiac cycle. Valvular clicks and snaps are similarly characterized.

Certain other tests of cardiac function and circulation are performed as indicated. A tilt test involves noting any change in the pulse when the patient is subjected to changes from a recumbent to a sitting position. Marked increase in pulse suggests hypovolemia and impending shock. In doubtful cases, a sphygmomanometer can be used to read a drop in arterial pressure.

Pulse pressure is arithmetical difference between systolic and diastolic pressure. Hence if the patient's blood pressure is 148/68, his pulse pressure is 80. On palpating, the peripheral pulses have a particularly bounding character, the so-called Corrigan or water-happer pulse. Capillary pulsations (Quincke's pulse) may be evident in the nail beds and elsewhere as rhythmic blushing synchronous with heart beat.

Examination of the Lungs

Physical assessment of the lungs naturally follows examination of the heart. Evaluation of the lungs is performed almost entirely by the techniques of auscultation and percussion. The passage of air into and out of the lungs during normal respiration procedures are characteristic sequence of sounds, as heard with the stethoscope through the chest wall. Structural changes in the lung due to disease or injury predictable changes in the quality and loudness of the breath sounds can induce abnormal sounds.

Certain abnormal conditions can superimpose abnormal sounds (rhonchi, rales, or rubs) on the inspiratory-expiratory breath sounds. A rhonchus is a continuous sound such of a whistle or horn. A rale is irregular and discontinuous, like bubbling fluid, crackling paper, or popping corn. Rhonchi result from narrowing of bronchiolar passages by bronchospasm (in asthma), swelling, thickened secretions, or tumor. In asthma, rhonchi of many different pitches may be heard together. Rales are due to passage of air through fluid-mucus, pus, edema fluid, or blood-or to sudden expansion of small air passages that have been plugged or sealed by mucus. The examiner carefully notes in what part of the chest and at what part of the breathing cycle rhonchi or rales are heard or are loudest.

Examination of the Abdomen, Groins, Rectum, Anus and Genitalia

The abdomen and pelvis comprise the lower half of the trunk, from the diaphragm to the perineum. Whereas the physician examines the thorax from all sides with the patient upright, he approaches the abdomen almost exclusively from the ventral surface and carries out most of the examination with the patient supine. The physician systematically goes over the entire abdomen, feeling in each area for possible enlargement of structure he knows to be there, and always looking for masses, pulsations and tenderness (pulsations of the aorta can normally be felt). The patient inhale deeply while he places his hand just below the right and left costal margin respectively. Descent of the diaphragm on inspiration will bring an enlarged liver or spleen down into contact with the examining hand. To enhance the sensitivity of the test he places his other hand under the patient's ribs on the same side and lifts gently as the patient inhales.

Examination of the Back and Extremities

The physician examines the back and extremities to detect abnormalities of the skin and subcutaneous tissues in these regions, injuries and diseases of the musculoskeletal system, disorders of the circulation, and evidence of central or peripheral nervous system disease. The examinations of the skin, bones, joints, muscles, and peripheral circulation are described in this chapter, and of the nervous system in the next.

The history and physical findings influence the scope and thoroughness of the examination in that, some special procedures are applied only when indicated. The hands and feet are examined particularly for cutaneous lesions, and the appearance of the nails are carefully noted. The physician looks for clubbing of fingers or toes, seen in chronic pulmonary disease and certain other conditions, and observes the nail beds for pallor or cyanosis.

Having considered the skin and the circulation, the examiner turns his attention to the bones, joints, muscles, and other connective and supporting structures. In performing the orthopedic examination, he looks for any developmental or traumatic deformities not previously noted and any evidence of generalized conditions such as muscle waste or weakness, stiffness, or tremors. The terms varus and valgus refer to abnormal deviations in joints of the extremities. In a varus deformity, the bones distal to the affected joint is deviated inward; hence genu varum means bowleg, valgus is outward deviation of the distal bone; hence genu valgum means knock knee.

Neurologic Examination

Most of the parts of the neurologic examination are carried out on a regional basis and interspersed with examinations of other systems. In analyzing and recording his findings, however, the physician classifies them according to anatomic and functional divisions of the nervous system. The central nervous system (CNS) comprises the brain and spinal cord; the peripheral nervous system, the cranial and spinal nerves. Peripheral nerve fibers are either motor (efferent) fibers carrying impulses to muscles, or sensory (afferent) fibers carrying impulses to the spinal cord or brainstem. Both kinds of fibers are often combined in a single nerve trunk.

The physician tests sensory functions by stimulating appropriate receptors and noting the corresponding responses. He tests motor functions by observing the patient's ability to perform certain actions. Even in an unconscious patient, by testing the deep tendon reflexes he can assess the integrity of the spinal reflex arcs, which consist of both sensory stretch receptor and motor nerve fibers. Evaluation of complex voluntary movements and muscle coordination requires the conscious collaboration of the patient. Assessment of cerebral functions (memory, orientation, thinking capacity, mood) is described in the next chapter.

If the patient is stuporous or unconscious the physician tries to determine the degree of central nervous system depression by noting the size and reactivity of the pupils, the rate and rhythm of breathing, the response to noxious stimuli such as loud noises and firm pressure over bony prominences, and the presence of certain primitive reflexes such as the corneal and gag reflex. In the doll's eye maneuver, the examiner rotates the patient's head from side to side and notes the effect on eye position. Normally, the eyes rotate in opposite to that in which the head is moved, tending to maintain the same direction of gaze. Failure of the eyes to rotate around this own vertical axes during this maneuver indicates brainstem damage.

The twelve pairs of cranial nerves emanate from the brainstem and pass through structures in head and neck. The first pair of cranial nerves (olfactory) are not routinely tested but, as noted in chapter 5, the subject's sense of smell can be evaluated by making him try to identify common substances (soap, tobacco) by their odors. The second pair (optic) are inspected during the fundoscopic examination and their function is checked through vision testing. The third, fourth and sixth pairs (oculomotor, trochlear and abducens) control ocular movement. The fifth pair (trigeminal) supply the face with motor and sensory branches. They are tested by noting the strength of jaw clenching and the sensitivity of the facial skin in various areas to gentle pinprick. The seventh pair (facial) innervate the muscles of the face and are tested by having the patient grimace, purse his lips, wrinkle his forehead, close his eyes tightly, and so on. The sense of taste on the anterior two-thirds of the tongue is also supplied by the seventh pair. This can be tested by touching the tongue with a drop of salt or sugar solution or vinegar. The eighth pair (acoustic) are the nerves of hearing and equilibrium. Testing the pharyngeal 9 gag reflex assesses both the ninth pair (glossopharyngeal), which carry the afferent side of this reflex are (as well as taste afferents from the posterior third of the tongue), and the tenth (vagus), which carry the efferent side. The eleventh pair (spinal accessory) send motor fibers to the sternocleido-mastoid muscles at the sides of the neck. These are tested by having the subject rotate his head against a resisting hand placed along his chin. The twelfth pair (hypoglossal) innervate the tongue and are tested by having the patient stretch out his tongue.

The spinal nerves emerge from the spinal cord in pairs, on right and one left, and supply the body from the occiput downward with sensory and motor fibers. A pair of spinal nerves is named from the vertebra above which (cervical region) or below which (other regions) it emerges. Thus, the L_2 pair emerge below the second lumbar vertebra. Sensory nerve-endings in the skin are distributed in segments called dermatomes, each corresponding to a pair of spinal nerves. Sensory and motor fibers to the limbs pass through complicated systems of branching and interconnection (brachial and lumbar plexi) before forming the main nerve trunks of the upper and lower extremities. The entire skin surface can be mapped as to the segmental origin of its sensory supply, and likewise the spinal segment or segments innervating each muscle are known. With this anatomical knowledge in hand, the physician can localize and characterize lesions of the spinal cord and peripheral nerves by precise study of sensory and motor deficits. In addition, lesion of the brain can be localized by their effect on coordination, stereognosis, and other complexed motor and sensory functions.

The examiner obtains some information about the motor system from his first view of the patient, and gains more as the examination proceeds. Generalized weakness, hemiparesis, disturbances of gait, posture, or speech, and abnormal movements such as tics and tremors are readily observed.

The orthopedic examination provides data about muscle mass, strength, tone and control. Paralyzed muscle eventually undergo contracture and atrophy. Paralysis due to peripheral nerve (lower motor neuron) disease is flaccid (muscle soft and limp). Paralysis due to cerebral (upper motor neuron) lesion is spastic (muscles tight, with rigid or jerky resistance to movement by the examiner) because of uninterrupted but no longer efficacious postural and checking signals from the basal ganglia of the brain.

In neurology, the term reflex refers to a muscular contraction in response to some stimulus, such as tapping the patellar tendon. For a reflex to occur, both sensory and motor limbs of the reflex are must be intact. A deep tendon reflex, such as the familiar knee jerk, is elicited by tapping the tendon smartly with a rubber reflex hammer. For some tendons, such as the biceps brachii, the examiner may place his thumb firmly over the tendon and then strike his thumb with the hammer. For some tendons, such as the biceps brachii, the examiner may place his thumb firmly over the tendon and then strike his thumb with the hammer. This does not feel very good but it vastly improves the accuracy of his aim. The examiner tests selected tendons (at a minimum, the biceps and triceps in the arm and the patellar and calcaneal in the leg) and notes the quality and strength of responses, comparing right and left. Normally, a sudden stretch of a voluntary muscle tendon elicits a prompt, brisk and transitory contraction of the muscle. In lower motor neuron lesions, the reflexes are reduced or absent. In upper motor neuron lesions, the reflexes are not only unimpaired but exaggerated. Besides deep tendon reflexes, superficial or cutaneous reflexes yield information about peripheral sensory and motor reflexes, elicited by stroking the relaxed abdomen, causing contraction of abdominal wall muscles, with movement of the umbilicus toward the area stroked. The *cremasteric* reflex causes the testicles to draw up when the physician strokes the skin of the inner thigh.

Certain reflexes are seen only with upper motor neuron damage (pathologic reflexes). These include the Babinski (upward deviation of the great toe on stroking the sole of the foot), the Hoffman (twitching of the thumb when the middle finger is snapped), and the palmomental (twitching of the chin on stimulation of the palm of the hand).

Motor coordination is tested by having the patient perform complex actions such as touching his nose with his eye closed, moving his heel up and down, the opposite shin bone while recumbent and making rapidly alternating movements with his hands. In the Gordon Holmes test, the patient pulls his fist towards his face against the physician's resistance. When the physician suddenly releases the fist, a patient with abnormal coordination may be unable to check himself in time keep from punching his own face (the physician, however, prevents this).

Abnormal movements vary from fine, ineffectual twitches of a few muscle fibers (fasciculation) to violent thrusting or hurling movements of the whole body. Tremors can be coarse of fine, local or generalized, worse at rest (resting tremor), with purposeful movement (intention tremor), or with position-holding (postural tremor). Asterixis is a coarse, flapping tremor that occurs when the patient attempts to hold his hands steady before him, palms down. Chorea denotes sudden, brief, involuntary jerking movements of the face or limbs; athetosis is a slow, continuous writhing. Often these two occur together.

The physician performs a basic sensory examination by noting the subject's ability to detect light touch (as from a soft brush or a wisp of cotton) and superficial pain (from a gentle pinprick) over various parts of the body surface, always comparing right and left. Sensitivity to temperature can be tested by applying cool and warm metal disks, or test tubes of cool and warm water to the skin. Vibratory sense is tested by placing the shank of a vibrating tuning fork against a superficially lying bone, such as a knuckle or shin. Proprioception is a form of sensation by which the brain monitors the position and degree of stretch of muscles. It is important for both balance sense and coordination. Proprioception can be tested by asking the patient to report the position in which fingers or toes are placed by the examiner.

Other sensory modalities that are tested in selected cases are two-point discrimination (the ability to distinguish two adjacent, simultaneous pinpricks), stereognosis (the ability to identify objects solely by feeling them), and graphesthesia (the ability to recognize letters or numbers traced on the skin).

Meningitis, inflammation of the covering membranes of the brain and spinal cord, is often accompanied by painful spasm of paraspinal and leg muscles. Marked stiffness of the neck (nuchal rigidity) is a cardinal finding in meningitis. In addition, two signs are often present.

Kernig's sign is inability of the knee to be extended when the hip is flexed. Brudzinski's sign is involuntary flexion of the hips and knees when the neck is flexed by the examiner.

Tertiary, a hyperirritable state of the neuromuscular system, can be induced by various drugs and metabolic states, particularly hypocalcemia. Sings of tetany are involuntary muscle twitches and spasms, including carpopedal spasm, risus sardonicus, and Trousseau's and Chvostek's signs. Chvostek's sign is spasm of facial muscle induced by tapping over the facial nerve in front of the ear. Trousseau's sign is spastic contraction of wrist and forearm muscles induced by inflation of a sphygmomanometer cuff above systolic pressure.

The Formal Mental Status Examination

If the patient displays psychiatric symptoms, the medical examination includes a more formal investigation of his mental status. A thorough assessment of a patient's psychiatric condition can take weeks or months, and in a sense is never complete. The mental status examination performed in conjunction with a physical examination is a brief survey of selected aspects of the patient's mental health that can be evaluated without prolonged and intensive interviewing.

Most of the data for this kind of examination are gathered during history recording. In addition to the basic historical interview, the examiner asks the subject questions specifically designed to test his mental status. The examiner records his findings and conclusions according to a fairly standard format. A psychiatrist or other physician with psychiatric learning may use highly specialized, not to say extravagant, terminology. The following is a typical format for recording the results of the mental status examination.

Appearance

The examiner records any peculiarities of dress or personal grooming.

Sensorium

This refers to the subject's receptiveness and responsiveness to external stimuli. The physician judges his alertness, attention span, and ability to receive and process visual, auditory and tactile stimuli.

Activity and Behavior

Gait, posture and general level of motor activity are assessed, and any bizarre or compulsive actions, mannerisms, or catatonic posturings are noted.

Method

The subject's emotional state and his response to being interviewed are observed and recorded.

Thought Content

The physician look for evidence of unconventional thoughts, fantasies, phobias, hallucinations, delusions, obsessive ideas, or lack of poor reasoning or IQ.

Intellectual Function

The physician tests the speed, coherence and relevance of the subject's abstract reasoning by asking him to simple mental arithmetic and to interpret proverbs such as "Birds of the feather flock together."

Orientation

The examiner ascertains the subject's awareness of time (time of day, day of week, date, season, year), place (state, city, exact present location), and person (who he is, identity of family or friends).

Memory

The subject's recall of recent and remote events is tested through questioning. The examiner also assesses his fund of information by asking about matters of general knowledge. Who discovered America?

Judgment

This term refers to the subject's competence of reliability in analyzing facts or situations and deriving conclusions and plans of action from them. (What would you do if you ran out of gas on the interstate ?)

Insight

In psychiatry, insight means a patient's awareness that he is ill and his recognition of the nature and implications of his illness.

Orientation, memory and judgment are often called the organic triad, because they are commonly affected in organic dementia. In addition to relatively unstructured interviewing, the subject may be given various formal, standardized tests of intelligence and personality.

PEDIATRIC HISTORY AND PHYSICAL EXAMINATION

The history and physical examination of an infant must be obtained from sources other than the patient. Parental factors and antenatal events emerge large in the history; indeed, a newborn has no other history. The physician must be alert for developmental anomalies and disturbances of nutrition, growth and maturation that are not diagnostic considerations in later life. On the other hand, degenerative diseases and most kinds of malignancy simply do not occur. Examination techniques are limited to those requiring no cooperation from the patient. Sizes, shapes, textures and levels of functions that would be abnormal in an adult may be perfectly normal in a baby and vice versa.

A newborn undergoes a thorough examination within a few hours after birth. Periodic well-baby checks are part of routine pediatric care. When an infant is admitted to the hospital, a history and physical examination will be done. Although, these examination vary in scope and emphasis, certain basic points of similarity can be noted. My purpose here is to sketch briefly the pediatric history and physical examination with emphasis to variations in diagnostic procedures used for older children and adults.

The physician precedes his record of the pediatric history with a note of his informant or informants, their relation to the child, and any emotional or other factors that may affect the accuracy of the information. The chief complaint and history of present illness for a small child are necessarily stated from the viewpoint of the informant. The past history begins before the childs conception with the health history of the parents and their families and of any elder siblings, particularly with respect to hereditary disease or abnormalities. Apgar score, the child's birth weight and evidence of congenital anomalies. The child's health state during the neonatal period is reviewed, with particular attention to jaundice, respiratory distress, feeding difficulties, fever, or seizures. The nutritional history (breast or bottle feeding, vitamin supplements, weight gain) is reviewed.

An important feature of pediatric history is an account of the child's growth and development. Any available data on height and weight at various ages are collected. Teething history is recorded. Psychomotor development is traced in terms of "milestones" such as acquisition of head control, speech, walking and toilet training. Social responses and adjustments of the older infant and toddler are evaluated.

The child's temperature is taken rectally and blood pressure is determined with suitably sized cuff. Height (length) and weight are recorded, as well as the circumferences of the head and the chest. Throughout the examination the physician is particularly alert for evidence of congenital or developmental abnormalities or signs of dehydration is noted and the fontanels are palpated. The eyes are examined for strabismus, congenital cataract and signs of infection. Vision can be tested in preschool children with an eye chart consisting entirely of 'E' printed in various positions.

Examination of ears, nose and throat is often a tiring experience for both examiner and subject. Assistance is essential. Auscultation of the lungs of a crying child may have to be confined to the inspiratory phase of respiration. The heart is examined for evidence of congenital anomalies. Palpation of the abdomen is performed carefully to detect malignant tumors, which occasionally occur in quite small children, and umbilical or inguinal hernias. Examination of the genitalia and rectum is generally limited to external inspection unless disease or injury of these structure are suspected.

In the orthopedic examination, the physician looks for evidence of congenital malformations or injuries. He pays special attention to the hip joints, legs and feet. The neurologic examination of small children includes tests for reflexes that are present in normal infants but not in older children or adults. These include the Moro (Startle), grasp, rooting, and tonic neck reflexes. Alertness, muscle tone and general responsiveness to stimuli are assessed with due consideration of the child's age.

DIAGNOSTIC FORMULATION

The performance of a history and physical examination is to assess diagnosis. The formulation of a diagnosis is the pivotal point in the doctor-patient interaction where investigation culminate and gives way to intervention. As described in the introduction, diagnosis in this context usually means the name of a disease.

When, as often happens, the history and physical examination are recorded before X-rays, laboratory tests, and other special procedures have supplied data for a firm and narrow diagnostic label, the physician may conclude the history and physical examination report with a tentative (provisional, working) diagnosis. For a patient just admitted to the hospital, this translates to admitting diagnosis. The physician's phrase to rule out, as in "to rule out myocardial infarction", is sometimes misunderstood. This expression does not mean that the diagnosis has been ruled out, but rather that, although less than probable, it remains enough of possibility to require further consideration. When such a possibility is confirmed after all, it is said , somewhat probability, to have been ruled in. At the conclusion of the diagnostic process a final diagnosis is recorded. In a hospital record this is called a discharge diagnosis (assuming that the patient leaves the hospital alive). In surgical cases, preoperative and postoperative diagnoses are recorded.

The choice of diagnostic language is presently governed by many factors extraneous to the purely practical question on a basis or starting point for treatment. Most healthcare institutions and third-party payers of medical expenses insist on a fairly standard nomenclature of disease. Most accept the terminological guidelines of the International Classification of Diseases (ICD) prepared and published under the auspices of World Health Organization. Besides being extremely well-organized, the ICD has the advantage of providing a number code for each diagnosis. Diagnostic labels are used by various committees and agencies for purposes of classification and analysis. To an increasing extent, third-party payers gear specific dollar limits on healthcare payment to specific diagnostic categories (Diagnosis related groups, DRG). Peer-review committee assessing the degree to which individual physician follow professional standards key to their investigations for specific admitting and discharge diagnoses in hospital charts. Hospital administrators and accrediting agencies compile statistics on the basis of recorded diagnoses.

Labels that specify particular injuries, diseases, or abnormalities (incised wound, myocardial infarction, sigmoid diverticulosis), physicians append many qualifying adjectives to indicate whether they are local or general, acute or chronic, constant or intermittent, symptomatic or asymptomatic, early or late in their course, typical or atypical. Etiologic terms are also added, particularly terms that distinguish primary from secondary conditions and organic from functional ones. It may be important to indicate that a condition is a complication or sequela of another condition.

Various types of classifications may be combined with diagnoses. A prognosis is a prediction of the outcome of the disease. For many diseases, stages have been established according to standard criteria. A common staging format for malignancies is the Tumor-node-metastasis (TNM) classification. For example, T2a, Nib, MO for a breast cancer means "primary tumor between 2 and 5 cm in size with no fixation to underlying pectoral fascia or muscle; movable axillary nodes on the same side, believed to contain cancer; no distant metastases known." The degree of disability arising from an illness or injury may be estimated in qualitative or quantitative terms as a part of diagnostic formulation. Such an estimate can have a bearing on the patient's employability or on compensation or disability payments.

GLOSSARY

Benign: Not malignant. Not diseased. Normal, not showing evidence of disease or abnormality.

Black hairy tongue: Discoloration and alteration of the surface texture of the tongue by fungal infection.

Blackout (lay term): Syncope; loss of consciousness.

Bleed: A hemorrhage, usually gastrointestinal.

Bull's eye lesion: A skin lesion consisting of concentric rings of erythema.

Butterflies in the stomach: A sensation of nausea or uneasiness in the upper abdomen, often due to anxiety.

Cauliflower ear: An external ear deformed by repeated or severe trauma, as in boxers and wrestlers.

Chart: The entire record of a patient's hospitalization.

Chronic: Persistent or prolonged, as in chronic bronchitis, chronic steroid therapy.

Compliance: A patient following of his physician's directions and advice regarding diet or medicinal treatment.

Goose-egg (lay term): Traumatic hematoma of the scalp.

Gravida: Pregnant. In medical jargon, the number of pregnancies a woman had.

Hypnotic: A drug used to induce sleep.

In extremis: At the point of death.

Lancinating: Stabbing, piercing (of a pain).

Maintain: To control or limit the effects of an illness or abnormal state with diet, medicine or other means.

Moribund: Dying state.

Morsicatio buccarum: The nervous habit of biting or chewing the buccal mucosa.

Para: Denotes the number of times a woman had delivered a child.

Parity: A woman's reproductive history.

Rabbit nose: Habitual repeated wrinkling of the nose by a person with itching of the nares due to allergic rhinitis.

Residual(s): Lasting effects of disease or injury.

Running: Producing abnormal or excessive secretions.

Sequela (usually used in pleural, sequelae)*:* A persistent effect of an illness or injury, such as paralysis after a stroke.

Toxic: Showing signs of toxemia or septicemia, such as fever, tachycardia, flushing and mental confusion.

Wean: To discontinue a medicine by gradually reducing the dose.

Workup: To perform a thorough diagnostic evaluation or workup.

Wrist drop: Passive flexion of the wrist due to paralysis of extensor muscles.

PART–II

Nursing, Allied Health Sciences and Diagnostics

15

Nursing Services

INTRODUCTION

Nursing is a *discipline*, profession, and an area of practice. As a discipline, nursing is centered-around knowledge development. As a profession, nursing has a social mandate to be responsible and accountable to the public it serves.

Nursing is *the integral part of the health care system*, and as such encompasses the promotion of health, prevention of illness, and care physically ill, mentally ill, and disabled people of all ages, in all health care and other community settings. Within this broad-spectrum of health care, the particular concern to nurses is individual, family and group "responses" to actual or potential health problems". The human responses range broadly from health-restoring reactions to an individual episode of illness to the development of policy in promoting the long-term health of a population.

Nursing is *both an art and science* involving the total patients, as promoting spiritual, mental and physical health; stressing health education and health preservation, ministering to the sick, caring for the patient environment and giving health service to the family, the community and the individual (Mother Olivia Gowan, 1943).

Nursing is a *profession in transition*. The trends and issues that underline this phenomenon hold important implications for the management of hospitals and other healthcare institutions and agencies. Nursing service is a critical component in fulfilling hospital, long-term care, and other health service organization objectives for patient care. The nursing profession exists in response to a need of a society and holds ideals related to man's health throughout his lifespan.

DEFINITIONS

Nursing Diagnosis

Nursing diagnosis is the process of assessing potential or actual health problems, including those pertaining to a family or community, that fall within the scope of nursing practice; also, a judgment or conclusion reached as a result of such assessment or derived from assessment data.

Nursing Audit

Nursing audit is a method of evaluating nursing practice by reviewing records that document the care provided to patients.

OBJECTIVES

- To provide professional care for patients' recovery and physical and mental health.
- To provide non-professional care for patients' comfort and safety such as bed making.
- To perform administrative duties such as safe-custody of drugs and maintenance of equipment and materials in satisfactory condition.
- To provide continuing education for professional nurses and nursing assistants.
- To undertake understanding, or assist with, research for improved nursing care.
- To provide, where necessary, clinical experience for student nurses.

POLICIES

- To restore patients to the highest level of health individually possible.
- To get patients' families to participate where appropriate, in tasks such as patients' feeding, washing, and dressing.
- To group patients in large wards by degree of illness with groups needing most care located nearest the Nurses' Station.
- To change locations in ward periodically for long stay patients' psychological benefit.

PROCEDURES

Patient Care

- Receiving admitted patients
- Administration of medication
- Assisting physicians
- Performing simple diagnostic procedures
- Collecting and sending specimens to laboratory
- Recording and maintaining medical records
- Recording of vital signs

- Performing gastric lavage and giving enema
- Preoperative preparations
- Delivering bedside nursing
- Coordinating patient care with other team members
- Maintaining clean and safe environment
- Bed making and providing privacy to patients.

Ward Management

- Supervising, directing and controlling staff
- Diet ordering
- Maintaining poisonous and narcotic drug controls and registers
- Communicating
- Maintaining records pertaining to patient care, investigation reports, inventory, medicolegal cases, etc.
- Nursing education
- Safe custody of patients' valuables
- Visitors control
- Discharge and bill settlement.

Operation Theater Management

- Aseptic environment maintenance
- Autoclaving
- Receiving patients from wards
- Coordinating trolley traffic
- Assisting surgeon and anesthetist
- Indenting and procuring surgical instruments and surgical sundries
- Maintaining records and reports
- Safe maintenance of theater equipment and apparatus.

Labor Room Management

- Preparation of expectant mother for aseptic safe delivery
- Conducting normal deliveries
- Assisting doctors in obstetrical emergencies
- Assisting difficult and abnormal deliveries
- Taking care of newborn and premature babies
- Indenting and procuring drugs, linen, etc.
- Maintaining records and reports pertaining to labor room.

Psychiatry Unit Management

- Assisting doctors in admission and discharges
- Preparing patients for ECT, therapies and other procedures

- Assisting management of aggressive patients and that with suicidal motives
- Maintaining records, reports and registers.

Postoperative/ICU/Burns Unit Management

- Indenting and procuring drugs, equipment and oxygen cylinders
- Operating ECG, EEG, cardiac resuscitation
- Assisting physicians in operating other high-tech equipment and apparatus.

Educational

- Orientation of new staff and students
- Teaching and guiding staff
- Teaching individual or group of patients
- Clinical teaching
- Demonstrating methods and procedures
- In-service education programs
- Assisting in research programs.

FUNCTIONS

Independent Functions

- The supervision of a patient involving the whole management of care, requiring the application of principles based upon the biological, physical and social sciences.
- The observations of symptoms and reactions, including symptoms of physical and conditions and needs, requiring evaluation or application of principles based upon the biological, the physical and social sciences.
- The accurate recording and reporting of facts, including evaluation of the whole care of the patient.
- The supervision of others, except physicians, contributing to the care of the patient.
- The application and the execution of nursing procedures and techniques.
- The direction and education to secure physical and mental care.

Dependent Function

The application and the execution of legal orders of physicians concerning treatments and medications with an understanding of cause thereof.

PROFESSIONAL NURSING PRACTICE

Professional nursing practice includes:
- Assessment, planning, intervention and evaluation of human responses to health and illness.
- Provision of nursing care to individuals to restore optimum health.
- Procurement, coordination and management of essential patient resources.
- Provision of health counseling and education.
- Establishment of standards of practice for nursing care.
- Development of policies, procedures and protocols.
- Supervision of those assist in the practice of nursing.
- Administration of medications and treatment as prescribed by qualified medical professionals.

ORGANIZATION (FLOW CHART 15.1)

Flow chart 15.1: Structure of organization

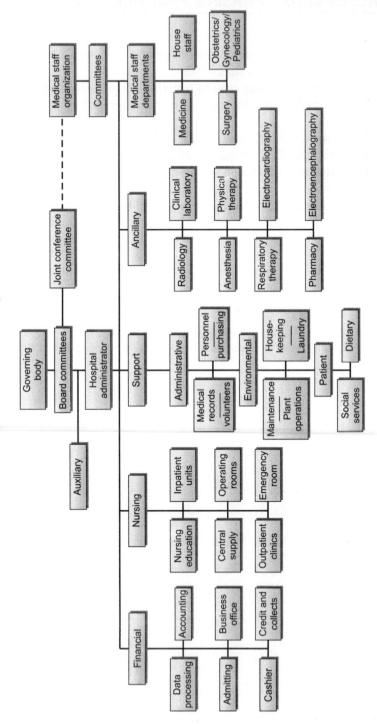

JOB RESPONSIBILITIES, QUALIFICATION AND TRAINING AND EXPERIENCE OF NURSING STAFF

Job	Responsibilities	Education, training and experience
Director of Nursing	• Directs and supervises all nursing staff and activities • Determines and implements nursing policies and procedures • Plans and directs nurses' introduction and in-service training • Evaluates quality of care	PhD/MSc in Nursing with 5 years nursing administration
Assistant Director of Nursing	• Assists Director of nursing and assumes most of the duties and authority during absence • Analyses and evaluates nursing care quality and corrective measures	PhD/MSc Degree in Nursing with 3 years nursing administration
Nursing Supervisor	• Oversees administration and nursing care for a group of Wards or a Special Care Unit and coordinates them with other departments	BSc degree in Nursing with 5 years experience as a Head Nurse
Night Supervisor	• Represents the Administrator at nights • Visits nursing areas, some patients and other departments • Admits and transfers patients when postponement to day time would be inadvisable	Senior staff-nurse with previous experience as a Head Nurse
Ward Sister	• Supervises and manages ward independently in teaching hospitals. Teaches nursing students in GNM and BSc level	BSc degree in nursing with 3 years experience
Senior Staff-nurse	• Functions as ward in charge, supervises junior staff nurses, auxiliary nurses/midwives and nursing aides	General Nursing and Midwifery trained with 5 years experience as staff nurse in a reputed hospital
Staff Nurses	• Provide nursing services in wards, OPD, A&E, Operation theaters, Labor room CSSD, Radiology, etc. under the supervision of Senior staff nurse/ ward sister/ nursing supervisor	General nursing and Midwifery trained
Auxiliary Nurses and Midwives	• Assist staff nurses in wards, OPD, A&E, CSSD, Labor room, Radiology, etc. under the supervision of senior staff nurse/ ward sister	Auxiliary Nursing and Midwifery (ANM) trained

Contd...

Contd...

Job	Responsibilities	Education, training and experience
Ward Aides/ Medical Orderlies	• Assist nurses, provides patient transportation / messenger services	Secondary School Certificate with formal training in a reputed hospital
Ward Clerks	• Inventory control, collection of patient records, laboratory results, responding admitting office queries, laundry, CSSD affairs, etc.	Secondary school Certificate with good handwriting

Specialized Nursing Fields

- Medical surgical
- Obstetrics and gynecology
- Pediatric
- Psychiatry
- Community
- Operation theater technique
- Intensive care unit
- Trauma care
- Coronary care.

Operational Fields of Nursing

- Accident and emergency
- Outpatient clinics
- Wards including special care units
- Delivery suites
- CSSD
- Operating rooms
- Radiology
- Public health
- Nursing education.

DOCUMENTATION OF RECORDS

A list of documents/records maintained in the wards is listed below:
- Day and night report book
- Treatment book/injection book
- Instructions book—the head nurse carries with her when she accompanies the medical officer during ward rounds
- Dangerous drugs register
- Dispatch book
- Inventory book

- Breakages account book
- Standing orders for patients
- Telephone message book (specially maintained for receiving laboratory results of serious patients when required urgently)
- Demand/indent book
- Maintenance/repairs request book.

A List of Medical Record Forms used by Nurses

1. Temperature, pulse, respiration form
2. Nursing progress record form
3. Operation/Special procedures consent form
4. Fluid balance sheet
5. Medication sheet
6. Laboratory mount sheet
7. Preoperative checklist
8. Intake output record
9. Nursing information sheet
10. Nursing care plan
11. 24 Hours bed turning
12. 24 Hours ward returns
13. Diet orders
14. Report form—absconded patient
15. Incident report form.

Approaches to Staff Development Programs

- Providing information about the current developments in nursing (by magazines, video program, inviting experts for lectures/demonstrations, continuing medical education programs)
- Formal programs
- Unit programs
- Workshops and conferences.

Quality of Nursing Care

The Head Nurse of each ward or special care unit controls the quality of nursing care, primarily, and in detail. Nursing Department Office staff make routine and may be unannounced, overall observations, of 'rounds' of ward activities. Remedial action is implemented through the Head Nurse. Such control may relate to the patients' condition (for controlled pain and anxiety), nurses' professional attitude (for example, attention to patients and families), nursing practices (for example, outdated medications returned to Pharmacy department and materials stored properly), and Medical Records (for example, Nurses' notes recorded up-to-date and without erasures). Other matters controlled by the Nursing Department Office include staff meetings (for example, discussions documented adequately and decisions implemented), and nursing environment (for example, corridors clean, equipment working satisfactorily and materials labeled properly.

Communications

Oral communication includes meetings with nursing staff groups for better use of resources and for better patient care. The public address system, using a coded message summons physicians and specially trained nurses to cardiac arrest patients.

Written communication includes the daily patients' census. The administration Manual should include guidance for the Night Supervisor to deal with situations such as power failures and with workers unfit to remain on duty.

Visual communication includes style and color of nurses' uniforms, caps, and belt to signify rank, and lapel pins to signify training school and own name.

Coordination

Coordination is needed:
- Between Nursing Department Office and wards for efficient use of nurses for effective care
- With Medical Staff, while accompanying physicians to patients' bedside
- With Admissions Department to provide accommodation to patients
- Patients selected for clinical lectures and bedside clinics must be available readily for Medical Staff.

Methods of Assigning Nursing Personnel

1. *Case method:* It is the set of activities undertaken by a single nurse to mobilize, monitor and evaluate all resources used by a patient during the episode of an illness.
2. *Functional nursing:* The responsibilities of the unit are assigned to selected people (Head Nurse) according to their expertise.
3. *Team nursing:* In team nursing, ancillary personnel collaborate in providing care to a group of patients under the direction of a professional nurse.
4. *Progressive patient care:* A method in which patient care areas provide various levels of care such as Intensive care unit, post intensive care unit, regular care units, convalescent unit and self-care unit
5. *Primary nursing:* The primary nurse assumes responsibility for planning the care of one or more patients from admittance to discharge.

6. *Modular nursing:* It is a method of nursing assignment in which each nurse is given total responsibility for planning, executing and evaluating nursing care for 4 to 6 patients.

Public Health Nursing—Functions

- To promote Maternal and Child Health Program (MCH)
- To promote health and nutrition education activities
- To coordinate the activities of health visitors in MCH, Family Planning and Health and Nutrition Education
- To coordinate and conduct Immunization programs
- To help in school health program in the district
- To ensure regular supply of equipment, records, registers, drugs, vaccines and other sundries for MCH program
- To ensure the maintenance of prescribed records and submission of periodical progress of MCH/Family Planning/Nutrition programs
- To help the Statistical Officer in compiling periodical progress reports of programs
- To review the progress of public health programs
- To supervise and give technical guidance and support to ANMs and Health Visitors
- To investigate complaints against public health workers
- To provide continuing education for public health workers
- To work with other functionaries of Social Welfare, Rural Development and voluntary organizations.

Utilization of Nursing Resources

- Nurses' time should be spent on nursing, example, providing direct patient care; adequate staffing levels of clinical and non-clinical support services are required.
- Staffing patterns should utilize levels of education, competence, and experience among nurses. Automated information systems and other labor saving devices should be developed and utilized.
- Costing, budgeting, reporting, and tracking nursing resource utilization should be developed and implemented.

Quality Control

Quality control refers to activities that evaluate, monitor, or regulate services rendered to patients, which can be achieved through the following steps:
- Determination of minimum standards
- Collection of information to determine whether standards are met
- Comparing collected information with established criteria
- Making judgment on quality
- Adopting corrective measures if the standards are not met.

Staff Development

Staff development activities include the following:

1. *Induction training:* Briefing philosophy, purpose policies and procedures during first two or three days of employment.
2. *Job orientation:* Intended to acquaint a new employee with job responsibilities, work place and routines.
3. *In-service education and training:* Ongoing on-the-job education given to enhance performance with advanced techniques.
4. *Continuing education:* Educational activity primarily designed to keep the nurses abreast of their field of interest/specialty by updating skills and knowledge.

Nurse Decision-making

- Policy-making and regulatory bodies that have an impact on health care should foster greater representation and active participation of the nursing profession
- Employers should ensure active nurse participation in governance, administration and management
- Employers of nurses and physicians should recognize the appropriate clinical decision-making authority of nurses in relationship to other health care professionals foster communication and collaboration among the health care team, and ensure that the appropriate provider delivers the necessary care; close cooperation and mutual respect between nursing and medicine is essential.

Standards

- *Standard* is a practice that enjoys general recognition and conformity among professionals or an authoritative statement by which the quality of practice, service or education can be judged
- *Standard* are an established rules or basis of comparison in measuring or judging capacity, quantity and value of other products in the same category
- *Standard* is a broad statement of quality
- *Standard* is an acknowledged measure of comparison for quantitative and qualitative values, criterion and norm
- *Standard* is a means of determining what something should be.

Nursing Care Standards

Planning a nursing care standard can be setting a target or a gauge. The following statements visualize the relationship of nursing care standards relating to planning and control devices:

An *objective* is a concrete statement of intention or goal. A *criterion* is the description of variable believed to be an indicator of patient care quality. A *norm* is the current level of performance of a specific criterion, determined by the description of the target population.

By means of objectives, criterion, and norms, the nursing policies and procedures shall be drawn and followed in letter and spirit to establish and maintain required nursing care standards.

Professional Issues

The environment within which every organization function is more stressful than it was in the past. Nursing, traditionally an occupation for women faces additional pressures from the changing opportunities and expectations for women. Nursing, as the largest health profession, has probably received the brunt of the rapid changes in health care services.

On the other hand, physicians delegate more responsibility to nurses. Nurses' responsibilities must be coordinated with many other professions. Organization management is much more aggressive in monitoring and controlling patient care practices.

One of the most persistent problems faced by nursing is that of defining what nursing is and what is distinctive about it. Although nurses understand nursing and perhaps most physicians understand nursing, the difficulty in translating nursing to hospital managers remains an enigma, and both nursing and patient care can suffer. This of course stems from the close historical relationship between medicine and nursing and their joint involvement in the clinical care of the patient. In trying to define the nurse's role in relation to the physician's role, some have suggested *nurse's primary emphasis is concerned with care while medicine is concerned with cure.*

Nursing care is not a series of tasks provided to, at, or for someone, but represents *holistic care* individually rendered and *based on needs* of the patient and family. Such nursing output is not easily measured. This lack of quantification can be a source of frustration for some managers. Long-term patient/family outcomes may be the ultimate evaluation of nursing care. But institutions are not directed to improved patient outcome; indeed the converse may be true; for example, under fee-for service reimbursement systems, there are additional financial rewards for complications, such as infection.

Another model suggested by nursing groups emphasizes a decision-making role for nurses. Although it designates a separate domain of expertise and practice, this approach views nursing interacting with the physicians and other health workers. It sees nursing separated into professional decision-making and leadership and technical (cure and care services) activities. This approach stems from increased emphasis on the behavioral sciences. It also represents a determined effort by the profession to develop a science of nursing that will permit accurate prediction and control of the outcomes of nursing intervention.

Negligence

Negligence is the failure to exercise that a prudent (shrewd in the management of practical affairs) person usually exercises marked by a carelessly easy manner.

A nurse may be held liable under negligence in the following incidents:
- Failure to use aseptic technique where required
- Leaving a foreign body inside a patient's body during surgery (mistakes in sponge, instrument or needle count in surgical cases
- Failing to respond promptly on patient symptoms, in critically ill conditions
- Failing to protect an unstable patient from falling or sustaining injuries by any other means
- Disclosure of patient's information to unauthorized persons/agency
- Administering wrong medicine or over dosage of right medicine.

Do it Absolutely Right and Safe

- Right patient
- Right site
- Right drug
- Right dosage
- Right time
- Right route.

Interdepartmental Relationships of Nursing Services

Being the largest department in any health care facility, they have relationship with each and every service unit of the hospital and they provide round the clock service to patients of all categories. Being the noblest profession of the world, their relationship starts right from the Enquiry Unit, labor-room Medical records, A&E, Wards, special care units, all outpatient clinics, operation theaters, laboratory, radiology CSSD, dietary, social service, laundry, pharmacy, engineering, transports, community health, public health, administrative and up to mortuary services in all levels with high tolerance, accuracy and neatness which is briefed below:

The nursing service is organized into patient care areas by services that include medicine, surgery, obstetrics and gynecology, pediatrics, psychiatry, operating room, outpatient and A&E services. In addition, there may be specialized areas such as cardiac unit, intensive care unit, and respiratory disease unit. The nurse acts as a coordinator of all patient care activities. She works closely with other professionals such as dietitians, medical social workers, pharmacists and others in supplying a comprehensive program of patient care. Good nursing service implies expert observations, which are recorded in the medical record, in medicolegal controversies, nurses' notes are of value as evidence of nursing care given and patient reactions to medical treatment.

The fact that the patient records are in the hands of nursing service throughout a patient's hospitalization brings about the need for a close relationship between medical record and nursing personnel. Prompt preparation and delivery of the medical record by nursing service upon discharge of the patient assist the medical record department in carrying out its many functions. Medical record personnel must understand both the nurses' responsibility in recording nursing treatments and observations, and the duties of ward/ unit clerks as they relate to chart arrangement and movement of records. Ward/unit clerks are usually considered to be members of the nursing service. However, in some hospitals, the ward/unit clerk is a member of the medical record department, and in some others, the ward/unit clerk is responsible to a unit manager directly responsible to administration rather than to nursing.

The medical record director, can be helpful to the nursing department in the development of general and special record forms required for recording nursing observations. He would also be involved in determining these forms are incorporated into the patient medical record. The medical record practitioner can assist the nursing department in the conduct of the nursing audit and in the orientation of new nursing personnel. Better understanding of the overall functions of the medical record department should result with cooperation between the medical record and nursing service departments. The nursing personnel deal with medical records in outpatient clinics, emergency service and in wards. In fact, the nursing personnel are the first to handle the records before the medical staff gets them. Proper maintenance of records in the outpatient clinics and emergency service rests mainly with the nursing staff. In case of missing records or reports are conveyed by the nursing staff, to the medical record staff for tracing and making available for patient care. In some hospitals, in the absence of medical record staff, nursing personnel take the responsibility of maintaining records. The nursing staff collects laboratory, X-ray and other reports and mounts them in the respective records and also X-rays are arranged and placed in the appropriate patient records. They take the responsibility of collecting and handing over the records to medical record department. During hospitalization of a patient, the in-charge nurse of the ward collects the investigation reports and mounts them in the concerned record. The X-rays of patients are also collected and kept safely and returned along with patient medical record to the MRD after discharge of the patient. The ward nurse collects and maintains medical record forms in the ward; She takes the responsibility for preparation of birth, death, and stillbirth notifications. The nursing staff also informs if any case happens to be medicolegal one. She helps in getting consent from the patient. The admission and discharge register maintained in the ward helps in preparing 'Daily Ward Census' of patients and also help in tracing out old records of patients. The nursing staff is an instrument in getting records completed by the medical staff and always assists the doctors in completing operation notes, discharge summary, final diagnosis and so on. The nursing staff has close relationship with the admitting office, and informs regularly the bed status of the ward. The nursing staff fixes for follow-up care. The nursing staff also helps in recording correct identification data in all the forms of the record.

PERFORMANCE APPRAISALS

1. *Trait rating scales:* Rating an individual against a set standard.
2. *Job dimension scales:* Rating factors are taken from written job description.
3. *Behaviorally anchored rating scales:* A technique that requires a separate rating form developed for each job classification.
4. *Checklists:* Composed of many behavior styles that indicate desirable behaviors. Score is based on behavior or attributes.
5. *Essays:* The appraiser describes the employee strengths and area where improvement or perfection is needed.

PROBLEMS

1. Time management
2. Frequent change of nurses between service units
3. Medication orders by physicians over telephone
4. Too many instructions from many sides
5. Answering everybody
6. Distractions and forgetting instructions
7. Controlling visitors.

Note

If any issue is managed with team spirit, considering the well being of patients, most of the problems can be easily avoided. Egoistic nature of professionals should not affect quality of patient care.

Date	Time	Temp	Pulse	Resp	BP	Pupils and Fundi	State of Consciousness	Breathing Control		Muscle Tone & Reflexes	Arterial Pulses			Color
								Coughing	Respirations		Ankl	G molar	Poplit	

SPECIFIC NURSING CARE, COMMENTS

NURSES OBSERVATION CHART

Bed No.: _____   Page No.: _____

Date	Time	Treat	Nurses Notes	Signature

Please Date and Sign each Entry

NURSES NOTES FORM

16 Pathology

INTRODUCTION

Pathology; *patho* means disease, *ology* means study of, hence pathology is study of diseases. It is a branch of medicine, concerned with the study of disease in all aspects, namely nature, causes, development, and consequence. Examination of pathologic condition is divided into several subspecialties like, clinical, cellular pathologies. Macroscopic and microscopic observations are made on body tissues, internal organs, and structures, following dissections. Gross specimens, by size, color, texture, and appearance, are examined, in addition, to analyzing gross and microscopic specimens, pathologists, are frequently called on to form a frozen section. Permanent sections are taken for routine microscopic examination to decide the pathologic conditions. The pathology department also performs autopsy (postmortem examination of the body including the internal organs and structures after dissection so as to determine the cause of death of or the nature of pathological nature which is also called necropsy.

Pathology is the study and diagnosis of disease through examination of organs, tissues, bodily fluids, and whole bodies (autopsies). Pathology also encompasses the related scientific study of disease processes, called General pathology.

Medical pathology is divided in two main branches, Anatomical pathology and Clinical pathology. Veterinary pathology is concerned with animal disease whereas Phytopathology is the study of plant diseases.

General pathology, also called investigative pathology, experimental pathology or theoretical pathology, is a broad and complex scientific field which seeks to understand the mechanisms of injury to cells and tissues, as well as the body's means of responding to and repairing injury. Areas of study include cellular adaptation to injury, necrosis, inflammation, wound healing and neoplasia. It forms the foundation of pathology, the application of this knowledge to diagnose diseases in humans and animals.

The term "general pathology" is also used to describe the practice of both anatomical and clinical pathology.

PATHOLOGY AS A MEDICAL SPECIALTY (FIG. 16.1)

Pathologists are physicians who diagnose and characterize disease in living patients by examining biopsies or bodily fluid. The vast majority of cancer diagnoses are made or confirmed by a pathologist. Pathologists may also conduct autopsies to investigate causes of death. Pathology is a core discipline of medical school and many pathologists are also teachers. As managers of medical laboratories which include chemistry, microbiology, cytology, the blood bank, etc. pathologists play an important role in the development of Laboratory information systems. Although the medical practice of pathology grew out of the tradition of investigative pathology, most modern pathologists do not perform original research.

Pathology is a medical specialty although pathologists typically do not see patients directly, but rather serves as consultants to other physicians (often referred to as "clinicians" within the pathology community). To be licensed, candidates must complete medical training, an approved residency program and be certified by an appropriate body. In the US, certification is by the American Board of Pathology or the American Osteopathic Board of Pathology. The organization of subspecialties within pathology varies between nations, but usually includes anatomical pathology and clinical pathology.

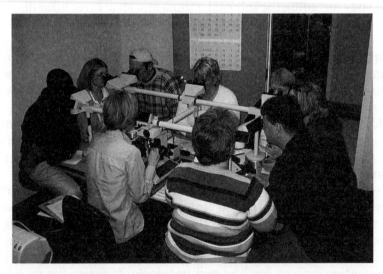

Fig. 16.1: Pathologist instructor and students of anatomical pathology
(*For color version, see Plate 1*)

Anatomical Pathology

Anatomical pathology (*Commonwealth*) or Anatomic pathology (*US*) is a medical specialty that is concerned with the diagnosis of disease based on the gross, microscopic, chemical, immunologic and molecular examination of organs, tissues and whole bodies (autopsy).

Anatomical pathology is itself divided in subspecialties, the main ones being surgical pathology, cytopathology and forensic pathology. To be licensed to practice pathology, one has to complete medical school and secure a license to practice medicine. An approved residency program and certification (in the US, the American board of Pathology or the American Osteopathic Board of Pathology) is usually required to obtain employment or hospital privileges.

Anatomical pathology is one of the two branches of pathology, the other being clinical pathology, the diagnosis of disease through the laboratory analysis of bodily fluids and/or tissues. Often, pathologists practice both anatomical and clinical pathology, a combination known as general pathology. The distinction between anatomic and clinical pathology is increasingly blurred by the introduction of technologies that require new expertize and the need to provide patients and referring physicians with integrated diagnostic reports. Similar specialties exist in veterinary pathology.

Clinical Pathology

Clinical pathology is a medical specialty that is concerned with the diagnosis of disease based on the laboratory analysis of bodily fluids such as blood and urine, and tissues using the tools of chemistry, microbiology, hematology and molecular pathology. Clinical pathologists work in close collaboration with medical technologists, hospital administrations and referring physicians to ensure the accuracy and optimal utilization of laboratory testing.

Clinical pathology is one of the two major divisions of pathology, the other being anatomical pathology. Often, pathologists practice both anatomical and clinical pathology, a combination sometimes known as general pathology.

Biomedical science which is a field of science, must not be confused with Pathology, a field of medicine.

Forensic Pathology

Forensic pathology is a branch of pathology concerned with determining the cause of death by examination of a cadaver. The autopsy is performed by the pathologist at the request of a coroner usually during the investigation of criminal law cases and civil law cases in some jurisdictions. Forensic pathologists are also frequently asked to confirm the identity of a cadaver (The word forensics is derived from the Latin *forçnsis* meaning *forum.*).

Veterinary Pathology

Veterinary pathologists are doctors of veterinary medicine who specialize in the diagnosis of diseases through the examination of animal tissue and body fluids. Like for medical pathology, veterinary pathology is divided in two branches, anatomical pathology and clinical pathology. Veterinary pathologists are critical participants in the drug development process.

Plant Pathology

Plant pathology (also Phytopathology) is the scientific study of plant diseases caused by pathogens (infectious diseases) and environmental conditions (physiological factors). Organisms that cause infectious disease include fungi, oomycetes, bacteria, viruses, viroids, virus-like organisms, phytoplasmas, protozoa, nematodes and parasitic plants. Not included are insects, mites, vertebrate or other pests that affect plant health by consumption of plant tissues. Plant pathology also involves the study of pathogen identification, disease etiology, disease cycles, economic impact, plant disease epidemiology, plant disease resistance, how plant diseases affect humans and animals, pathosystem genetics, and management of plant diseases.

The *"Disease triangle"* is a central concept of plant pathology. It is based on the principle that infectious diseases develop, or do not develop, based on three-way interactions between the host, the pathogen and environmental conditions.

Molecular Pathology

Molecular pathology is an emerging discipline within pathology which is focused in the study and diagnosis of disease through the examination of molecules within organs, tissues or bodily fluids. Molecular pathology shares some aspects of practice with both anatomic pathology and clinical pathology, molecular biology, biochemistry, proteomics and genetics, and is sometimes considered a "crossover" discipline. It is multi-disciplinary in nature and focuses mainly on the sub-microscopic aspects of disease and unknown illnesses with strange causes.

It is a scientific discipline that encompasses the development of molecular and genetic approaches to the diagnosis and classification of human tumors, the design and validation of predictive biomarkers for treatment response and disease progression, the susceptibility of individuals of different genetic constitution to develop cancer and the environmental and lifestyle factors implicated in carcinogenesis.

Bed No.: _____   Diagnosis: _____

Specimen: ☐ Blood ☐ Urine ☐ CSF ☐ Other   Date & Time Requested:
☐ Routine ☐ Urgent ☐ Preop ☐ Stat   Requested by:

Alb/glob	gm/dl	(3.8-4.8/2.4-3.5)	O ZIT	KU	(2-12)
Urea N B	mg/dl	(7-22)	O COT	IU/L	(8-33)
U	mg/dl		O GPT	IU/L	(3-36)
Creatining B	mg/dl	(0.4-1.5)	O Alk P-tase	IU/L	(2.5-9.7)
U	mg/dl		O LDH	IU/L	(100-190)
Uric acid B	mg/dl	(M.3.8-7.1/F.2.6-5.6)	O Bilirubin T.	mg/dl	(1.5)
U	mg/dl		O D	mg/dl	(0.36)
Mg	mg/dl	(1.8-2.4)	O BSP 45 min	%	(5)
Ca	mg/dl	(9-11)	O LLDH	IU/L	(0-20)
P	mg/dl	(2.5-4.9)	O r-GT	IL/L	(M.15.85/F.5.55)
Na	mmol/l	(135-145)	O CPK	IU/L	(50-180)
K	mmol/l	(3.8-5.0)	O HBDH	IU/L	(170-300)
Cl	mmol/l	(96-108)	O Lactic acid	mEq/L	(0.5-2.2)
Li	mmol/l	(0.4-2.0)	O Total protein	mg/dl	
Ammonia	umol/L	(11-35)	O Sugar AC	mg/dl	(70-110)
Fe	ug/dl	(42-135)	O PC	mg/dl	
TIBC	ug/dl	(280-400)	O GTT		
Amylase	U	(5-75)	O Electrophoresis		
Acid P-taste	IU/L	(0-0.8)	O Salicylate	mg/dl	(29)
Mucoprotein	mg/dl	(75-135)	O Blood pH/gas		
Cholesterol	mg/dl	(120-280)	Blood O Arterial, O Venous		
Triglyceride	mg/dl	(30-200)	Breathing O Air, _____ % O_2		
T4	ug/dl	(4-12)	pH _____		(7.31-7.45)
T3	ug/dl	(80-200)	PCO_2		(33-48)
			_____ mm Hg		
T3 uptake	%	(24-36)	PO_2		(80-104)
			_____ mm Hg		
TSH	uU/ml	(10)	HCO_3		(21-25)
			_____ mEq/L		
			Base		(M 2.4-2.3)
			excess _____ mEq/L		(F 3.3-1.2)

Specimen Description:

Hemolysis: + ++ +++

Lactescene: + ++ +++

Remark: Check by   Examiner   Date

CHEMISTRY/BLOOD GAS FORM

Hospital _____
Unit/Clinic _____

No. _____
Name _____
Sex _____
D.O.B _____
I.D. No. _____

Bed No _____ Diagnosis _____

☐ Routine ☐ Urgent
☐ Preop   ☐ Stat

Date & Time Requested:
Requested By:

• Hb gm%	• ESR 1" mm 2" mm	• RBC morphology
• RBC x10⁴/cmm	• Bleeding time min	Anisocytosis
• Hct %	• Clotting time min	Poikilocytosis
• MCV u	• Prothrombin time sec control sec	Polychromatophilia ( )
• MCH uug	• PTT sec control sec	Target cell ( )
• MCHC %	• TGT	• Sickle cell ( )
• Retic %	• Fetal Hb %	• Bone marrow exam
• Platelet /cmm	• Osmotic fragility test	• L-E prep
• WBC /cmm	Initial %	• Fibrinogen mg/dl
• Blood type ( )	Complete %	• Others (Specify)
• Rh Type ( )		

• Differential	Mybl	Pro	Myelo	Meta	Band	Seg	Eos	Baso	Mono	Lymph		
%												

Remarks   Checked by   Examiner   Date

HEMATOLOGY FORM (26)

• Latex RA	• VDRL
• C-Reactive Protein	• TPHA
• Coombs' test: Direct	• Hb₅ Ag
Indirect ( )	
• ASO Titer	• Echinococcus Ah. Titer
• Cold Hemagglutinin	• Shistosoma Ab. Titer
• Anti A Titer	• Brucella Ab. Titer
• Anti B Titer	
• Mono test	
• IgG mg/dl	
• IgA mg/dl	• Salmonella Ab. Titer
• IgM mg/dl	
• IgD mg/dl	
• Fetoprotein	
Remarks	

Abort	Melit	Suis

A	B	C	D	E	F	G	H	ox19	ox2	oxk

Check by   Examiner   Date

SEROLOGY FORM (27)

Appearnce: plain, light, dark, yellow, brownish, reddish, greenish, bloody, clear, turbid   • Sp. gr. _____

• Combur:
    • pH( )   • Protein( )   • Glucose   • Ketone( )
    • Bilirubin( )   • Urobilinogen( )   • Occult Blood( )

• Sediment:
RBC(/HPF), WBC(/HPF), Epith cell(/HPF), Cast(/HPF), Crystal(/HPF),
Others:

• Microorganisms:
• Pregnancy Test:

Remarks   Check by   Examiner   Date

URINALYSIS FORM (28)

• Routine
  Apperance   Transparent, hazy, fainty, turbid, purulent, colorless, yellow, reddish
                Bloody( ), coagulation( ), pellicles( ), sediment( )
  Protein   Pandy( ), Nonne-Apelt( ),
  Glucose   mg/dl
  Cell count   Differential count: Polymorpho   % Mono   %

• Gram's stain
• Acid-fast stain
• Others (Specify)

Remarks   Check by   Examiner   Date

CSF ANALYSIS FORM

	No.: —————————————————
	Name: ———————————————
Hospital: ———————————————————	Sex: —————————————————
Unit/Clinic: ———————————————————	D.O.B. —————————————————
	I.D. No: ———————————————

Bed No.: ————————— Diagnosis: ————————————————————————

Specimen: ☐ Routine ☐ Urgent	Date and Time Requested:
☐ Preop ☐ Stat	Requested By:

0 Routine
  Appearance: Clear, opalescent, turbid, light, straw, yellow-green, greenish, reddish.
              bloody (   ), Chylous (   ), coagulation (   )
  Sp. gr. (   ),Rivalta (   ) Cell count:
  Differential count: Polymorpho   % mono   %, Abnormal cells (   ).
0 Gram's stain
0 Loeffler's stain
0 Acid-fast stain
0 Others (Specify)
  Remarks: Check by: Examiner: Date:

BODY FLUID ANALYSIS FORM (30)

Character: Fluid, semifluid, soft, formed, hard, yellow, brown, green, black tarry,
            red, clay; mucus(   ), pus (   ), blood(   ), fat(   ), gas bubbles (   ),

0 Occult blood:	0 Neutral fat
0 Parasites and ova	0 Fatty acid
0 Ameba	0 Starch
0 Others (Specify)	

  Remarks: Check by: Examiner: Date:

STOOL ANALYSIS FORM (31)

Appearance: serous, mucous, purulent, bloody, chessy
            microscopic   elastic fiber (   ), crystal (   ).
0 Acid - fast stain (Negative, Positive   /F).
0 Paragonims ova (Negative, Positive   /F).
0 Loeffler's stain
0 Gram's stain

  Remarks: Check by: Examiner: Date:

SPUTUM ANALYSIS FORM (32)

Request:

Result:

Remarks:

                 Check by: Examiner: Date:

MULTIPURPOSE USE FORM

17 | Laboratory Investigation Cookbook

INTRODUCTION

The author has taken care to incorporate this chapter especially for the benefit of users of the *Paramedics 6-in-1 Handbook*. When we talk of general and special investigations that includes test of laboratories such as pathology, microbiology, serology, biochemistry, radiology, diagnostic therapies, ECG, EEG, ultrasound, CT scan and MRI. Investigations as such are vital part of dynamic medicine. Without these tests detecting, proper diagnoses would not have happened and without established diagnoses, there would not be in any remedial treatment. Precisely, appropriate investigation carried out in patient on time would reveal the health problem of the patient that will help the doctors and medical care providers to plan and treat the disease/injury promptly that remedies the sick and injured not only saves live but also prevents further aggravation and complications. It is hard to measure dimension and role of investigation.

The role of investigations have tremendously increased in curing preventing, promoting and rehabilitating the sick and injured despite of medical education, sophisticated equipment, supersonic technology and extensive global medical research. Hence, investigations find a place in vital part of health care delivery system and the professionals especially nursing and paramedical should have a good background picture of names of investigations that are required to establish accurate diagnosis /injuries.

Almost all-important investigations are classified and presented in the following manner to serve as quick "cook book" to users:

1. Description of some investigations commonly used to establish diagnoses
2. Selected diagnoses and required investigations

3. Variations of investigations (increase and decrease) with normal values and resulting diagnoses
4. List of normal values of investigations in alphabetical order.

This list will be of great value for all those who are involved in analysis of ambulatory, discharge record analysis, quality assurance, case mix studies, diagnostic related group, cost calculation for investigation and justification of diagnoses, and deviation of investigation studies, etc.

DESCRIPTION OF THE LABORATORY AND RADIOLOGICAL INVESTIGATIONS (SYSTEMWISE)

Blood and Lymphatic System

S.No.	Name of the test	Description
1.	Hemoglobin	Measurement of the amount of hemoglobin in blood sample
2.	Hematocrit	Percentage of erythrocytes (RBC) in a volume of blood
3.	White blood cell count	Number of white blood cells or leukocytes per cubic millimeter
4.	White blood cell differential count	Numbers of different types of leukocytes (immature and mature forms)
5.	Platelet count	Number of platelets per cubic millimeter of blood
6.	Red blood cell count	Number of erythrocytes per cubic millimeter of blood
7.	Erythrocyte sedimentation	Speed at which erythrocytes settle out of plasma
8.	Prothrombin time	Ability of the blood to clot
9.	Partial thromboplastin time	Determination of the presence of important clotting factors in the blood
10.	Antiglobulin test	This test demonstrates whether the patient's erythrocytes are coated with antibody and is useful in determining the presence of antibodies in infants or "RH" women
11.	Bleeding time	A small stab wound is made in the earlobe or forearm and the time required for it to stop bleeding is recorded. This test evaluates the vascular and platelet factors associated with hemostasis. Failure of either of these components leads to a prolonged bleeding time. An increase in noted in thrombocytopenia, ingestion of anti-inflammatory drugs, and infiltration of bone marrow by primary or metastatic tumors
12.	Alpha-fetoprotein (AFP)	A plasma protein found normally in some embryonic tissue. It is also present in the blood of adults with hepatocellular carcinoma and germ cell neoplasms. The AFP levels are used to monitor the effectiveness of cancer therapy in patients with these types of malignancies

Musculoskeletal System

S.No.	Name of the test	Description
1.	Rheumatoid factor	The serum of a patient with rheumatoid arthritis contains this antibody in elevated levels. The test, however, is not specific since rheumatoid factor is present in aging, scleroderma, acute pulmonary tuberculosis, systemic lupus erythematosus, and other disorders

Skin

S.No.	Name of the test	Description
1.	Bacterial analysis	Sample of purulent (pus-filled) material or exudates (fluid which accumulates in a space or passes out of tissues) is sent to the laboratory for examination to determine what type of bacteria is present
2.	Fungal tests	Scrapings from skin lesions are placed on a growth medium for several weeks and then examined microscopically for evidence for fungal growth

Endocrine System

S.No.	Name of the test	Description
1.	Serum tests	The measurement of the following substances in serum (blood) is important in diagnosing endocrine disorders:

Substance	Endocrine gland gunction
Calcium	Parathyroid gland
Cortisol	Adrenal cortex
Electrolytes	Adrenal cortex
Estradiol (estrogen)	Ovaries
FSH	Adenohypophysis
HGH	Adenohypophysis
Insulin	Pancreas
LH	Adenohypophysis
Parathyroid hormone	Parathyroid gland
Prolactin	Adenohypophysis
T3	Thyroid gland
Free thyroxin (not bound to protein)	Thyroid gland
Testosterone	Testis
TSH	Adenohypophysis

The following substances are measured in the urine as indicators of endocrine function:

Substance	Endocrine gland function
Calcium	Parathyroid gland
Catecholamines	Adrenal medulla
Free cortisol	Adrenal cortex
Electrolytes	Adrenal cortex
17-hydroxycorticosteroids	Adrenal cortex
17-ketosteroids	Adrenal cortex

Contd...

Contd...

S.No.	Name of the test	Description
1.		Ketones Pancreas Glucose Pancreas
	Blood sugar	Blood sugar determination helps to estimate the amount of glucose in the blood when the patient is fasting and after the food is consumed. High percent of glucose in the blood indicate the presence of diabetes mellitus and low percent indicates hypoglycemia. Blood sugar determination helps to estimate the amount of glucose in the blood when the patient is fasting and after the food is consumed. High percent of glucose in the blood indicate the presence of diabetes mellitus and low percent indicates hypoglycemia
2.	Fasting blood sugar	Used to detect abnormalities of glucose metabolism. The level of glucose in the blood is determined after the patient has fasted for 8 hours
3.	Glucose tolerance test	This test measures the glucose level in a blood sample from a fasting patient (fasting blood sugar) and in specimens taken 50 minutes, 1 hour, 2 hours, and 3 hours after ingestion of 100 gm of glucose
4.	Radioimmunoassay	This test measures hormone levels in plasma

Cardiovascular System

S.No.	Name of the test	Description
1.	Serum enzyme tests	During a myocardial infarction, enzymes released into the bloodstream from the heart muscle can be measured and found as evidence of an infarction
2.	Lipid tests	Lipids are fatty substances found in food and in the bloodstream. Lipid tests measure the amounts of these substances in a blood sample
3.	Lipoprotein electrophoresis	Lipoproteins are fats (lipids) and protein molecules bound together. Protein electrophoresis is the process of physically separating lipoproteins from a blood sample

Respiratory System

S.No.	Name of the test	Description
1.	Pulmonary function tests	This group of tests evaluates ventilation capabilities of the lungs
2.	Tuberculin test	Antigens such as PPDC (purified protein derivative) are applied to the skin with multiple punctures (tine tests) or intradermally (matoux test). A local inflammatory reaction is observed in infected persons after 48 to 96 hours
3.	Sputum culture and sensitivity (CS)	Bacteriological procedure used to isolate the organism causing disease, especially pneumonia. When the caustic organism is isolated, this test determines which antibiotic will be effective for treatment

Digestive System

S.No.	Name of the test	Description
1.	Liver function tests	SGOT (serum glutamic oxyacetic transaminase) SGPT (serum glutamic pyruvic transaminase) These tests reveal the levels of enzymes (SGOT and SGPT) in the blood serum. Enzyme levels are elevated when there is damage to liver cells
2.	ALP (alkaline phosphate)	This is another enzyme test done on serum. An increased level of alkaline phosphatase is found in liver disease
3.	Serum bilirubin	High level of bilirubin in the blood produces a jaundiced condition in the patient. This test indicates excessive hemolysis, hepatic disorders, or obstructive conditions of the bile ducts. Serum bilirubin is formed from the breakdown of hemoglobin. In the liver, bilirubin is secreted into the bile and then excreted into the intestinal tract through the bile ducts
4.	Stool culture	Feces are placed in a growth medium to test for the presence of microorganisms
5.	Occult blood	Determines bleeding in gastrointestinal disorders. Because this test is so sensitive, the patient is instructed to have a meat-free diet for 3 days before the test. The presence of undigested mean can give a false-positive reading
6.	Stool guaiac	Guaiac is added to a stool sample to reveal the presence of blood in the feces

Urinary System

S.No.	Name of the test	Description
1.	Blood urea nitrogen (BUN)	This test measures the amount of urea in the blood. Normally the urea level is low since urea is excreted in the urine continuously. When the kidney is diseased or fails, however, urea accumulates in the blood and this can lead to unconsciousness and death
2.	Urinalysis	One of the most widely used laboratory tests. It provides general information regarding the health of the body as a whole as well as specific information on the conditions of the urinary structures
3.	Creatinine clearance test	This test measures the ability of the kidney to remove creatinine from the blood. A blood sample is drawn and the amount of creatinine concentration is compared with the amount of creatinine excreted in the urine during a 24-hour period. If the kidney is not functioning well in its job of clearing creatinine from the blood, there will be a disproportionate amount of creatinine in the blood, compared with the urine

Female Reproductive System

S.No.	Name of the test	Description
1.	Pap test	Microscopic analysis of the cell smear (spread on a glass slide) can detect the presence of cervical or vaginal carcinoma
2.	Pregnancy test	This test detects the presence or human chorionic gonadotropin (HCG) in the urine or blood
3.	Endometrial biopsy	Used in screening high-risk patients for endometrial cancer. This test is done as an office procedure during the gynecologic examination. Following the administration of a small amount of anesthetic, a thin, hollow curette is used to remove endometrial tissue for laboratory analysis

Male Reproductive System

S.No	Name of the test	Description
1.	Semen analysis	This test is done for fertility analysis and is also to establish the effectiveness of vasectomy. Sperm cells are counted and examined for motility and shape
2.	VDRL (venereal disease research laboratory) test	This test is for syphilis. The patient's blood (serum) is placed with the syphilis antigen (spirochete)
3.	FTA-ABS Test	This is more specific test for syphilis. The syphilis bacterium is actually searched for under the microscope

Cancer Medicine

S.No	Name of the test	Description
1.	CEA test (carcino-embryonic antigen) test	Carcinoembryonic antigen can be found in the bloodstream of patients with a variety of tumors of gastrointestinal origin. Measurements of levels in the bloodstream can lead to early identification, resection, and possible cure of some cases
2.	Alpha-fetoprotein test	This test detects the presence of the protein antigen (alpha-fetoprotein) in the serum of patients with liver and testicular cancer
3.	Beta-HCG (human chorionic gonadotropin) Test	This blood test detects the presence of a portion of human chorionic gonadotropin (HCG) in the serum of patients with testicular cancer and is used as a marker for the presence of tumor cells in the body
4.	Estrogen (estradiol) receptor assay	This test measures the concentration of estrogen receptor site on tumor cells of breast cancer patients

SELECTED DIAGNOSIS WITH REQUIRED INVESTIGATIONS

S.No.	Diagnosis	System	Investigations
1.	Achalasia cardia	Gastrointestinal	X-ray, fluoroscopy
2.	Acne vulgaris	Skin	Skin test
3.	Acoustic neuroma	ENT	ENT examination, lumbar puncture—CSF culture
4.	Acute alcohol intoxication	General	Toxicology test, BP, pupil examination, blood Gas analysis, blood examination, blood alcohol level, urine analysis, stool test
5.	Acute bronchitis	Respiratory	Chest X-ray, blood gas analysis, sputum culture
6.	Acute cholecystitis	Gastrointestinal	WBC differential, X-ray
7.	Acute gastritis	Gastrointestinal	Endoscopy
8.	Acute glomerulonephritis	Nephrology	Renal funtion test, electrolytic examination, ESR, BP, 24 hours urine volume, blood culture, hyaline test, specific gravity, urine analysis,
9.	Acute leukemia	Hematology	Hematological examination, total WBC, differential WBC, bone marrow test, lymph node examination
10.	Acute mesenteric lymphadenitis	Gastrointestinal	Lymph node aspiration or culture
11.	Acute mesenteric vascular occlusion	Gastrointestinal	WBC differential, hemoglobin
12.	Acute morphine poisoning	General	Toxicology test, BP, pupil examination, blood gas analysis, blood examination, stool test, urine analysis
13.	Acute organic small bowel obstruction	Gastrointestinal	WBC differential, X-ray
14.	Acute otitis media	ENT	ENT examination, ESR, swap culture, audiometry test
15.	Acute pancreatitis	Gastrointestinal	WBC differential, serum amylase, urine amylase, lipase
16.	Acute pyelonephritis	Nephrology	Renal function test, electrolytic examination, ESR, BP, 24 hours urine volume, blood culture, hyaline test, specific gravity, urine analysis and culture,
17.	Acute renal failure	Nephrology	Renal function test, electrolytic examination, ESR, BP, 24 hours urine volume, blood culture, hyaline test, specific gravity, urine analysis and culture,
18.	Acute respiratory failure	Respiratory	BP, chest X-ray, blood gas analysis, ESR, ECG, blood examination, blood and urine culture
19.	Acute retention of urine	Nephrology	Cystoscopy, ultrasound kidney, intravenous pylogram, X-ray kidney, ureter, bladder
20.	Acute rheumatic fever	Pediatric	Pediatric examination, cardilogical consultation, ESR, chest X-ray, differential WBC, ECG, RH factor titer
21.	Addison's disease	Nephrology	BP, total and differential WBC, hematological study, 17 hydroxy corticoids level
22.	Adult respiratory distress syndrome	Respiratory	WBC total, ESR, X-ray
23.	Agranulocytosis	General	Total WBC, differential WBC, ESR, lymph node examination
24.	Alcoholic hepatitis	Gastrointestinal	Alkaline phosphatase, SGOT, liver biopsy, prothrombin time
25.	Amenorrhea	Gynecological	Irregular menstrual cycle, pregnancy test, tubercline test, Hb count

Contd...

Contd...

S.No.	Diagnosis	System	Investigations
26.	Amoebiasis	Gastrointestinal	Stool, sigmoidoscopy
27.	Anaemia	Pediatric	Pediatric examination, Hb count, ESR, LFT, ultrasound spleen
28.	Anal fissure	Gastrointestinal	Stool, sigmoidoscopy
29.	Anaphylitic shock	General	Toxicology test, BP, pupil examination, blood examination, stool test, urine analysis
30.	Anemia	General	Hemoglobin, RBC, hematocrit
31.	Angina pectoris	Cardiovascular	ECG, angiography, radioisotope
32.	Aortic regurgitation	Pediatric	Pediatric examination, cardiological consultation, chest X-ray, barium X-ray, sputum culture, RH factor titer, hematological study
33.	Aortic stenosis	Pediatric	Pediatric examination, cardiological consultation, chest X-ray, ECG
34.	Aortic stenosis	Cardiovascular	ECG, X-ray, Doppler echocardiography
35.	Appendicitis	Gastrointestinal	WBC differential, X-ray abdomen, liver function test
36.	Arsenic poisoning	General	Toxicology test, BP, pupil examination, blood gas analysis, blood examination, stool test, urine analysis
37.	Ascites	Gastrointestinal	Diagnostic paracentesis, protein analysis, blood count, blood culture, AFT, amylase, WBC total, WBC differential, LFT
38.	Atelectasis	Respiratory	X-ray, CT scan
39.	Atypical pneumonia	Respiratory	WBC total, sputum culture, X-ray
40.	Bacillary dysentery	Gastrointestinal	Stool culture
41.	Barbiturate poisoning	General	Toxicology test, BP, pupil examination, blood examination, stool test, urine analysis
42.	Bee sting	General	Skin test
43.	Bell's palsy	Neurology	Nervous conduction test, EMG, phenatine assay test
44.	Bronchopneumonia	Pediatric	Pediatric examination, chest X-ray, stool test, electrolytic test
45.	Bronchial adenoma	Respiratory	Bronchoscopy
46.	Bronchial asthma	Respiratory	WBC total, WBC differential, ESR, sputum culture, blood gas analysis, PFT, X-ray chest, allergic skin test
47.	Bronchiectasis	Respiratory	WBC total, sputum culture, X-ray, bronchogram
48.	Bronchiolar carcinoma	Respiratory	Sputum, chest X-ray, bronchoscopy, biopsy
49.	Bronchopneumonia	Respiratory	Blood culture, WBC differential, X-ray
50.	Burns	General	Electrolytic analysis, skin test, BP, blood examination
51.	Cancer cervix	Gynecological	Hb count, ESR, differential WBC count, blood culture, lymph biopsy
52.	Cancer colon	Gastrointestinal	Hemoglobin, sigmoidoscopic and X-ray
53.	Cancer oesophagus	Gastrointestinal	Hemoglobin, barium swallow
54.	Candidiasis (Thrush)	Gastrointestinal	Skin test
55.	Carcinoma of body of uterus	Gynecological	ESR, urine analysis, Hb count, differential WBC count, pap smear, biopsy cervix, lymph node

Contd...

Contd...

S.No.	Diagnosis	System	Investigations
56.	Carcinoma of liver	Gastrointestinal	Hemoglobin, liver function test, ultrasound and CT scan, liver scan
57.	Carcinoma of stomach	Gastrointestinal	Hemoglobin, stool, gastroscopic and X-ray
58.	Cardiac arrest	Cardiovascular	BP, ECG, chest X-ray, pupil examination, blood gas analysis, blood examination
59.	Cardiogenic shock	Cardiovascular	BP, ECG, chest X-ray, pupil examination, blood gas analysis, blood examination
60.	Cardiogenic shock	Cardiovascular	Urine flow, blood gas analysis, blood pressure, ECG
61.	Cervicitis	Gynecological	Biopsy cervix, histological study, urine analysis, culture
62.	Choledocholithiasis	Gastrointestinal	WBC differential, liver function test, platelet count
63.	Cholera	Gastrointestinal	Stool culture
64.	Cholesteatoma	ENT	ENT examination, audiometry test, PNS X-ray
65.	Chronic bronchitis	Respiratory	Sputum, X-ray
66.	Chronic cholecystitis	Gastrointestinal	X-ray
67.	Chronic bastritis	Gastrointestinal	WBC differential, gastroscopy
68.	Chronic lymphatic leukemia	Hematology	Total and differential WBC, HB count, bone marrow test, lymph node examination, hematological study
69.	Chronic obstructive	Respiratory pulmonary disease	Chest X-ray, planogram, CT scan-lungs, WBC total, differential, RBC, spirometry
70.	Chronic simple otitis media	ENT	ENT examination, audiometry test, PNS X-ray
71.	Chronic myeloid leukemia	Hematology	Total and differential WBC, Hb count, lymph node examination, hematological study, bone marrow test
72.	Congenital syphilis	Pediatric	Paediatric examination, Hb count, weight loss, LFT, X-ray of fore and hind bone
73.	Congestive cardiac failure	Cardiovascular	BP, ECG, echocardiogram, chest X-ray, cardiac enzyme test, lipid profile,LFT, serum potassium level
74.	Contact dermatitis	Skin	Skin scrach test
75.	Cushing's syndrome	Endocrine	Plasma cortisol test, ACTH
76.	Deafness	ENT	ENT examination, audiometry test,
77.	Dehydration	General	Electrolytic analysis, skin test, BP
78.	Delaying menstruation	Gynecological	Irregular, menstrual cycle, Hb count
79.	Dermatophytosis	Skin	Scaling skin test
80.	Deviated nasal septum	ENT	ENT examination, PNS X-ray
81.	Dhaturia poisoning	General	Toxicology test, BP, ECG, pupil examination, skint test, blood gas analysis, blood examination, photosensitivity test, urine analysis, stool analysis
82.	Diabetes insipidus	Endocrine	24 urine volume, ADH test,
83.	Diabetes mellitus	Endocrine	24 Urine volume, ADH test, GTT, sugar level, blood sugar level—fasting and postprandial, urine sugar level,
84.	Diabetic ketoacidosis	Endocrine	Blood sugar level—fasting and postprandial, electrolytic analysis, ketone test, urine sugar and ketone test, urine analysis
85.	Diphtheria	Pediatric	Pediatric examination, swap culture, ESR

Contd...

Contd...

S.No.	Diagnosis	System	Investigations
86.	Discharge from ear	ENT	ENT examination, swap culture test,
87.	Diverticular disease of colon	Gastrointestinal	X-ray, barium enema
88.	Drowning	General	BP, ECG, chest X-ray, pupil examination, blood gas analysis, blood examination
89.	Dumping syndrome	Gastrointestinal	
90.	Duodenal ulcer	Gastrointestinal	Endoscopy
91.	Dysfunctional uterine bleeding		Gynecological Hb count, ESR, differential WBC count, blood culture, lymph biopsy, psychoanalytical test
92.	Dysmenorrhea	Gynecological	Urine analysis, culture, ESR, Hb count
93.	Ectopic pregnancy	Gynecological	Ultrasound uterus, fallopian tube, PV examination
94.	Eczema	Skin	Skin test
95.	Emphysema	Respiratory	Pulmonary function test, X-ray
96.	Empyema	Respiratory	Pus culture
97.	Endocarditis	Cardiovascular	Blood culture, echocardiogram, ECG, ESR, WBC differential, blood culture
98.	Epilepsy	Neurology	Pupil examination, BP, EEG, phenatine assey test, blood gas analysis, blood examination.
99.	Epistaxis	ENT	ENT examination, BP test, ECG, differential WBC, ESR, HB count, prothrombine time
100.	Exfoliative dermatitis	Skin	Skin test
101.	Filaria	General	ESR, blood examination, lymph node test, blood culture, gland biopsy
102.	Frost bite	General	Skin test, BP, ECG, blood gas analysis, blood examination, extremity test, ESR
103.	Gastric ulcer	Gastrointestinal	Barium meal and X-ray, gastroscopy
104.	Gonorrhea	Skin	Urine analysis, urine culture
105.	Habitual abortion	Gynecological	Rh- incompatibility test, VDRL, thyroid function test, blood sugar
106.	Hemoptysis	Respiratory	Sputum culture, blood culture
107.	Hemorrhoids	Gastrointestinal	Colonoscopy
108.	Hemothorax	Respiratory	
109.	Heat Stroke	General	Skin test, BP, blood gas analysis, blood examination
110.	Hemophilia	Hematology	Prothrombin time (PTT), specific assays factor - VIII and IX
111.	Hepatitis	Gastrointestinal	
112.	Hepatitis	Gastrointestinal	Amino transferase, AST-SGOT, ALT-SGPT, WBC count
113.	Herpes zoster	Skin	
114.	Herpetic stomatitis	Gastrointestinal	WBC differential, blood culture
115.	Hiccup	Gastrointestinal	
116.	Hodgkin's disease		ESR, blood examination, total and differential WBC, serum copper, serum alkaline phosphate, serum haptoglobin, lymph node biopsy, ultrasound spleen
117.	Hookworm infestation	General	BP, ECG, chest X -ray, blood examination, ESR, skin test, stool test

Contd...

Contd...

S.No	Diagnosis	System	Investigations
118.	Hydrothorax	Respiratory	
119.	Hyperemis gravidarum	Gynecological	Electrolytic analysis
120.	Hyperkalemia	General	BP, ECG, blood examination, skin test, serum Potassium level, ADH test
121.	Hypertension	Cardiovascular	BP measurement, ECG, chest X-ray, RBC count, blood urea nitrogen, serum creatinine, potassium level, 17 hydroxycorticosteroids
122.	Hyperthyroidism	Endocrine	Thyroid function test, thyroid scan
123.	Hypoglycemia	Endocrine	Blood sugar level examination, corticosteroids level
124.	Hypothermia	General	Skin test, BP, ECG, blood gas analysis
125.	Hypothyroidism	Endocrine	Thyroid function test, thyroid scan
126.	Incomplete abortion	Gynecological	Ultrasound scanning, Hb count, ESR, differential, total WBC
127.	Indian childhood cirrhosis	Pediatric	Pediatric examination, liver function test, ESR
128.	Inevitable abortion	Gynecological	Ultrasound scanning, Hb count, ESR, differential, total WBC
129.	Infantile diarrhea	Pediatric	Pediatric examination, stool examination, ENT examination, oral examination,
130.	Infantile echema	Skin	Skin test, X-ray
131.	Infective arthritis	Musculoskeletal	WBC total, WBC differential, synovial fluid, blood glucose ratio, uric acid, synovial biopsy and culture
132.	Infective polyneuritis	General	ESR, X-ray KUB, blood and urine culture, CSF analysis, ACTH test
133.	Injuries to vulva and vagina	Gynecological	Hb count, ESR, blood examination, vaginal examination, urine analysis
134.	Intestinal tuberculosis	Gastrointestinal	Stool culture, X-ray, barium swallow
135.	Intracerebral hemorrhage	Neurology	BP, ESR, coma scale, blood examination, blood gas analysis, pupil examination, X-ray skull, CT scan
136.	Intracranial tumor	Neurology	BP, ESR, coma scale, blood examination, blood gas analysis, pupil examination, X-ray skull, CT scan
137.	Irritable bowel syndrome	Gastrointestinal	Stool analysis
138.	Kwashiorkor	Pediatric	Pediatric examination, skin test, hair examination (pigmentation test), stool examination
139	Lactic acidosis		BP, ESR, blood examination, blood gas analysis, plasma level
140.	Left ventricular failure	Cardiovascular	BP, ECG, echocardiogram, chest X-ray, cardiac enzyme test, lipid profile, LFT, serum potassium level
141.	Left ventricular failure	Cardiovascular	ECG, chest X-ray, sputum, blood gas analysis
142.	Leukorrhea	Gynecological	Urine analysis, culture pap smear
143.	Leukemias	Hematology	WBC total, WBC differential, bone marrow aspiration, bone biopsy
144.	Lobar pneumonia	Respiratory	WBC differential, sputum culture, chest X-ray
145.	Localized otitis externa	ENT	ENT examination, ESR, swap culture, audiometry test

Contd...

Contd...

S.No.	Diagnosis	System	Investigations
146.	Lung abscess	Respiratory	Hemoglobin, WBC differential, sputum culture, X-ray
147.	Malaria	General	ESR, blood examination and culture for MP
148.	Marasmus	Pediatric	Paediatric examination, weight loss
149.	Mediastinal tumor	Respiratory	Barium swallow, chest X-ray
150.	Menopause	Gynecological	LDH, FSH test, PAP smear, Hb count
151.	Migraine	Neurology	Skull, PNS X-ray, EEG, audiogram, ENT, neurological examination
152.	Mitral regurgitation	Pediatric	Paediatric examination, cardiological consultation, chest X-ray, ECG
153.	Mitral regurgitation	Cardiovascular	ECG, chest X-ray, echocardiogram, BP
154.	Mitral stenosis	Pediatric	Pediatric examination, cardiological consultation, chest X-ray, barium X-ray, sputum culture, RH factor titer, hematological study
155.	Mitral stenosis	Cardiovascular	ECG, chest X-ray, echocardiogram, cardiac catheterization
156.	Mitral value disease	Cardiovascular	ECG, echocardiogram, stress test
157.	Monilial vaginitis	Gynecological	Urine culture, pap smear, ESR, skin scaling test
158.	Multiple myeloma	Neurology	ESR, total and differntial WBC, bone morrow test, bence jones protein test, bone scan, BUN, serum creatinine, serum uric acid, serum calcium, X-ray bone
159.	Myasthenia gravis		Muse tone test (EMG), edrophonium and neostigmine test
160.	Myocardial infarction	Cardiovascular	ECG, differential WBC, ESR, CPK - MB, SGOT, LDH, radioisotopes
161.	Nausea and vomiting	Gastrointestinal	Chloride
162.	Nephrotic syndrome	Nephrology	24 hours protein urine, urine albumin, Hb count, lipid profile, LFT
163.	Nodular cirrhosis	Gastrointestinal	Hemoglobin, LDH, SGOT, alkaline phosphates, bilirubin, albumin, liver biopsy
164.	Non-specific ulcerative colitis	Gastrointestinal	WBC differential, barium enema and X-ray, sigmoidoscopy
165.	Non-Hodgkin's lymphoma	Cancer Medicine	ERS, blood examination, lymph node biopsy, total and differential WBC count
166.	Organophosphorus poisoning	General	BP, ECG, pupil examination, blood examination, gastric lavage test, urine analysis, stool analysis
167.	Osteoarthritis	Musculoskeletal	ESR, RA factor, radiological study, arthroscopy
168.	Osteomyelitis	Musculoskeletal	Blood culture, X-ray, ESR, WBC, bone marrow test
169.	Pancreatitis	Gastrointestinal	Serum amylase, serum lipase concentration, WBC total, WBC differential, serum calcium concentration, serum albumin, chest x-ray, ultrasonography, CT-pancrease, cholangiography
170.	Paralytic ileus	Gastrointestinal	X-ray
171.	Parkinson's disease	General	Nerve conduction test, ECG, EEG, CT scan and MRI
172.	Pemphigus	Skin	Skin test

Contd...

Contd...

S.No.	Diagnosis	System	Investigations
173.	Peptic oesophagitis	Gastrointestinal	X-ray, biopsy
174.	Peptic ulcer	Gastrointestinal	Endoscopy, fluoroscopy, gastric analysis
175.	Pleural effusion	Respiratory	X-ray, thoracocentesis-definite procedure
176.	Pneumonia	Respiratory	WBC differential, blood gas analysis, sputum culture, X-ray findings, lung scan
177.	Poisoning	General	Toxicology test, BP, pupil examination, blood gas analysis, blood examination, stool test, urine analysis
178.	Premenstrual tension	Gynecological	Breast Examination, ECG, BP, psychoanalytical test
179.	Primary billiary cirrhosis	Gastrointestinal	Alkaline phosphatase, liver function test
180.	Profuse vaginal hemorrhage	Gynecological	BP, Hb count, blood examination, ultrasound pelvic, vaginal examination
181.	Psoriasis	Skin	Scaling skin test
182.	Pulmonary edema	Respiratory	X-ray
183.	Pulmonary thromboembolism	Respiratory	X-ray, lung scan, ecg, pulmonary angiography
184.	Pulmonay embolism	Respiratory	X-ray, ECG, CBC, serum enzyme (AST, LDH), serum bilirubin, lung scan, ultrasound-lungs
185.	Pulmonary tuberculosis	Respiratory	Tuberculin skin test, mantoux test, sputum culture AFB, chest X-ray
186.	Raised intracranial tension	Neurology	BP, ECG, pupil examination, CT scan, skull X-ray
187.	Rectal polyp	Gastrointestinal	
188.	Regional enteritis (Crohn's disease)		Gastrointestinal WBC differential, calcium
189.	Renal Colic	Nephrology	ESR, cystoscopy, ultrasound kidney, intravenous pylogram, X-ray kidney, ureter, bladder, urine examination
190.	Rheumatic fever	Cardiovascular	ESR, rheumatoid factro, antistreptolysin-o' titer
191.	Rheumatoid arthritis	Musculoskeletal	Hb count, U/S spleen, ESR, rheumatoid factor (RFS), WBC total and differential, X-ray joint, arthroscopy
192.	Rickets	Pediatric	Pediatric examination, fore limb X-ray, vitamin D deficiency
193.	Ringworm	Skin	Skin test
194.	Roundworm	General	ESR, blood examination, total and differential WBC count, stool test
195.	Sarcoidosis	Respiratory	Chest X-ray, sputum culture- AFB, limb biopsy
196.	Scabies	Skin	Skin test
197.	Scurvey	Pediatric	Pediatric examination, oral-gum and teeth examination, hind limb X-ray, vitamin C deficiency
198.	Seborrhoeic dermatitis	Skin	Scaling skin test
199.	Secondary biliary cirrhosis	Gastrointestinal	Liver function test
200.	Secondary otitis media	ENT	ENT examination, tuning fork test, audiometry test
201.	Senile vaginitis	Gynecological	Skin test, urine culture, cervical biopsy, cervical cytological test
202.	Sickle cell anemia	Hematology	RBC count, Hb, WBC differential, erythropoetic study

Contd...

Contd...

S.No.	Diagnosis	System	Investigations
203.	Snake bite	General	Toxicology test, BP, ECG, pupil examination, skint test, blood gas analysis, blood examination, Photosensitivity Test, Urine Analysis, Stool Analysis
204.	Spontaneous pneumothorax	Respiratory	Chest X-ray
205.	Spontaneous pneumothorax	Respiratory	BP, chest X-ray
206.	Sprue syndrome	Gastrointestinal	Stool culture, vitamin deficiency, X-ray
207.	Stroke	General	BP, prothrombin test, EEG, CT scan, blood examination, ECG
208.	Subacute bacterial endocarditis		Cardiovascular blood culture, urine analysis, Hb count
209.	Sucidal behavior	Psychiatry	BP, psychoanalytical test, previous history investigation
210.	Syncope	Cardiovascular	ECG, tredmill test, echocardiogram, fasting sugar
211.	Syphilis	Skin	Urine analysis, urine culture, lymph node test
212.	Tapeworm infestation	General	ESR, stool test
213.	Tension pneumothorax	Respiratory	Chest X-ray
214.	Thalassemias	Hematology	Hb, hematocrit, RBC count, serum bilirubin, serum ferritin, bone marrow study
215.	Threadworm	General	ESR, stool test,
216.	Threatened abortion	Gynecological	Hb count, ESR, urine analysis, culture, beta HCG liter
217.	Tinitus	ENT	ENT examination, audiometry test
218.	Transfusion reaction	General	BP, skin test, lymph node examination, corticosteroid level
219.	Traumatic pneumothorax	Respiratory	Emergency surgical procedure is required
220.	Trichomonas vaginitis	Gynecological	Urine analysis, ESR, skin test, Hb count
221.	Typhoid fever	Gastrointestinal	Widal test, stool
222.	Upper gastrointestinal hemorrhage	Gastrointestinal	WBC differential, stool, liver function test
223.	Uremia	Urology	Urine analysis, skin test, serum creatinine level, chloride level
224.	Vaginitis	Gynecological	Urine analysis, culture, ESR, Hb count, skin test
225.	Vertigo	ENT	ENT examination
226.	Vertigo due to Meniers diseases	ENT	ENT examination, audometry test
227.	Vincent's stomatitis	Gastrointestinal	
228.	Viral hepatitis	Gastrointestinal	SGOT, SGPT, LDH, liver biopsy
229.	Viral pneumonia	Respiratory	Sputum culture, chest X-ray
230.	Wilson's disease	Gastrointestinal	Liver function test, ceruloplasmin

NORMAL VALUES FOR LABORATORY INVESTIGATIONS

S.No.	Test	Conventional units	SI units
1.	Acid hemolysis test	No hemolysis	No hemolysis
2.	Alkaline phosphatase	Total score 14 to 100	Total score 14 to 100
3.	Cell Counts Erythrocytes		
	Males	4.6 to 6.2 million/mm³	4.6 to 6.2 × 10¹²/L
	Females	4.2 to 5.4 million/mm³	4.2 to 5.2 × 10¹²/L
	Children	4.5 to 5.1 million/mm³	4.5 to 5.1 × 10¹²/L
	Leukocytes, total	4500 to 11,000/mm³	4.5 to 11.0 × 10⁹/L
4.	Leukocytes, differential		
	Myelocytes	0/mm³	O/L
	Band neutrophils	150 to 400/mm³	150 to 400 × 10⁶ / L
	Segmented neutrophils	3000 to 5800/mm³	3000 to 5800 × 10⁶ / L
	Lymphocytes	1500 to 3000/mm³	1500 to 3000 × 10⁶ / L
	Monocytes	300 to 500/mm³	300 to 500 × 10⁶ / L
	Eosinophils	50 to 250/mm³	50 to 250 × 10⁶ / L
	Basophils	15 to 50/mm³	15 to 50 × 10⁶/ L
	Platelets	150,000 to 350,000/mm³	150 to 350 × 10⁹/L
	Reticulocytes	25,000 to 75,000/mm³ 0.5 to 1.5 % of erythrocytes	25 to 75 × 10⁹/ L
5.	Coagulation tests		
	Bleeding time (template)	2.75 to 8.0 min	2.75 to 8.0 min
	Coagulation time (glass tubes)	5 to 15 min	5 to 15 min
	Factor VIII and other coagulation factors	50 to 150% of normal	0.5 to 1.5 of normal
	Fibrin split products (Thrombo-Welco test)	<10 µg/ml	<10 mg/L
	Fibrinogen	200 to 400 mg / dl	2.0 to 4.0 g/L
	Partial thromboplastic time (PTT)	20 to 35 sec	20 to 35 sec
	Prothrombin time (PT)	12.0 to 14.0 sec	12.0 to 14.0 sec
6.	Coombs test		
	Direct	Negative	Negative
	Indirect	Negative	Negative
7.	Corpuscular Values of erythrocytes		
	Mean corpuscular hemoglobin (MCH)	26 to 34 pg	0.40 to 0.53 fmol
	Mean corpuscular volume (MCV)	80 to 96 µm³	80 to 96 fL
	Mean corpuscular hemoglobin Concentration	32 to 36%	0.32 to 0.36%
8.	Hepatoglobin	26 to 185 mg/dl	260 to 1850 mg/L
9.	Hematocrit		
	Males	40 to 54 ml/dl	0.40 to 0.54 volume fraction
	Females	37 to 47 ml/dl	0.37 to 0.47 volume fraction
	Newborns	49 to 54 ml/dl	0.49 to 0.54 volume fraction
	Children	35 to 49 ml/dl	0.35 to 0.49 volume fraction
10.	Hemoglobin		
	Males	14.0 to 18.0 g/dl	2.17 to 2.79 mmol/L
	Females	12.0 to 16.0 g/dl	1.86 to 2.48 mmol/L
	Newborns	16.5 to 19.5 g/dl	2.56 to 3.02 mmol/L
	Children (varies with age)	11.2 to 16.5 g/dl	1.74 to 2.56 mmol/L
11.	Hemoglobin, fetal	<1.0% of total	<0.01% of total
12.	Hemoglobin A$_{1c}$	3 to 5% of total	0.03 to 0.05% of total
13.	Hemoglobin A$_2$	1.5 to 3.0% of total	0.015 to 0.03% of total
14.	Hemoglobin, plasma	0 to 5.0 mg/dl	0 to 0.8 µmol/L

Contd...

Contd...

S.No.	Test	Conventional units	SI units
15.	Methemoglobin	30 to 130 mg/dl	4.7 to 20 µmol/L
16.	Sedimentation rate (ESR)		
	Males	0 to 5 mm/hr	0 to 5 mm/hr
	Females	0 to 15 mm/hr	0 to 15 mm/hr
	Westergren		
	Males	0 to 15 mm/hr	0 to 15 mm/hr
	Females	0 to 20 mm/hr	0 to 20 mm/hr
17.	Acetoacetate plus acetone		
	Qualitative	Negative	Negative
	Quantitative	0.3 to 2.0 mg/dl	3 to 20 mg/L
18.	Acid phosphatase, serum (thymolphthalein monophosphate substrate)	0.11 to 0.60 U/L	0.11 to 0.60 U/L
19.	Adrenocorticotropin, plasma (ACTH)		
	6.00 am	10 to 80 pg/ml	10 to 80 ng/L
	6.00 pm	< 50 pg/ml	<50 ng/L
20.	Alanine aminotransferase, serum (ALT, SGPT)	7 to 35 U/L	7 tp 35 U/L
21.	Albumin, serum	3.5 to 5.5 g/dl	35 to 55 g/L
22.	Aldolase, serum	1.5 to 12.0 U/L	1.5 to 12.0 U/L
23.	Aldosterone, plasma		
	Supine	3 to 10 ng/dl	0.08 to 0.30 nmol/L
	Standing		
	Males	6 to 22 ng/dl	0.17 to 0.61 nmol/L
	Females	5 to 30 ng/dl	0.14 to 0.83 nmol/L
24.	Alkaline phosphatase, serum (ALP)	20 to 90 U/L (30° C)	20 to 90 U/L/ (30°C)
25.	Ammonia nitrogen, plasma	15 to 49 µg/dl	11 to 35 µmol/L
26.	Amylase, serum	25 to 125 U/L	25 to 125 U/L
27.	Anion gap	8 to 16 mEq/L	8 to 16 mmol/L
28.	Ascorbic acid, blood	0.4 to 1.5 mg/dl	23 to 85 µmol/L
29.	Aspartate aminotransferase, serum (AST, SGOT)	7 to 40 U/L	7 to 40 U/L
30.	Base excess, blood	0 + 2 mEq/L	0 + 2 mmol/L
31.	Bicarbonate		
	Venous plasma	23 to 29 mEq/L	23 to 29 mmol/L
	Arterial blood	18 to 23 mEq/L	18 to 23 mmol/L
32.	Bile acids, serum	0.3 to 3.0 mg/dl	3 to 30 mg/L
33.	Bilirubin, serum		
	Conjugated	0.1 to 0.4 mg/dl	1.7 to 6.8 µmol/L
	Unconjugated	0.2 to 0.7 mg/dl	3.4 to 12 µmol/L
	Total	0.3 to 1.1 mg/dl	5.1 to 19 µmol/L
34.	Calcium, serum	9.0 to 11.0 mg/dl	2.25 to 2.75 mmol/L
35.	Calcium, ionized, serum	4.25 to 5.25 mg/dl	1.05 to 1.30 mmol/L
36.	Carbon-dioxide, total, serum or plasma	24 to 30 mEq/L	24 to 30 mmol/L
37.	Carbon-dioxide tension, blood PCO_2	35 to 45 mm Hg	35 to 45 mm Hg
38.	ß-Carotene serum	40 to 200 µg/dl	0.74 to 3.72 µmol/L
39.	Catecholamines, plasma		
	Epinephrine	15 to 55 pg/ml	82 to 300 pmol/L
	Norepinephrine	65 to 400 pg/ml	384 to 2364 pmol/L
40.	Ceruloplasmin, serum	23 to 44 mg/dl	230 to 440 mg/L

Contd...

Contd...

S.No.	Test	Conventional units	SI units
41.	Chloride, serum or plasma	96 to 106 mEq/L	96 to 106 mmol/L
42.	Cholesterol, serum or EDTA plasma		
	Desirable range	< 200 mg/dl	<5.18 mmol/L
	LDL Cholesterol	60 to 180 mgdl	600 to 1800 mg/L
	HDL Cholesterol	30 to 80 mg/dl	300 to 800 mg/L
43.	Copper		
	Males	70 to 140 µg/dl	11 to 22 µmol/L
	Females	85 to 155 µg/dl	13 to 24 µmol/L
44.	Cortisol, plasma		
	8.00 AM	6 to 23 µg/dl	170 to 635 nmol/L
	4.00 PM	3 to 15 µg/dl	82 to 413 nmol/l
	10.00 PM	<50% of 8 AM value	< 0.5 % of 8 AM value
45.	Creatine, serum	0.2 to 0.8 mg/dl	15 to 61 umol/L
46.	Creatine kinase, serum (CK, CPK)		
	Males	55 to 170 U/L	55 to 170 U/L
	Females	30 to 135 U/L	30 to 135 U/L
47.	Creatine kinase MB Isozyme, serum	0.0 to 4.7 ng/ml	0.0 to 4.7 µg/L
48.	Creatinine, serum	0.6 to 1.2 mg/dl	53 to 108 µmol/L
49.	Ferritin, serum	20 to 200 ng/ml	20 to 200 µg/L
50.	Fibrinogen, plasma	200 to 400 mg/dl	2.0 to 4.0 g/L
51.	Folate		
	Serum	1.8 to 9.0 ng/ml	4.1 to 20.4 nmol/L
	Erythrocytes	150 to 450 ng/ml	340 to 1020 nmol/L
52.	Follicle-stimulating hormone, plasma (FSH)		
	Males	4 to 25 mU/ml	4 to 25 U/L
	Females	4 to 30 mU/ml	4 to 30 U/L
	Postmenopausal	40 to 250 mU/ml	40 to 250 U/L
53.	Y-Glutamyltransferase, serum		
	Males	5 to 38 U/L	5 to 38 U/L
	Females	5 to 29 U/L	5 to 29 U/L
54.	Gastrin, serum	0 to 200 pg/ml	0 to 200 ng/L
55.	Glucose (fasting), plasma or serum	70 to 115 mg/dl	3.89 to 6.38 mmol/L
56.	Growth hormone, plasma (HGH)	0 to 10 ng/ml	0 to 10 µg/L
57.	Haptoglobin, serum	26 to 185 mg/dl	260 to 1850 mg/L
58.	Immunoglobulins, serum		
	IgG	550 to 1900 mg/dl	5.5 to 19.0 g/L
	IgA	60 to 333 mg/dl	0.60 to 3.3 g/L
	IgM	45 to 145 mg/dl	0.45 to 1.5 g/L
	IgD	0.5 to 3.0 mg/dl	5 to 30 mg/L
	IgE	< 500 ng/ml	< 500 µg/L
59.	Insulin (fasting), plasma	5 to 25 µU/ml	36 to 179 pmol/L
60.	Iron, serum	75 to 175 ng/dl	13 to 31 umol/L
61.	Iron-binding capacity, serum		
	Total	250 to 410 µg/dl	45 to 73 µmol/L
	Saturation	20% to 55%	0.20 to 0.55
62.	Lactate		
	Venous blood	4.5 to 19.8 mg/dl	0.50 to 2.2 mmol/L
	Arterial blood	4.5 to 14.4 mg/dl	0.50 to 1.6 mmol/L
63.	Lactate dehydrogenase, serum (LD, LDH)	100 to 190 U/L	100 to 190 U/L

Contd...

Contd...

S.No.	Test	Conventional units	SI units
64.	Lipase, serum	10 to 140 U/L	10 to 140 U/L
65.	Lipids, total, serum	450 to 850 mg/dl	4.5 to 8.5 g/L
66.	Luteinizing hormone, serum (LH)		
	Males	6 to 18 mU/ml	6 to 18 U/L
	Females		
	Premenopausal	5 to 22 mU/ml	5 to 22 U/L
	Midcycle	3 × baseline	3 × baseline
	Postmenopausal	>30 mU/ml	>30 U/L
67.	Magnesium, serum	1.8 to 3.0 mg/dl	0.75 to 1.25 mmol/L
68.	Osmolality	286 to 295 mOsm/kg H_2O	2.85 to 2.95 mOsm/kg H_2O
69.	Oxygen blood		
	Capacity	16 to 24 Vol %	7.14 to 10.7 mmol/L
	Content, arterial	15 to 23 Vol %	6.69 to 10.3 mmol/L
	Saturation, arterial	94 to 100%	0.94 to 1.00
	Tension, Po_2	75 to 100 mm Hg	75 to 100 mm Hg
70.	P_{50}	26 to 27 mm Hg	26 to 27 mm Hg
71.	pH, arterial blood	7.35 to 7.45	7.35 to 7.45
72.	Phenylalanine, serum	<3 mg/dl	<0.18 mmol/L
73.	Phosphate, inorganic, serum	3.0 to 4.5 mg/dl	1.0 to 1.5 mmol/L
74.	Potassium, serum or plasma	3.5 to 5.0 mEq/l	3.5 to 5.0 mmol/L
75.	Prolactin, serum		
	Males	1 to 20 ng/ml	1 to 20 µg/L
	Females	1 to 25 ng/ml	1 to 25 µg/L
76.	Protein, serum		
	Total	6.0 to 8.0 g/dl	60 to 80 g/L
	Albumin	3.5 to 5.5 g/dl	35 to 55 g/L
	α1-Globulin	0.2 to 0.4 g/dl	2 to 4 g/L
	α2-Globulin	0.5 to 0.9 g/dl	5 to 9 g/L
	β-Globulin	0.6 to 1.1 g/dl	6 to 11 g/L
	γ-Globulin	0.7 to 1.7 g/dl	7 to 17 g/L
77.	Pyruvate, blood	0.3 to 0.9 mg/dl	0.03 to 0.10 mmol/L
78.	Sodium, serum or plasma	136 to 145 mEq/L	136 to 145 mmol/L
79.	Testosterone, plasma		
	Males	275 to 875 ng/dl	9.0 to 10.0 nmol/L
	Females	23 to 75 ng/dl	0.8 to 2.6 nmol/L
	pregnant	38 to 190 ng/dl	1.3 to 6.6 nmol/L
80.	Thyroid stimulating hormone, serum(TSH)	0 to 7 µU/ml	0 to 7 mU/L
81.	Thyroxine, free, serum (FT_4)	1.0 to 2.1 ng/dl	13 to 27 pmol/L
82.	Thyroxine, serum (T_4)	4.4 to 9.9 ug/dl	57 to 128 nmol/L
83.	Triglycerides, serum	40 to 150 mg/dl	0.4 to 1.5 g/L
84.	Triiodothyronine, serum (T_3)	150 to 250 ng/dl	2.3 to 3.9 nmol/L
85.	Triiodothyronine uptake, resin (T_3RU)	25 to 38% uptake	0.25 to 0.38 uptake
86.	Urate		
	Males	2.5 to 8.0 mg/dl	0.15 to 0.48 mmol/L
	Females	1.5 to 7.0 mg/dl	0.09 to 0.42 mmol/L
87.	Urea, serum or plasma	24 to 49 mg/dl	4.0 to 8.2 mmol/L
88.	Urea nitrogen, serum or plasma	11 to 23 mg/dl	3.9 to 8.2 mmol/L

Contd...

Contd...

S.No.	Test	Conventional units	SI units
89.	Viscosity, serum	1.4 to 1.8 × water	1.4 to 1.8 × water
90.	Vitamin A, serum	20 to 80 µg/dl	0.70 to 2.80 µmol/L
91.	Vitamin B$_{12}$, serum	180 to 900 pg/ml	133 to 664 pmol/L

URINE INVESTIGATIONS

S.No.	Test	Conventional units	SI units
1.	Acetone and acetoacetate, qualitative	Negative	Negative
2.	Albumin		
	Quantitative	Negative	Negative
	Qualitative	10 to 100 mg/24 hrs	10 to 100 mg/24 hrs
3.	Aldosterone	3 to 20 µg/24 hrs	8.3 to 55 nmol/24 hrs
4.	δ-Aminolevulinic acid	1.3 to 7.0 mg/24 hrs	10 to 53 µmol/24 hrs
5.	Amylase	3 to 20 U/hr	3 to 20 U/hr
6.	Amylase/Creatinine clearance ratio	1 to 4%	0.01 to 0.04%
7.	Bilirubin, qualitative	Negative	Negative
8.	Calcium (usual diet)	<250 mg/24 hrs	< 6.3 mmol/24 hrs
9.	Catecholamines		
	Epinephrine	<10 µg/24 hrs	<55 nmol/24 hrs
	Norepinephrine	<100 µg/24 hrs	< 590 nmol/24 hrs
	Total free catecholamines	4 to 126 µg/24 hrs	24 to 745 nmol/24 hrs
	Total metanephrines	0.1 to 1.6 µg/24 hrs	0.5 to 8.1 µmol/24 hrs
10.	Chloride (varies with intake)	110 to 250 mEq/24 hrs	110 to 250 nmol/24 hrs
11.	Copper	0 to 50 µg/24 hrs	0 to 0.80 µmol/24 hrs
12.	Cortisol, free	10 to 100 µg/24 hrs	27.6 to 276 nmol/24 hrs
13.	Creatinine	15 to 25 mg/kg body weight/24 hrs	0.13 to 0.22 mmol/kg
14.	Creatinine clearance (corrected to 1.73 m^2 body surface area)		
	Males	110 to 150 ml/min	110 to 150 ml/min
	Females	105 to 132 ml/min	105 to 132 ml/min
15.	Dehydroepiandrosterone		
	Males	0.2 to 2.0 mg/24 hrs	0.7 to 6.9 µmol/24 hrs
	Females	0.2 1.8 mg/24 hrs	0.7 to 6.2 µmol/24 hrs
16.	Estrogens, total		
	Males	4 to 25 mg/24 hrs	14 to 90 nmol/24 hrs
	Females	5 to 100 mg/24 hrs	18 to 360 nmol/24 hrs
17.	Glucose (as reducing substance)	< 250 mg/24 hrs	< 250 mg/24 hrs
18.	Hemoglobin and myoglobin, qualitative	Negative	Negative
19.	17-Hydroxycorticosteroids		
	Males	3 to 9 mg/24 hrs	8.3 to 25 umol/24 hrs
	Females	2 to 8 mg/24 hrs	5.5 to 22 umol/24 hrs
20.	5-Hydroxyindoleacetic acid		
	Qualitative	Negative	Negative
	Quantitative	<9 mg/24 hrs	< 47 µmol/24 hrs
21.	17-Ketosteroids		
	Males	6 to 18 mg/24 hrs	21 to 62 µmol/24 hrs
	Females	4 to 13 mg/24 hrs	14 to 45 µmol/24 hrs
22.	Magnesium	6.0 to 8.5 mEq/24 hrs	3.0 to 4.2 µmol/24 hrs
23.	Osmolality	38 to 1400 mOsm/kg H$_2$O	38 to 1400 mOsm/kg H$_2$O
24.	pH	4.6 to 8.0	4.6 to 8.0
25.	Phenylpyruvic acid, qualitative	Negative	Negative
26.	Phosphate	0.9 to 1.3 g/24 hrs	29 to 42 mmol/24 hrs

Contd...

Contd...

S.No.	Test	Conventional units	SI units
27.	Porphobilinogen		
	Qualitative	Negative	Negative
	Quantitative	<2.0 mg/24 hrs	< 9 µmol/24 hrs
28.	Porphyrins		
	Coproporphyrin	50 to 250 µg/24 hrs	77 to 380 nmol/24 hrs
	Uroporphyrin	10 to 30 µg/24 hrs	12 to 36 nmol/24 hrs
29.	Potassium	25 to 100 mEq/24 hrs	25 to 100 mmol/24 hrs
30.	Pregnanediol		
	Males	0.4 to 1.4 mg/24 hrs	1.2 to 4.4 umol/24 hrs
	Females		
	Proliferative phase	0.5 to 1.5 mg/24 hrs	1.6 to 4.7 µmol/24 hrs
	Luteal Phase	2.0 to 7.0 mg/24 hrs	6.2 to 22 µmol/24 hrs
	Postmenopausal	0.2 to 1.0 mg/24 hrs	0.6 to 3.1 µmol/24 hrs
31.	Pregnanetriol	<2.5 mg/24 hrs	< 7.4 mmol/24 hrs
32.	Protein		
	Qualitative	Negative	Negative
	Quantitative	10 to 150 mg/24 hrs	10 to 150 mg/24 hrs
33.	Sodium	130 to 260 mEq/24 hrs	130 to 260 mmol/24 hrs
34.	Specific gravity	1.003 to 1.030	1.003 to 1.030
35.	Urate	200 to 500 mg/24 hrs	1.2 to 3.0 mmol/24 hrs
36.	Urobilinogen	<4.0 mg/24 hrs	< 6.8 µmol/24 hrs
37.	Vanillylmandelic acid (VMA)		
	(4-hydroxy-3methoxymandelic acid)	1 to 8 mg/24 hrs	5 to 40 µmol/24 hrs

SEMEN ANALYSIS

S.No.	Test	Conventional units	SI units
1.	Volume	2 to 5 ml	2 to 5 ml
2.	Liquefaction	Complete in 15 min	Complete in 15 min
3.	Leukocytes	Occasional or absent	Occasional or absent
4.	Count	60 to 150 million/ml	60 to 150 × 10^6/ml
5.	Motility	> 80% motile	> 0.80 motile
6.	Morphology	80 to 90% normal forms	0.80 to 0.90 normal forms
7.	Fructose	> 150 mg/dl	> 8.33 mmol/L

CEREBROSPINAL FLUID

S.No.	Test	Conventional units	SI units
1.	Cells	< 5/mm 3	< 5 × 10^6/L
2.	Electrophoresis	All mononuclear	All mononuclear
3.	Glucose	to 75 mg/dl	2.8 to 4.2 mmol/L
		(20 mg/dl less than serum)	(1.1 mmol/L less than serum)
4.	IgG		
5.	Children < 14 years	< 8% of total protein	< 0.08 of total protein
6.	Adults	< 14% of total protein	< 0.14 of total protein
7.	Ig Index	0.3 to 0.6	0.3 to 0.6
8.	CSF/serum IgG ratio		
9.	Oligoclonal banding on electrophoresis	Absent	Absent
10.	Pressure	70 to 180 mm H$_2$O	70 to 180 mm H$_2$O
11.	Protein, total	15 to 45 mg/dl	150 to 450 mg/L

VARIATIONS OF INVESTIGATION VALUES WITH NORMAL VALUES AND RESULTING DIAGNOSES

S.No.	Test name	Normal values	Increasing condition	Decreasing condition
1.	Acetone	Negative	Acetone (Ketone bodies) are found in the urine when the body's fat is metabolized for energy, producing an excess of metabolic end products. This occurs in an uncontrolled diabetes, starvation, severe infection accompanied by vomiting and diarrhea, pregnancy and lactation	
2.	Acid phosphatase	1 to 3 KA units/dl	Increased level of acid phosphatase indicates prostatic carcinoma, advanced Paget's disease, and hyperparathyroidism	
3.	Alkaline phasphatase	5 to 11 KA units/dl	Alkaline phosphatase is raised when there is an increase in the osteoblastic activity of bone, rickets, Paget's disease, myeloid leukemia, hyperparathyroidism, liver diseases, pregnancy and following ingestion of larger amounts of vitamin D	Hypothyroidism
4.	Amino (nitrogen) acids in blood	3.5 to 5.5 mg/dl	Liver disease	Severe burns
5.	Ammonia	80–110 μ mg	Hepatic necrosis	Terminal portal cirrhosis
6.	Aspartate transaminase (AST) (or) Serum glutamic Orxaloacetic transaminase (SGOT) Aianine transaminase (ALT) (or) Serum glutamic Pyruvic transaminase (SGPT)	Less than 40 IU/l	Both AST and ALT are released from damaged hepatic, cardiac and kidney muscles cells as seen in myocardial infarction and liver diseases	
7.	Australia antigen	Negative	Positive results indicates viral hepatitis B	
8.	Bacteria	Nil	Presence of bacteria represents infection within the urinary tract	
9.	Basal metabolic rate (BMR)		Hyperthyroidism	Hypothyroidism
10.	Basophils	0–1 %	Chronic myloid leukemia, polycythemia, vera, cirrhosis of liver, measkes, chickenpox	

Contd...

Contd...

S.No.	Test name	Normal values	Increasing condition	Decreasing condition
11.	Bence Jones protein in urine	Nil	Bence Jones protein is precipitated between 40° to 60°C, and it disappears when boiling point is reached. Bence Jones protein is present in cases of multiple myeloma	
12.	Bicarbonates	23 to 31 mmol/l 23 to 31 mEq/l	Abnormal increase in the bicarbonates leads to metabolic alkalosis and a decrease in the hydrogen ion concentration of the plasma with a resultant rise in blood pH Increased in respiratory acidosis, emphysema of pneumonia	Abnormal decrease in the bicarbonates result in the decrease of blood pH due to metabolic acidosis. Metabolic acidosis is commonly seen in diabetes mellitus, hyperthyroidism, starvation, severe infections with fever, excessive vomiting which results in the accumulation of ketone bodies Decreased in respiratory alkalosis (Excessive respiration)
13.	Bilirubin	0.3 to 1.1 mg/100 ml	Biliary obstruction (jaundice), chronic hepatitis	
14.	Bleeding time (BT)	1 to 6 minutes in adults	Prolonged bleeding time occurs in vascular purpuras, thrombocytopenia, chloroform and phosphorus poisoning, and after ingestion of aspirin tablets	
15.	Blood pH (hydrogen iron concentration)	7.35 to 7.45	Blood pH value is raised in vomiting, hyperpnea, fever, intestinal obstruction etc.	It is decreased in uremia, acidosis, hemorrhage, nephritis, etc.
16.	Blood picture	Anisocytosis - nil Poikilocytosis - nil Microcytes - nil Macrocytes - nil Hypochromic cells - nil Nucleated - nil Erythrocytes - nil Sickle cells - nil Spherocytes - nil	Anisocytosis—nil anisocytosis—erythrocytes vary in size from normal—is seen in anemias Poikilocytosis tear shaped or club shape RBC seen in severe anemias Microcytes RBC small in size than normal and are seen in microcytic anemia and thalassemia major Macrocytes RBC large in size than normal and are seen in pernicious anemia and folic acid deficiency anemia Hypochromic cells—the RBC with abnormally low Hb content as seen in iron deficiency anemia Nucleated erythrocytes are seen in severe anemia Sickle cells are sickle shaped. RBC are found in sickle cell anemia	

Contd...

Contd...

S.No.	Test name	Normal values	Increasing condition	Decreasing condition
17.	Blood sugar fasting	55 to 110 mg/dl postprandial (2 hours) 65 to 140 mg/dl	Spherocytes—erythrocytes are relatively small and round rather than biconcave in shape and are seen in thalassemia major. Blood sugar level is increased in nephritis, hyperthyroidism, pregnancy, uremia, infections, cerebral lesions, etc.	Blood sugar level is decreased in hyperinsulinism, hypothyroidism. Addison's diseases, extensive hepatic damage
18.	Blood urea	2.5 to 6.5 mmol/l (or) 20 to 40 mg/dl (or) 3.5 to 5.5 mmol/l	Increase in the blood urea indicates an impairment of renal functions	
19.	Bromsulphthalein test	Less than 5% retention of the dye at 45 minutes	Based on hepatic fuction	
20.	Casts	Nil	Presence of cast indicates tubular or glomerular diseases	
21.	Cereloplasmin in serum	23 to 44 mg/dl		Wilson's disease (hepatocellular degeneration)
22.	Chlorides	96 to 106 mEq/L	Acidosis	Vomiting
23.	Chronic gonadotrophin (pregnancy test)	Negative	Positive results are seen in pregnancy, chorionepithelioma and hydatiliform mole	
24.	Coagulation time (CT)	5 to 18 minutes in adults	The coagulation time is prolonged whenever there is a defect in the clotting mechanism. The important coagulation disorders are hemophilia, liver disases, vitamin K deficiency, thrombocytopenia, hypofibrinogenemia, and in patients who receive anticoagulants	Coagulation time is reduced in typhoid, endocarditis
25.	Coomb's test	Direct Coomb's test— negative Indirect Coomb's test negative	Direct Coomb's test is used to test blood from the umbilical cord for the possible presence of erythroblastosis fetalis and to diagnose acquired hemolytic anemia. Indirect Coomb's test is to identify antibodies to erythrocyte antigens in the pregnant mother's serum or in patients developing transfusion reaction against Rh positive blood	
26.	CPK (creatinine phosphokinase)	Male: 5–55 mu/mL Female: 5–35 mu/mL	Myocardial infarction	Muscular dystrophy

Contd...

S.No.	Test name	Normal values	Increasing condition	Decreasing condition
27.	Creatinine	18 mmol/24 hrs 0.8 to 2 gm/24 hrs	Increased levels are seen in typhoid fever, *Salmonella* infections, and tetanus Renal - Diabetes, Cushing's syndrome	Decreased in muscular atrophy, anemia, leukemia and advanced degeneration of kidney
28.	Differential WBC count	Polymorphonuclear cells: 50–70 % Lymphocytes: 20–40% Monocytes: 4–8 % Eosinophils: 0–2 % Basophils: 0–1 % Band forms: 3–5 %	Neutrophilia (increased neutrophils) is found in pyogenic bacterial infections. The severity of the infection and the degree of response of the body are indicated by the degree of increase in neutrophils Lymphocytosis (increased lymphocytes) are seen in children, in certain infections (whooping cough, mumps, measles, influenza, syphilis, TB, typhoid, etc) and in lymphatic leukemia. Monocytosis are found in kala azar, typhoid, TB, subacute bacterial endocarditis and malaria Eosinophilia is found in parasitic infestations, allergic conditions and leukemia Agranulocytosis (a marked decrease in the number of polymorpho-nuclear cells) is found in suppression of the bone marrow by drugs and radiation Asthma, drug allergy, urticaria, bilharziasis, eczema, exfoliative dermatitis, Hodgkins' disease	Neutropenia (decreased neutrophils) are found in certain infections (typhoid, measles, influenza, etc.), anemia, and suppression of the bone marrow by various drugs and radiation Lymphocytopenia (decreased lymphocytes) are seen in acute stages of infection and excessive radiation Esonopenia—aplastic anemia, Systemic lupus erythematosus, Cushing's diseases, acromegaly
29.	Erythrocyte sedimentation rate (ESR)	Males: 0 to 9 mm/1st hour Females: 1 to 20 mm/1st hour	The ESR is increased in tissue destruction, whether inflammatory, or degenerative and during menstruation, pregnancy and in acute febrile disease	Polycythemia vera, congestive cardiac failure, whooping cough, dehydration
30.	Erythrocytes	4.5 to 5.5 million/cmm	Erythrocyte count is increased in polycythemia vera, in cardiac and pulmonary disorders that are characterized by cyanosis	It is decreased in anemias
31.	Glucose (Fasting)	70–110 mg/100 ml	Diabetes, shock	Hypoglycemia, carcinoma of pancreas
32.	Glucose in CSF	50 to 75 mg/dl	Encephalitis, syphilis of CNS	Tuberculous, sarcoma, lymphoma
33.	Glucose tolerance test (GTT) oral	Fasting 55 to 110 mgm/dl 1/2 hour—30 to 60 mgm (above fasting) 1 hour—20 to 50 mgm above fasting	Flat or inverted curve are seen in hyperinsulinism, adrenal cortical insufficiency, hypothyroidism, sprue and celiac diseases, anterior pituitary hypofunctioning	High or porlonged curve suggests diabetes mellitous, hyperthyroidism, adrenal cortical tumor, severe anemia, etc.

Contd...

Contd...

S.No.	Test name	Normal values	Increasing condition	Decreasing condition
34.	Hemoglobin in plasma	2 hours—5 to 15 mgm above fasting 3 hours—fasting level or below Men 13 to 16 gm% Women 12 to 15 gm%	Hb is increased in sickle cell anemia, polycythemias and dehydration	Hb is decreased in anemias and hemodilution especially in Thalassemia
35.	Icterus index iodine, protein bound (PBI)	1 to 6 units 4.0 to 8.0 ug/dl	Increased in biliary obstruction, hemolytic anemias and hyperthyroidism	Decreased in hypothyroidism
36.	Idorganic phosphate in plasma		Renal failure, diabetic ketosis	Fancoris syndrome
37.	Iodine	3.5 to 8 mcg/100 ml	Pregnancy, hyperthyroidism	Hypothyroidism
38.	Iron	75 to 175 mcg/100 ml	Aplastic anemia, hemosiderosis, pernicious anemia	Iron deficiency anemia, nephrosis, chronic renal insufficiency
39.	Lactic acid in blood	<1.2 mmol/liter	Anemia	Diabetes
40.	Lactate dehydrogenase (LDH)	100 to 140 U/L	Myocardial infarction	Acute hepatitis
41.	Leukocytes	4000 to 11000/cu mm of blood	Myloic leukemia, emotional disturbances, bacterial infections, gout, diabetic coma, cirrhosis of liver, intestinal obstructions, uremia, malignant tumors, myocardial infarction.	Typhoid fever, paratyphoid fever, brucellosis, miliary tuberculosis, measles, infective hepatitis, malaria, kala azar, relapsing fever, aplastic anemia, megaloblastic anemia, multiple myeloma
42.	Lipase	0.2 to 1.5 units/ml	Increased in acute and chronic pancreatitis, biliary obstruction, cirrhosis, hepatitis and peptic ulcer	
43.	Lipids (total)	450 to 850 mg/dl	Diabetes	
44.	Lithium in serum	Therapeutic: 0.5 to 1.4 mmol/L Toxic: < 2.0 mmol/L	Psychiatric conditions	

Contd....

Contd...

S.No.	Test name	Normal values	Increasing condition	Decreasing condition
45.	Lymphocytes	20 to 35%	Chronic lymphatic leukemia, tuberculosis, syphilis, infective hepatitis, mumps, measles, chickenpox	Typhoid fever, subacute bacterial endocarditis, malaria, kala azar, amebiasis, Hodgkin's disease
46.	Malarial parasite (MP)	Negative	Thin and thick smears are used for ditecting malarial parasite and microfilaria	
47.	Mean corpuscular hemoglobin (MCH)	27 to 32 pg	Macrocytic anemia	Hypochromic anemia
48.	Microfilaria (MF)	Negative		
49.	Non-protein nitrogen (NPN)		Acute and chronic nephritis	
50.	Packed cell volume (PCV) or hematocrit	Men 40 to 54% Women 36 to 47%	Hematocrit is increased in polycythemia vera and in hemoconcentration resulting from blood loss, dehydration and shock	It is decreased in severe anemias, anemia of pregnancy, acute massive blood loss
51.	Phosphorus	0.8 to 1.4 mmol/l (or) 2.5 to 4.5 mg/dl	Phosphorus is elevated in hypoparathyroidism, chronic nephritis, uremia, and alkalosis. There is an inverse relationship between serum calcium and serum phosphorus	Phosphorus is decreased in hyperparathyroidism, rickets, osteomalacia, steatorrhea
52.	Platelet count	1 to 3.5 lacks/cmm	Thrombocytosis is usually a symptomatic	Thrombocytopenia is found in acute leukemia, aplastic anemia, in idiopathic thrombocytopenic purpura and during cancer therapy
53.	Protein (urine albumin)	Negative	Albuminuria may be found in nephritis and nephrosis, febrile conditions, poisoning, eclampsia, hypertension, and some forms of cardiovascular diseases	
54.	Protein bound iodine (PBI)		Hyperthyroidism	Hypothyroidism
55.	Prothrombin time (PT)	60 to 100% of control blood 12 to 16 seconds	Prothrombin time is increased in liver diseases, vitamin K deficiency, fibrinogen deficiency, other hemorrhagic diseases and in cirrhosis, hepatic, and acute toxic necrosis of the liver. It is also prolonged in decumerol therapy	

Contd...

Contd...

S.No.	Test name	Normal values	Increasing condition	Decreasing condition
56.	RBC	Nil	Hematuria often indicates pathology. It is found in glomerulonephritis, tuberculosis of the kidney, renal calculi, sickle cell anemia, tumors of the kidney, systemic lupus erythematosus, anticogulation therapy, excessive use of analgesics, etc.	
57.	Reticulocyte count	Adults—0.2 to 2% of the total erythrocyte count Infants—2 to 6% of the total erythrocyte count	Increase with any condition stimulating increase in bone marrow activity, i.e. infection, blood loss, following iron therapy in iron deficiency anemia, erythroblastosis fetalis	Decreased with any condition depressing bone marrow activity, such as leukemia, late stages of anemias
58.	Rheumatoid factor	Negative	The presence of rehumatoid factor may suggests the presence of rheumatoid arthritis, but it is not specific test for rheumatoid arthritis since they are found in other conditions also. A high titer of RF is indicative of a poor prognosis	
59.	Serum albumin	3.5 to 5.5. gm/100 ml	Dehytration, hemoconcentration	Glomerulonephritis, leukemia, malnutrition, starvation
60.	Serum amylase	80 to 200 units/dl	When the serum amylase is elevated over 300 units, it indicates acute pancreatitis. It is also elevated in carcinoma of the head of pancreas, duodenal ulcer, mumps, etc. Elevation is not directly correlated with severity	Decreased in chronic pancreatitis, pancreatic fibrosis and atrophy, cirrhosis of liver, acute alcoholism and toxemia of pregnancy
61.	Serum calcium	2.1 to 2.7 mmol/l 9 to 11 mg/dl	Calcium excess may be seen in cases of tumor or hyperplasia of parathyroid, hyperparathyroidism, multiple myeloma, hypervita-mirosis-D, nephritis with uremia, etc. When the blood calcium levels become high, the serum phosphorus levels become low	Calcium deficit may occur in acute pancreatitis, accidental removal of parathyroid glands following thyroidectomy, diarrhea, celiac diseases, rickets, osteomalacia, malnutrition, nephrosis, renal disorders, pregnancy and lactation hypocalcemia is characterized by tetany

Contd...

Contd...

S.No.	Test name	Normal values	Increasing condition	Decreasing condition
62.	Serum chloride	98 to 108 mmol/l 98 to 108 mEq/l	Chloride is elevated in nephritis, cardiac decompensation, urinary obstruction, etc.	Decreased in diarrhea, vomiting, Cushing's syndrome, burns, intestinal obstructions, febrile conditions, etc.
63.	Serum cholesterol	3.5 to 7.8 mmol/l 100 to 300 mg/dl	Cholesterol is elevated in cases of myxedema, hypothyroidism, arteriosclerosis and bile duct obstruction, physiological in pregnancy, obesity, nephrotic syndrome	Cholesterol is reduced when severe liver damage reduced the ability of the body to synthesize cholesterol, hyperthyroidism, anemia
64.	Serum creatinine	55 to 125 umol/l 1 to 2 mg/dl	Increased serum levels of creatinine indicate decreased renal functions. It is more accurate indicator of renal functions tests	Testosterone treatment
65.	Serum fibrinogen	0.2 to 0.4 gm/100 ml	Rheumatic fever, arthritis, glomerulonephritis	Typhoid, anemia, eclampsia of pregnancy, hypofibrinogenemia, liver failure, carcinoma of prostate
66.	Serum globulin	1.5 to 3 gm/130 ml	Multiple myeloma, infective hepatitis	Lymphatic leukemia
67.	Serum mangesium	108 to 3.0 mg/dl	Renal failure, liver disease	Chronic alcoholism, chronic hepatitis, hypervitaminosis D
68.	Serum potassium	3.4 to 5.4 mmol/l 3.4 to 5.4 mEq/l	Elevated potassium is seen in patients with renal failure, post-operative patients with a poor renal output, those with adreno-cortical deficiency and intestinal obstruction with vomiting	Potassium deficit is seen in patients with poor dietary intake, excessive potassium loss due to diuretics, laxatives, gastric and intestinal suction, drainage from colostomies, excessive vomiting and diarrheas, fistulas of small and large intestines
69.	Serum proteins	6.0 to 8.0 g/dl		Liver disease
70.	Serum sodium	135 to 146 mmol/l 135 to 146 mEq/l	Elevated serum sodium value (hypernatremia) indicates a state of hyperosmolality. It results from a water deficit or an extracellular solute overload	Lower sodium indicates hypo-osmality. It results from excessive water intake, excessive infusions, inability of the kidneys to excrete water, poor salt intake and excessive use of diuretics

Contd...

S.No.	Test name	Normal values	Increasing condition	Decreasing condition
71.	Serum thyroxine (T4)	4.5 to 11.5 ug/dl 70 to 160 nmol/l	Increased in hyperthyroidism, thyroiditis administration of oral contraceptives and pregnancy	Decreased in hypoproteinemia nephrotic syndrome, primary and pituitary hypothyroidism, administration of androgenic and anabolic steroids, and mercurial diuretics
72.	Sodium, chloride, and potassium in sweat	Nil	To confirm cystic fibrosis of pancreas	
73.	Thrombocytes	Below 150,000/cu mm	Polycythemia vera, thrombocythemia	Aplastic anemia, multiple myeloma, hypersplenism, megaloblastic anemia
74.	Thymol turbidity	1 to 4.5 units/ml	Increased in liver diseases, infectious diseases with antibody production	
75.	Total bilirubin	1.7 to 15.4 umol (or) 0.1 to 1.0 mg/dl 0.1 to 0.2 mg/dl (direct) 0.1 to 0.8 mg/dl (indirect)	Increased level of bilirubin is seen in case hemolytic anemia, obstructive jaundice, infective hepatitis, pernicious anemia, hemolytic disease of the newborn and eclampsia. In cases of infective hepatitis and obstructive jaundice, the direct bilirubin is high	
76.	Total protein, albumin, globulin A/G ratio	6 to 8 gm/dl 3.5 to 5.5 gm/dl 1.5 to 3 gm/dl 1.5 : 1 to 2.5 : 1	A change in the A/G ratio indicates chronic hepatitis	Decreased level of plasma proteins indicates malnutrition, hemorrhage, loss of plasma from burns, proteinuria and liver damage
77.	Total WBC count	4500 to 11,000/mm³	Leukocytosis (above 10,000/cmm) is found in children, in pregnancy, pyrexia infections, infestations, hemorrhage, and in leukemia	Leukopenia (less than 4,000/cmm) is found in certain infections (such as typhoid, influenza, TB etc.) anemia, bone marrow depression and in cases of leukemic leukemia
78.	Triglycerides	0.3 to 1.7 mmol/l 25 to 150 mg/dl	Hypothyroidism, diabetes mellitus, nephrotic syndrome, biliary obstruction	Malabsorption, malnutrition
79.	Tri-iodothyronine (T3)	1.1 to 2.6 nmol/l (or) 60 to 150 ng/dl		

Contd...

Contd...

S.No.	Test name	Normal values	Increasing condition	Decreasing condition
80.	Urea (blood)	21 to 43 mg/100 ml	Renal failure	
81.	Uric acid	0.1 to 0.4 mmol/l 2.5 to 8 mg/dl	Increased in gouty arthritis, acute leukemia, lymphomas treated by chemotherapy, and toxemias of pregnancy	Decreased in xanthinuria and defective tubular reabsorption
82.	Urine crystals	Nil	Presence of crystals in the urine is an important predisposing factor in calculus formation	
83.	Urine sugar	Negative	Sugar in the urine (glycosuria) is found in uncontrolled diabetes mellitus, pancreatic disorders and impaired tubular reabsorption Glycosuria may normally result from eating a heavy meal or from emotional stress. IV infusions of glucose also may	
84.	Urobilinogen	Random urine less than 25 mg/dl 24 hours urine in 6.7 umol/24 hrs	Increased level are seen in liver diseases, biliary tract diseases and hemolytic anemias. Reduced excretions are seen in complete or nearly complete biliary obstruction, diarrhea, renal insufficiency	
85.	WBC (urine)	Nil	The presence of WBC in the urine designates an infectious process somewhere in the urinary tract	
86.	Widal test	Typhoid 'O' negative Typhoid 'H' negative Typhoid 'A' negative Typhoid 'B' negative	Typhoid positive titer is 1:160 or more and paratyphoid positive titer is 1:80 or more	Lower titers may be regarded as negative
87.	17-hydroxycorticoids in urine	Male: 3 to 9 mg/24 hrs Female: 2 to 8 mg/24 hrs	Cushing' syndrome	

18 Radiology

INTRODUCTION

Radiology is the medical specialty concerned with the study of parts and functions of body by means of X-rays. Nuclear medicine (NM) is a specialty that deals with the characteristics and uses of radioactive substances in the diagnosis and treatment of diseases. Imaging is the latest form of visualizing the part of the body by means of ultrasonography (USG), computerized tomography (CT) and magnetic resonance imaging (MRI). X-rays are a special type of rays which can be absorbed by the body substance (e.g. calcium in bones), they do not reach the photographic plate held behind the patient, and white areas are left in the X-ray film. A substance is said to be radio lucent, if it permits most of the X-rays (lung tissue). Radiopaque substances (bones) are those absorb most of the X-rays.

X-RAYS

In the process of clinical diagnosis X-rays are used to assess the nature of bone fractures, dislocations, vertebral disk prolapse, cardiomegaly, pathological cavities in lungs, by plain X-rays. Radiopaque substances are used to diagnose bowel conditions, and blood vessels (barium enema, angiogram, and intravenous pyelogram).

Special Diagnostic Techniques

Fluoroscopy

This procedure uses a fluorescent screen instead of photographic plate to derive a visual image from the X-rays through the patient. Internal organs like heart, and digestive tracts can be absorbed in motion.

Contrast Technique

Radiopaque fluids of iodine compounds are used in special procedures namely cardioangiogram, arteriogram, venogram, bronchogram and cholecystogram.

Dye Injection

Radiopaque dyes are used in procedures like hysterosalpingogram, intravenous cholangiogram (IVC), intravenous pyelogram (IVP), lymph angiogram, myelogram, retrograde pyelogram and sialogram.

Imaging

Modern developments in biomedical technology have gifted latest diagnosis methods like ultrasonography, computed axial tomography scanning and magnetic resonance imaging.

Tomography

Tomography is a technique for taking series of X-ray pictures, so that X-rays of a desired layer of the body are obtained while at the same time structure in front of and behind that layer are blurred out. Computed tomography is a revolutionary technique in radiological diagnosis. CT scanners attached to computers synthesizes all information in many views in a single composite picture of a specific slide.

Magnetic Resonance Imaging

Sound waves and magnetic field images the parts of the body with high accuracy three dimensionally, the same as CT scan. It is widely used in investigating the disorders of brain and spinal cord.

Mammography

Mammography is used for identifying the malignant and hormonal disorders of breasts.

Ultrasonography

Sound waves are transmitted into specific parts of the human body, and it is imaged into live telecast of the functioning especially, uterus, liver, gallbladder, etc. to examine fetal conditions, abscess of the liver and lithiasis of gallbladder. The ultrasonography is the safe method free from radiation.

Nuclear Medicine

Alpha particles, beta particles, and gamma rays are used in nuclear medicine. Bone scanning Iodine^{131}I uptakes are important nuclear medicine investigations. Nuclear medicines are therapeutically used to destroy tissues and stop the growth of malignant cells. Bone scanning is a specialty of nuclear medicine.

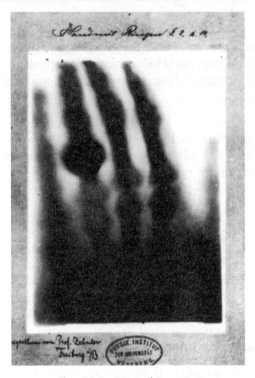

Fig. 18.1: Disambiguation

X-RADIATION

This article is about the form of radiation. For the method of imaging, *see* Radiography. For imaging in a medical context, *see* Radiology. For other uses, *see* X-ray (disambiguation) (Fig. 18.1).

Hand mit Ringen **(Hand with rings):** Print of Roentgen's first "medical" X-ray, of his wife's hand, taken on 22 December 1895 and presented to Professor Ludwig Zehnder of the Physik Institut, University of Freiburg, on 1 January 1896.

X-radiation (composed of X-rays) is a form of electromagnetic radiation. X-rays have a wavelength in the range of 10 to 0.01 nanometers, corresponding to frequencies in the range 30 pet hertz to 30 exahertz (3×10^{16} Hz to 3×10^{19} Hz) and energies in the range 120 eV to 120 keV. They are shorter in wavelength than UV rays. In many languages, X-radiation is called Roetgen radiation after Wilhelm Conrad Roentgen, who is generally credited as their discoverer, and who had called them X-rays to signify an unknown type of radiation.

X-rays can penetrate solid objects, and their largest use is to take images of the inside of objects in diagnostic radiography and crystallography. As a result, the term X-ray is metonymically used to refer to a radiographic image produced using this method, in addition to the method itself. X-rays are a form of ionizing radiation, and exposure to them can be a health hazard.

X-rays from about 0.12 to 12 keV (10 to 0.10 nm wavelength), are classified as soft X-rays, and from about 12 to 120 keV (0.10 to 0.010 nm wavelength) as hard X-rays, due to their penetrating abilities.

The distinction between X-rays and gamma rays has changed in recent decades. Originally, the electromagnetic radiation emitted by X-ray tubes had a longer wavelength than the radiation emitted by radioactive nuclei (gamma rays). So older literature distinguished between X- and gamma radiation on the basis of wavelength, with radiation shorter than some arbitrary wavelength, such as 10^{-11} m, defined as gamma rays. However, as shorter wavelength continuous spectrum "X-ray" sources such as linear accelerators and longer wavelength "gamma ray" emitters were discovered, the wavelength bands largely overlapped. The two types of radiation are now usually distinguished by their origin: X-rays are emitted by electrons outside the nucleus, while gamma rays are emitted by the nucleus.

Units of Measure and Exposure

The measure of X-rays ionizing ability is called the exposure:
* The coulomb per kilogram (C/kg) is the SI unit of ionizing radiation exposure, and is the amount of radiation required to create 1 coulomb of charge of each polarity in 1 kilogram of matter.
* The roentgen (R) is an obsolete traditional unit of exposure, which represented the amount of radiation required to create 1 esu of charge of each polarity in 1 cubic centimeter of dry air. 1 roentgen = 2.58×10^{-4} C/kg

  However, the effect of ionizing radiation on matter (especially living tissue) is more closely related to the amount of energy deposited rather than the charge. This is called the absorbed dose:
* The gray (Gy), which has units of (J/kg), is the SI unit of absorbed dose, and is the amount of radiation required to deposit 1 joule of energy in 1 kilogram of any kind of matter.
* The rad is the (obsolete) corresponding traditional unit, equal to 0.01 J deposited per kg 100 rad = 1 Gy.

  The equivalent dose is the measure of the biological effect of radiation on human tissue. For X-rays it is equal to the absorbed dose.
* The sievert (Sv) is the SI unit of equivalent dose, which for X-rays is numerically equal to the gray (Gy).
* The rem is the traditional unit of equivalent dose. For X-rays it is equal to the rad or 0.01 J of energy deposited per kg. 1 Sv = 100 rem.

Medical X-rays are a major source of *manmade* radiation exposure, accounting for 58 percent in the USA in 1987, but since most radiation exposure is natural (82%) it only accounts for 10 percent of total USA radiation exposure.

Reported dosage due to dental X-rays seems to vary significantly. Depending on the source, a typical dental X-ray of a human results in an exposure of perhaps, 3, 40, 300, or as many as 900 mrems (30 to 9,000 μSv).

Medical Physics

X-ray K-series spectral line wavelengths (nm) for some common target materials.

Target	Kβ	Kβ	Kα	Kα
Fe	0.17566	0.17442	0.193604	0.193998
Co	0.162079	0.160891	0.178897	0.179285
Ni	0.15001	0.14886	0.165791	0.166175
Cu	0.139222	0.138109	0.154056	0.154439
Zr	0.070173	0.068993	0.078593	0.079015
Mo	0.063229	0.062099	0.070930	0.071359

X-rays are generated by an X-ray tube, a vacuum tube that uses a high voltage to accelerate electrons released by a hot cathode to a high velocity. The high velocity electrons collide with a metal target, the anode, creating the X-rays. In medical X-ray tubes the target is usually tungsten or a more crack-resistant alloy of rhenium (5%) and tungsten (95%), but sometimes molybdenum for more specialized applications, such as when soft X-rays are needed as in mammography. In crystallography, a copper target is most common, with cobalt often being used when fluorescence from iron content in the sample might otherwise present a problem.

The maximum energy of the produced X-ray photon is limited by the energy of the incident electron, which is equal to the voltage on the tube, so an 80 kV tube cannot create X-rays with energy greater than 80 keV. When the electrons hit the target, X-rays are created by two different atomic processes:

1. *X-ray fluorescence:* If the electron has enough energy it can knock an orbital electron out of the inner shell of a metal atom, and as a result electrons from higher energy levels then fill-up the vacancy and X-ray photons are emitted. This process produces a discrete spectrum of X-ray frequencies, called spectral lines. The spectral lines generated depend on the target (anode) element used and thus are called characteristic lines. Usually these are transitions from upper shells into K shell (called K lines), into L shell (called L lines) and so on.

2. *Bremsstrahlung:* This is radiation given off by the electrons as they are scattered by the strong electric field near the high-Z

(proton number) nuclei. These X-rays have a continuous spectrum. The intensity of the X-rays increases linearly with decreasing frequency, from zero at the energy of the incident electrons, the voltage on the X-ray tube.

So the resulting output of a tube consists of a continuous Bremsstrahlung spectrum falling off to zero at the tube voltage, plus several spikes at the characteristic lines. The voltages used in diagnostic X-ray tubes, and thus the highest energies of the X-rays, range from roughly 20 to 150 kV.

In medical diagnostic applications, the low energy (soft) X-rays are unwanted, since they are totally absorbed by the body, increasing the dose. So a thin metal (often aluminum, but can be one of many X-ray filters) sheet is placed over the window of the X-ray tube, filtering out the low energy end of the spectrum. This is called *hardening* the beam.

Both X-ray production processes are extremely inefficient (~1%) and thus to produce a usable flux of X-rays plenty of energy has to be wasted into heat, which has to be removed from the X-ray tube.

Radiographs obtained using X-rays can be used to identify a wide spectrum of pathologies. Due to their short wavelength, in medical applications, X-rays act more like a particle than a wave. This is in contrast to their application in crystallography, where their wave-like nature is most important.

To take an X-ray of the bones, short X-ray pulses are shot through a body with radiographic film behind. The bones absorb the most photons by the photoelectric process, because they are more electron-dense. The X-rays leave a latent image in the photographic film; when it is subsequently developed, the parts of the image corresponding to higher X-ray exposure are dark, leaving a white shadow of bones on the film.

To generate an image of the cardiovascular system, including the arteries and veins (angiography) an initial image is taken of the anatomical region of interest. A second image is then taken of the same region after iodinated contrast material has been injected into the blood vessels within this area. These two images are then digitally subtracted, leaving an image of only the iodinated contrast outlining the blood vessels. The radiologist or surgeon then compares the image obtained to normal anatomical images to determine if there is any damage or blockage of the vessel.

A specialized source of X-rays which is becoming widely used in research is synchrotron radiation, which is generated by particle accelerators. Its unique features are brightness many orders of magnitude greater than X-ray tubes, wide spectrum, high collimation, and linear polarization.

Detectors

Photographic Plate

The detection of X-rays is based on various methods. The most commonly known methods are a photographic plate, X-ray film in a cassette, and rare earth screens. Regardless of what is "catching" the image, they are all categorized as "Image Receptors" (IR).

Before computers and before digital imaging, a photographic plate was used to produce radiographic images. The images were produced right on the glass plates. Film replaced these plates and was used in hospitals to produce images. Now computed and digital radiography has started to replace film in medicine, though film technology remains in use in industrial radiography processes (e.g. to inspect welded seams). Photographic plates are a thing of history, and their replacement (intensifying screens) is now becoming part of that same history. Silver (necessary to the radiographic and photographic industry) is a non-renewable resource, that has now been replaced by digital (DR) and computed (CR) technology. Where film required wet processing facilities, these new technologies do not. Archiving of these new technologies also saves space.

Since photographic plates are sensitive to X-rays, they provide a means of recording the image, but require a lot of exposure (to the patient), so intensifying screens were devised. They allow a lower dose to the patient, because the screens take the X-ray information and intensify it so that it can be recorded on film positioned next to the intensifying screen.

The part of the patient to be X-rayed is placed between the X-ray source and the image receptor to produce a shadow of the internal structure of that particular part of the body. X-rays are partially blocked ("attenuated") by dense tissues such as bone, and pass more easily through soft tissues. Areas where the X-rays strike darkens when developed, causing bones to appear lighter than the surrounding soft tissue.

Contrast compounds containing barium or iodine, which are radiopaque, can be ingested in the gastrointestinal tract (barium) or injected in the artery or veins to highlight these vessels. The contrast compounds have high atomic numbered elements in them that (like bone) essentially block the X-rays and hence the once hollow organ or vessel can be more readily seen. In the pursuit of a nontoxic contrast material, many types of high atomic number elements were evaluated.

For example, the first time the forefathers used contrast it was chalk, and was used on a cadaver's vessels. Unfortunately, some elements chosen proved to be harmful—for example, thorium was once used as a contrast medium (Thorotrast)—which turned out to be toxic in some cases (causing injury and occasionally death from the effects of thorium poisoning). Modern contrast material has improved, and while there is no way to determine who may have sensitivity to the contrast, the incidence of "allergic-type reactions" is low. The risk is comparable to that associated with penicillin.

PHOTOSTIMULABLE PHOSPHORS

An increasingly common method is the use of photostimulated luminescence (PSL), pioneered by Fuji in the 1980s. In modern hospitals a photostimulable phosphor plate (PSP plate) is used in place of the photographic plate. After the plate is X-rayed, excited electrons in the phosphor material remain "trapped" in "color centers" in the crystal lattice until stimulated by a laser beam passed over the plate surface. The light given off during laser stimulation is collected by a photomultiplier tube and the resulting signal is converted into a digital image by computer technology, which gives this process its common name, computed radiography (also referred to as digital radiography). The PSP plate can be reused, and existing X-ray equipment requires no modification to use them.

Geiger Counter

Initially, most common detection methods were based on the ionization of gases, as in the Geiger-Müller counter: a sealed volume, usually a cylinder, with a mica, polymer or thin metal window contains a gas, a cylindrical cathode and a wire anode; a high voltage is applied between the cathode and the anode. When an X-ray photon enters the cylinder, it ionizes the gas and forms ions and electrons. Electrons accelerate toward the anode, in the process causing further ionization along their trajectory. This process, known as a Townsend avalanche, is detected as a sudden current, called a "count" or "event".

In order to gain energy spectrum information, a diffracting crystal may be used to first separate the different photons. The method is called wavelength dispersive X-ray spectroscopy (WDX or WDS). Position-sensitive detectors are often used in conjunction with dispersive elements. Other detection equipment that is inherently energy-resolving may be used, such as the aforementioned proportional counters. In

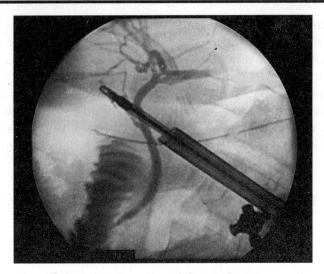

Fig. 18.2: X-ray during cholecystectomy

either case, use of suitable pulse-processing (MCA) equipment allows digital spectra to be created for later analysis.

For many applications, counters are not sealed but are constantly fed with purified gas, thus reducing problems of contamination or gas aging. These are called "flow counters".

Scintillators

Some materials such as sodium iodide (NaI) can "convert" an X-ray photon to a visible photon; an electronic detector can be built by adding a photomultiplier. These detectors are called "scintillators", film screens or "scintillation counters". The main advantage of using these is that an adequate image can be obtained while subjecting the patient to a much lower dose of X-rays.

Image Intensification (Fig. 18.2)

X-rays are also used in "real-time" procedures such as angiography or contrast studies of the hollow organs (e.g. barium enema of the small or large intestine) using fluoroscopy acquired using an X-ray image intensifier. Angioplasty, medical interventions of the arterial system rely heavily on X-ray-sensitive contrast to identify potentially treatable lesions.

Direct Semiconductor Detectors

Since the 1970s, new semiconductor detectors have been developed (silicon or germanium doped with lithium, Si (Li) or Ge (Li)). X-ray photons are converted to electron-hole pairs in the semiconductor and are collected to detect the X-rays. When the temperature is low enough (the detector is cooled by Peltier effect or even cooler liquid nitrogen), it is possible to directly determine the X-ray energy spectrum; this method is called energy dispersive X-ray spectroscopy (EDX or EDS); it is often used in small X-ray fluorescence spectrometers. These detectors are sometimes called "solid state detectors". Detectors based on cadmium telluride (CdTe) and its alloy with zinc, cadmium zinc telluride, have an increased sensitivity, which allows lower doses of X-rays to be used.

Practical application in medical imaging started in the 1990s. Currently amorphous selenium is used in commercial large area flat panel X-ray detectors for mammography and chest radiography. Current research and development is focused around pixel detectors, such as CERN's energy resolving Medipix detector.

Note: A standard semiconductor diode, such as a 1N4007, will produce a small amount of current when placed in an X-ray beam. A test device once used by Medical Imaging Service personnel was a small project box that contained several diodes of this type in series, which could be connected to an oscilloscope as a quick diagnostic.

Silicon drift detectors (SDDs)—produced by conventional semiconductor fabrication, now provide a cost-effective and high resolving power radiation measurement. Unlike conventional X-ray detectors, such as Si (Li)s, they do not need to be cooled with liquid nitrogen.

Scintillators Plus Semiconductor Detectors (Indirect Detection)

With the advent of large semiconductor array detectors it has become possible to design detector systems using a scintillators screen to convert from X-rays to visible light which is then converted to electrical signals in an array detector. Indirect Flat Panel Detectors (FPD) are in widespread use today in medical, dental, veterinary and industrial applications.

The array technology is a variant on the amorphous silicon TFT arrays used in many flat panel displays, like the ones in computer laptops. The array consists of a sheet of glass covered with a thin layer of silicon that is in an amorphous or disordered state. At a microscopic scale, the silicon has been imprinted with millions of transistors arranged in a highly ordered array, like the grid on a sheet of graph paper. Each of these thin film transistors (TFT) is attached to a light-absorbing photodiode making-up an individual pixel (picture element). Photons striking the photodiode are converted into two carriers of electrical charge, called electron-hole pairs. Since the number of charge carriers produced will vary with the intensity of incoming light photons, an electrical pattern is created that can be swiftly converted to a voltage and then a digital signal, which is interpreted by a computer to produce a digital image.

Although silicon has outstanding electronic properties, it is not a particularly good absorber of X-ray photons. For this reason, X-rays first impinge upon scintillators made from, e.g. gadolinium oxysulfide or cesium iodide. The scintillators absorbs the X-rays and converts them into visible light photons that then pass onto the photodiode array.

Visibility to the Human Eye

While generally considered invisible to the human eye, in special circumstances X-rays can be visible. Brandes in an experiment a short time after Roentgen's landmark 1895 paper, reported after dark adaptation and placing his eye close to an X-ray tube seeing a faint "blue-gray" glow which seemed to originate within the eye itself. Upon hearing this, Roentgen reviewed his record books and found he too had seen the effect. When placing an X-ray tube on the opposite side of a wooden door Roentgen had noted the same blue glow, seeming to emanate from the eye itself, but thought his observations to be spurious because he only saw the effect when he used one type of tube. Later he realized that the tube which had created the effect was the only one powerful enough to make the glow plainly visible and the experiment was thereafter readily repeatable. The knowledge that X-rays are actually faintly visible to the dark-adapted naked eye has largely been forgotten today; this is probably due to the desire not to repeat what would now be seen as a recklessly dangerous and potentially harmful experiment with ionizing radiation. It is not known what exact mechanism in the eye produces the visibility: it could be due to conventional detection (excitation of rhodopsin molecules in the retina), direct excitation of retinal nerve cells, or secondary detection via, for instance, X-ray induction of phosphorescence in the eyeball with conventional retinal detection of the secondarily produced visible light.

Though X-rays are otherwise invisible it is possible to see the ionization of the air molecules if the intensity of the X-ray beam is high enough. The beam line from the wiggler at the ID11 at ESRF is one example of such high intensity.

Medical Uses (Figs 18.3 and 18.4)

Since Roentgen's discovery that X-rays can identify bone structures, X-rays have been developed for their use in medical imaging. Radiology is a specialized field of medicine. Radiologists employ radiography and other techniques for diagnostic imaging. This is probably the most common use of X-ray technology.

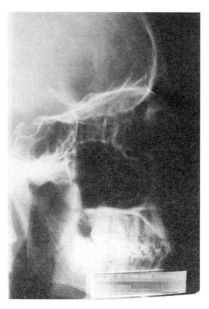

Fig. 18.3: X-ray image of the paranasal sinuses, lateral projection

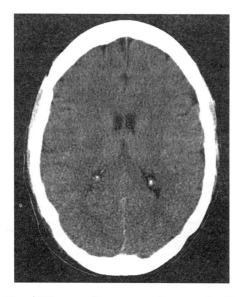

Fig. 18.4: Head CT scan slice—a modern application of X-rays

X-rays are especially useful in the detection of pathology of the skeletal system, but are also useful for detecting some disease processes in soft tissue. Some notable examples are the very common chest X-ray, which can be used to identify lung diseases such as pneumonia, lung cancer or pulmonary edema, and the abdominal X-ray, which can detect intestinal obstruction, free air (from visceral perforations) and free fluid (in ascites). X-rays may also be used to detect pathology such as gallstones (which are rarely radiopaque) or kidney stones which are often (but not always) visible. Traditional plain X-rays are less useful in the imaging of soft tissues such as the brain or muscle. Imaging alternatives for soft tissues are computed axial tomography (CAT or CT scanning), magnetic resonance imaging (MRI) or ultrasound. Since 2005, X-rays are listed as a carcinogen by the US government. The use of X-rays as a treatment is known as radiotherapy and is largely used for the management (including palliation) of cancer; it requires higher radiation energies than for imaging alone.

X-rays are a relatively safe method of investigation and the radiation exposure is low. But in pregnant patients, the benefits of the investigation (X-ray) should be balanced with the potential hazards to the unborn fetus.

Shielding Against X-rays

Lead is the most common shield against X-rays because of its high density (11340 kg/m³), stopping power, ease of installation and low cost. The maximum range of a high-energy photon such as an X-ray in matter is infinite; at every point in the matter traversed by the photon, there is a probability of interaction. Thus there is a very small probability of no interaction over very large distances. The shielding of photon beam is, therefore, exponential (with an attenuation length being close to the radiation length of the material); doubling the thickness of shielding will square the shielding effect.

Table 18.1 shows the recommended thickness of lead shielding in function of X-ray energy, from the recommendations by the Second International Congress of Radiology:

Table 18.1: Function of X-ray energy–recommended thickness of lead shielding

X-rays generated by peak voltages not exceeding	Minimum thickness of lead
75 kV	1.0 mm
100 kV	1.5 mm
125 kV	2.0 mm
150 kV	2.5 mm
175 kV	3.0 mm
200 kV	4.0 mm
225 kV	5.0 mm
300 kV	9.0 mm
400 kV	15.0 mm
500 kV	22.0 mm
600 kV	34.0 mm
900 kV	51.0 mm

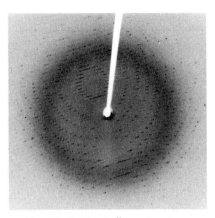

Fig. 18.5: Crystalline structure

Other Uses (Fig. 18.5)

Each dot, called a reflection, in this diffraction pattern forms from the constructive interference of scattered X-rays passing through a crystal. The data can be used to determine the crystalline structure.

Other Notable Uses of X-rays

• X-ray crystallography in which the pattern produced by the diffraction of X-rays through the closely spaced lattice of atoms in a crystal is recorded and then analyzed to reveal the nature of that lattice. A related technique, fiber diffraction, was used by Rosalind Franklin to discover the double helical structure of DNA.

• X-ray astronomy, which is an observational branch of astronomy, which deals with the study of X-ray emission from celestial objects.

• X-ray microscopic analysis, which uses electromagnetic radiation in the soft X-ray band to produce images of very small objects.

• X-ray fluorescence, a technique in which X-rays are generated within a specimen and detected. The outgoing energy of the X-ray can be used to identify the composition of the sample.

• Industrial radiography uses X-rays for inspection of industrial parts, particularly welds.

• Paintings are often X-rayed to reveal the under drawing and pentimenti or alterations in the course of painting, or by later restorers. Many pigments such as lead white show well in X-ray photographs.

• Airport security luggage scanners use X-rays for inspecting the interior of luggage for security threats before loading on aircraft.

• X-ray fine art photography.

• Roentgen Stereophotogrammetry is used to track movement of bones based on the implantation of markers.

• X-ray photoelectron spectroscopy is a chemical analysis technique relying on the photoelectric effect, usually employed in surface science.

Age   **Date**

Type of Request: Routine ☐ Emergency ☐   **Transport:** Wheelchair ☐ Trolley ☐

Allergies: Iodine ☐   Others _____

LNMP_____   **Contraceptive Pill:** Yes ☐ No ☐   **Pregnant:** Yes ☐ No ☐

Examination Required:

Brief Clinical Description: Date and Time

                                                          of X-ray

                                                          Appointment

Provisional Diagnosis

Previous X-ray

Patients Next Appointment with Clinic

Physician   Signature   Date

For Use of X-ray Department

Radiographer   Screening Time   X-ray No.

Checked by

Position		KV		Mas		Total No of Films	
35 × 43	35 × 35	35 × 40	24 × 30	18 × 24	ENTAL	OCC	

Report

Radiologist   Signature   Date

X-ray Request and Report

Age: _____ Nationality: _____ Date and Time of Admission: _____

LMP (Arabic) _____

English _____ Cycle _____ Pill _____ Parity _____

Past History ☐

                 ☐   ☐   ☐

                Twins   Cong Abnor   Type

Family History ☐   ☐   ☐

Present History ☐ Diabetes   ☐ Rh   ☐ Heart disease   ☐ APII _____

           ☐ Pre-eclampsia   ☐ Others

           Uterus by Date   Presentation

           Uterus by Size   ☐ F H H

Palpation ☐ F M F   ☐ Others

           ☐ Others

Other Exam Required

Information Requested

Physician _____ Signature _____ Date _____

Serial/Repeat Scan Request		**Appointment**		
Date	Signature	Date	Time	Signature
		1. _____		
		2. _____		
		3. _____		
		4. _____		

Report

_____

_____

_____

_____

_____

Physician _____ Signature _____ Date _____

ULTRASOUND EXAM FORM

RADIOLOGIC CONSULTATION REQUEST/REPORT
(Radiology/Nuclear Medicine/Ultrasound/Computer Tomography Examinations)

Examination Requested	Age	sex	SSN (Sponsor)	Ward/Clinic	Register No.
	Film No.				Pregnant ☐ Yes ☐ No
	Requested by (print)				Telephone/Page No.
	Signature of Requestor				Date Requested

Specific Reason for Request (Complaints and findings)

Date of Examination (Month, day, year)	Date of Report (Month, day, year)	Date of Transaction (Month, day, year)

Radiologic Report

Patients Identification (For typed or written entries give Name - last, first, middle, medical facility)	Location of Medical Records
	Location of Radiologic Facility
	Signature

Radiological Consultation
Request/Report

2 - Physician

19 | Radiation Therapy

Radiation therapy (in North America), or *radiotherapy* (in the UK and Australia) also called *radiation oncology*, and sometimes abbreviated to XRT, is the medical use of ionizing radiation as part of cancer treatment to control malignant cells (not to be confused with radiology, the use of radiation in medical imaging and diagnosis). Radiotherapy may be used for curative or adjuvant cancer treatment. It is used as palliative treatment (where cure is not possible and the aim is for local disease control or symptomatic relief) or as therapeutic treatment (where the therapy has survival benefit and it can be curative). Total body irradiation (TBI) is a radiotherapy technique used to prepare the body to receive a bone marrow transplant. Radiotherapy has several applications in non-malignant conditions, such as the treatment of trigeminal neuralgia, severe thyroid eye disease, pterygium, pigmented villonodular synovitis, prevention of keloid scar growth, and prevention of heterotopic ossification. The use of radiotherapy in non-malignant conditions is limited partly by worries about the risk of radiation-induced cancers.

Radiotherapy is used for the treatment of malignant tumors (cancer), and may be used as the primary therapy. It is also common to combine radiotherapy with surgery, chemotherapy, hormone therapy or some mixture of the three. Most common cancer types can be treated with radiotherapy in some way. The precise treatment intent (curative, adjuvant, neoadjuvant, therapeutic, or palliative) will depend on the tumor type, location, and stage, as well as the general health of the patient.

Radiation therapy is commonly applied to the cancerous tumor. The radiation fields may also include the draining lymph nodes if they are clinically or radio logically involved with tumor, or if there is thought to be a risk of subclinical malignant spread. It is necessary to include a margin of normal tissue around the tumor to allow for uncertainties in daily set-up and internal tumor motion. These uncertainties can be caused by internal movement (for example, respiration and bladder filling) and movement of external skin marks relative to the tumor position.

To spare normal tissues (such as skin or organs which radiation must pass through in order to treat the tumor), shaped radiation beams are aimed from several angles of exposure to intersect at the tumor, providing a much larger absorbed dose there than in the surrounding, healthy tissue.

Varian Clinac 2100C Linear Accelerator which is mostly widely selected medical accelerator in the world, treating thousands of patients everyday for treatment of radiology oncology practices. Clinicians around the world depend on Varian system to deliver treatment at the right-time-the instant the tumor is on target. The variant clinac delivers the exact prescribed dose to the patient in the lowest number of monitor units (MUs) possible. Whether it is day-to-day repositioning of the patient or managing motion during treatment. With this machine, clinicians can personalize each patient's care based on their needs and individual clinical protocol (Fig. 19.1).

MECHANISM OF ACTION

Radiation therapy works by damaging the DNA of cells. The damage is caused by a photon, electron, proton, neutron, or ion beam directly or indirectly ionizing the atoms which make up the DNA chain. Indirect ionization happens as a result of the ionization of water, forming free radicals, notably hydroxyl radicals, which then damage the DNA. In the most common forms of radiation therapy, most of the radiation effect is through free radicals. Because cells have mechanisms for repairing DNA damage, breaking the DNA on both strands proves to be the most significant technique in modifying cell characteristics. Because cancer cells generally are undifferentiated and stem cell-like,

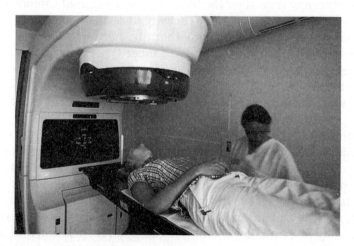

Fig. 19.1: Varian Clinac 2100C linear accelerator (*For color version, see Plate 1*).

they reproduce more, and have a diminished ability to repair sub-lethal damage compared to most healthy differentiated cells. The DNA damage is inherited through cell division, accumulating damage to the cancer cells, causing them to die or reproduce more slowly.

One of the major limitations of radiotherapy is that the cells of solid tumors become deficient in oxygen. Solid tumors can outgrow their blood supply, causing a low-oxygen state known as hypoxia. Oxygen is a potent radiosensitizer, increasing the effectiveness of a given dose of radiation by forming DNA-damaging free radicals. Tumor cells in a hypoxic environment may be as much as 2 to 3 times more resistant to radiation damage than those in a normal oxygen environment. Much research has been devoted to overcoming this problem including the use of high pressure oxygen tanks, blood substitutes that carry increased oxygen, hypoxic cell radio sensitizers such as misonidazole and metronidazole, and hypoxic cytotoxins, such as tirapazamine. There is also interest in the fact that high-LET (linear energy transfer) particles such as carbon or neon ions may have an anti-tumor effect which is less dependent of tumor oxygen because these particles act mostly via direct damage.

Dose

The amount of radiation used in radiation therapy is measured in gray (Gy), and varies depending on the type and stage of cancer being treated. For curative cases, the typical dose for a solid epithelial tumor ranges from 60 to 80 Gy, while lymphoma tumors are treated with 20 to 40 Gy.

Preventive (adjuvant) doses are typically around 45 to 60 Gy in 1.8 to 2 Gy fractions (for Breast, Head and Neck cancers respectively.) Many other factors are considered by radiation oncologists when selecting a dose, including whether the patient is receiving chemotherapy, whether radiation therapy is being administered before or after surgery, and the degree of success of surgery.

Radiation therapy plans are often evaluated using dose-volume histograms, which allow the clinician to assess the uniformity of the dose to the diseased tissue (tumor) and how well healthy structures are spared.

Fractionation

The total dose is fractionated (spread out over time) for several important reasons. Fractionation allows normal cells time to recover, while tumor cells are generally less efficient in repair between fractions. Fractionation also allows tumor cells that were in a relatively radio-resistant phase of the cell cycle during one treatment to cycle into a sensitive phase of the cycle before the next fraction is given. Similarly, tumor cells that were chronically or acutely hypoxic (and therefore more radio resistant) may reoxygenate between fractions, improving the tumor cell kill. Fractionation regimes are individualized between different radiotherapy centers and even between individual doctors. In North America, Australia, and Europe, the typical fractionation schedule for adults is 1.8 to 2 Gy per day, five days a week. In the northern United Kingdom, fractions are more commonly 2.67 to 2.75 Gy per day, which eases the burden on thinly spread resources in the National Health Service. In some cancer types, prolongation of the fraction schedule over too long can allow for the tumor to begin repopulating, and for these tumor types, including head-and-neck and cervical squamous cell cancers, radiation treatment is preferably completed within a certain amount of time. For children, a typical fraction size may be 1.5 to 1.8 Gy per day, as smaller fraction sizes are associated with reduced incidence and severity of late-onset side effects in normal tissues.

In some cases, two fractions per day are used near the end of a course of treatment. This schedule, known as a concomitant boost regimen or hyper fractionation, is used on tumors that regenerate more quickly when they are smaller. In particular, tumors in the head-and-neck demonstrate this behavior.

One of the best-known alternative fractionation schedules is Continuous Hyper fractionated Accelerated Radiotherapy (CHART). CHART, used to treat lung cancer, consists of three smaller fractions per day. Although reasonably successful, CHART can be a strain on radiation therapy departments.

Implants can be fractionated over minutes or hours, or they can be permanent seeds which slowly deliver radiation until they become inactive.

EFFECT ON DIFFERENT TYPES OF CANCER

Different cancers respond differently to radiation therapy. The response of a cancer to radiation is described by its radio sensitivity. Highly radiosensitive cancer cells are rapidly killed by modest doses of radiation. These include leukemia's, most lymphomas and germ cell tumors. The majority of epithelial cancers are only moderately radiosensitive, and require a significantly higher dose of radiation (60–70 Gy) to achieve a radical cure. Some types of cancer are notably radio resistant, that is, much higher doses are required to produce a radical cure than may be safe in clinical practice. Renal cell cancer and melanoma are generally considered to be radio resistant.

It is important to distinguish the radio sensitivity of a particular tumor, which to some extent is a laboratory measure, from the radiation "curability" of a cancer in actual clinical practice. For example, leukemia's are not generally curable with radiotherapy, because they are disseminated though the body. Lymphoma may be radically curable if it is localized to one area of the body. Similarly, many of the common, moderately radio responsive tumors are routinely treated with curative doses of radiotherapy if they are at an early stage. For example, non-melanoma skin cancer, head and neck cancer, non-small cell lung cancer, cervical cancer, anal cancer, prostate cancer. Metastatic cancers are generally incurable with radiotherapy because it is not possible to treat the whole body.

Before treatment, a CT scan is often performed to identify the tumor and surrounding normal structures. The patient is then sent for a simulation so that molds can be created to be used during treatment. The patient receives small skin marks to guide the placement of treatment fields.

The response of a tumor to radiotherapy is also related to its size. For complex reasons, very large tumors respond less well to radiation than smaller tumors or microscopic disease. Various strategies are used to overcome this effect. The most common technique is surgical resection prior to radiotherapy. This is most commonly seen in the treatment of breast cancer with wide local excision or mastectomy followed by adjuvant radiotherapy. Another method is to shrink the tumor with neoadjuvant chemotherapy prior to radical radiotherapy. A third technique is to enhance the radio sensitivity of the cancer by giving certain drugs during a course of radiotherapy. Examples of radiosensitizing drugs include: Cisplatin, Nimorazole and Cetuximab.

TYPES OF RADIATION THERAPY

Historically, the three main divisions of radiotherapy are external beam radiotherapy (EBRT or XBRT) or teletherapy, brachytherapy or sealed source radiotherapy, and systemic radioisotope therapy or unsealed source radiotherapy. The differences relate to the position of the radiation source; external is outside the body, brachytherapy uses sealed radioactive sources placed precisely in the area under treatment, and systemic radioisotopes are given by infusion or oral ingestion. Brachytherapy can use temporary or permanent placement of radioactive sources. The temporary sources are usually placed by a technique called after loading. In after loading a hollow tube or applicator is placed surgically in the organ to be treated, and the sources are loaded into the applicator after the applicator is implanted. This minimizes radiation exposure to health care personnel. Particle therapy is a special case of external beam radiotherapy where the particles are protons or heavier ions. Interpretative radiotherapy is a special type of radiotherapy that is delivered immediately after surgical removal of the cancer. This method has been employed in breast cancer (targeted interpretative radiotherapy), brain tumor and rectal cancers.

External Beam Radiotherapy

The following three sections refer to treatment using X-rays:

Conventional External Beam Radiotherapy

Conventional external beam radiotherapy (2DXRT) is delivered via two-dimensional beams using linear accelerator machines. 2DXRT mainly consists of a single beam of radiation delivered to the patient from several directions: often front or back, and both sides. *Conventional* refers to the way the treatment is *planned* or *simulated* on a specially calibrated diagnostic X-ray machine known as a simulator because it recreates the linear accelerator actions (or sometimes by eye), and to the usually well-established arrangements of the radiation beams to achieve a desired *plan*. The aim of simulation is to accurately target or localize the volume which is to be treated. This technique is well established and is generally quick and reliable. The worry is that some high-dose treatments may be limited by the radiation toxicity capacity of healthy tissues which lay close to the target tumor volume. An example of this problem is seen in radiation of the prostate gland, where the sensitivity of the adjacent rectum limited the A detector system for imaging radio therapeutic dose distributions in 4D dose which could be safely prescribed using 2DXRT planning to such an extent that tumor control may not be easily achievable. Prior to the invention of the CT, physicians and physicists had limited knowledge about the true radiation dosage delivered to both cancerous and healthy tissue. For this reason, 3-dimensional conformal radiotherapy is becoming the standard treatment for a number of tumor sites.

Stereotactic Radiation

Stereotactic radiation is a specialized type of external beam radiation therapy. It uses focused radiation beams targeting a well-defined tumor using extremely detailed imaging scans. Radiation oncologists perform stereo tactic treatments, often with the help of a neurosurgeon for tumors in the brain or spine.

There are two types of stereotactic radiation. Stereotactic radio surgery (SRS) is when doctors use a single or several stereotactic radiation treatments of the brain or spine. *Stereotactic body radiation therapy* (SBRT) refers to one or several stereotactic radiation treatments with the body, such as the lungs.

Some doctors say an advantage to stereo tactic treatments are they deliver the right amount of radiation to the cancer in a shorter amount of time than traditional treatments, which can often take 6 to 11 weeks. Plus treatments are given with extreme accuracy, which should limit the effect of the radiation on healthy tissues. One problem with stereotactic treatments is that they are only suitable for certain small tumors.

Stereotactic treatments can be confusing because many hospitals call the treatments by the name of the manufacturer rather than calling it SRS or SBRT. Brand names for these treatments include axesse, cyber knife, Gamma knife, novalis, prim atom, synergy, X-knife, tomo therapy and trilogy. This list changes as equipment manufacturers continue to develop new, specialized technologies to treat cancers.

Virtual Simulation, Three-Dimensional Conformal Radiotherapy, and Intensity-modulated Radiotherapy

The planning of radiotherapy treatment has been revolutionized by the ability to delineate tumors and adjacent normal structures in three dimensions using specialized CT and/or MRI scanners and planning software.

Virtual simulation, the most basic form of planning, allows more accurate placement of radiation beams than is possible using conventional X-rays, where soft-tissue structures are often difficult to assess and normal tissues difficult to protect.

An enhancement of virtual simulation is 3-Dimensional Conformal Radiotherapy (3DCRT), in which the profile of each radiation beam is shaped to fit the profile of the target from a beam's eye view (BEV) using a multileaf collimator (MLC) and a variable number of beams. When the treatment volume conforms to the shape of the tumor, the relative toxicity of radiation to the surrounding normal tissues is reduced, allowing a higher dose of radiation to be delivered to the tumor than conventional techniques would allow.

Intensity-modulated radiation therapy (IMRT) is an advanced type of high-precision radiation that is the next generation of 3DCRT. IMRT also improves the ability to conform the treatment volume to concave tumor shapes, for example when the tumor is wrapped around a vulnerable structure such as the spinal cord or a major organ or blood vessel. Computer-controlled X-ray accelerators distribute precise radiation doses to malignant tumors or specific areas within the tumor. The pattern of radiation delivery is determined using highly-tailored computing applications to perform optimization and treatment simulation (treatment planning). The radiation dose is consistent with the 3-D shape of the tumor by controlling, or modulating, the radiation beam's intensity. The radiation dose intensity is elevated near the gross tumor volume while radiation among the neighboring normal tissue is decreased or avoided completely. The customized radiation dose is intended to maximize tumor dose while simultaneously protecting the surrounding normal tissue. This may result in better tumor targeting, lessened side effects, and improved treatment outcomes than even 3DCRT.

3DCRT is still used extensively for many body sites but the use of IMRT is growing in more complicated body sites such as CNS, head and neck, prostate, breast and lung. Unfortunately, IMRT is limited by its need for additional time from experienced medical personnel. This is because physicians must manually delineate the tumors one CT image at a time through the entire disease site which can take much longer than 3DCRT preparation. Then, medical physicists and dosimetrists must be engaged to create a viable treatment plan. Also, the IMRT technology has only been used commercially since the late 1990s even at the most advanced cancer centers, so radiation oncologists who did not learn it as part of their residency program must find additional sources of education before implementing IMRT.

Proof of improved survival benefit from either of these two techniques over conventional radiotherapy (2DXRT) is growing for many tumor sites, but the ability to reduce toxicity is generally accepted. Both techniques enable dose escalation, potentially increasing usefulness. There has been some concern, particularly with 3DCRT, about increased exposure of normal tissue to radiation and the consequent potential for secondary malignancy. Overconfidence in the accuracy of imaging may increase the chance of missing lesions that are invisible on the planning scans (and therefore not included in the treatment plan) or that move between or during a treatment (for example, due to respiration or inadequate patient immobilization). New techniques are being developed to better control this uncertainty—for example, real-time imaging combined with real-time adjustment of the therapeutic beams. This new technology is called image-guided radiation therapy (IGRT) or four-dimensional radiotherapy.

Particle Therapy

In particle therapy (Proton therapy), energetic ionizing particles (protons or carbon ions) are directed at the target tumor. The dose increases while the particle penetrates the tissue, up to a maximum (the Bragg peak) that occurs near the end of the particle's range, and it then drops to (almost) zero. The advantage of this energy deposition profile is that less energy is deposited into the healthy tissue surrounding the target tissue.

Radioisotope Therapy (RIT)

Systemic radioisotope therapy is a form of targeted therapy. Targeting can be due to the chemical properties of the isotope such as radioiodine which is specifically absorbed by the thyroid gland a thousand fold better than other bodily organs. Targeting can also be achieved by attaching the radioisotope to another molecule or antibody to guide it to the target tissue. The radioisotopes are delivered through infusion (into the bloodstream) or ingestion. Examples are the infusion of metaiodobenzylguanidine (MIBG) to treat neuroblastoma, of oral iodine-131 to treat thyroid cancer or thyrotoxicosis, and of hormone-bound lutetium-177 and yttrium-90 to treat neuroendocrine tumors (peptide receptor radionuclide therapy). Another example is the injection of radioactive glass or resin micro spheres into the hepatic artery to radioembolize liver tumors or liver metastases.

A major use of systemic radioisotope therapy is in the treatment of bone metastasis from cancer. The radioisotopes travel selectively to areas of damaged bone, and spare normal undamaged bone. Isotopes commonly used in the treatment of bone metastasis are strontium-89 and samarium [153]Smlexidronam. In 2002, the United States Food and Drug Administration (FDA) approved ibritumomab tiuxetan (Zevalin), which is an anti-CD20 monoclonal antibody conjugated to yttrium-90. In 2003, the FDA approved the tositumomab/iodine (^{131}I) tositumomab regimen (Bexxar), which is a combination of an iodine-131 labeled and an unlabelled anti-CD20 monoclonal antibody. These medications were the first agents of what is known as radio immunotherapy, and they were approved for the treatment of refractory non-Hodgkin's lymphoma.

Side Effects

Radiation therapy is in itself painless. Many low-dose palliative treatments (for example, radiotherapy to bony metastases) cause minimal or no side effects, although short-term pain flare up can be experienced in the days following treatment due to edema compressing nerves in the treated area. Treatment to higher doses causes varying side effects during treatment (acute side effects), in the months or years following treatment (long-term side effects), or after re-treatment (cumulative side effects). The nature, severity, and longevity of side effects depends on the organs that receive the radiation, the treatment itself (type of radiation, dose, fractionation, concurrent chemotherapy), and the patient.

Most side effects are predictable and expected. Side effects from radiation are usually limited to the area of the patient's body that is under treatment. One of the aims of modern radiotherapy is to reduce side effects to a minimum, and to help the patient to understand and to deal with those side effects which are unavoidable.

The main side effects reported are fatigue and skin irritation, like a mild to moderate sun burn. The fatigue often sets in during the middle of a course of treatment and can last for weeks after treatment ends. The skin irritation will also go away, but it may not be as elastic as it was before. Patients should ask their radiation oncologist or radiation oncology nurse about possible products and medications that can help with side effects.

Acute Side Effects

Damage to the epithelial surfaces: Epithelial surfaces may sustain damage from radiation therapy. Depending on the area being treated, this may include the skin, oral mucosa, pharyngeal, bowel mucosa and ureter. The rates of onset of damage and recovery from it depend upon the turnover rate of epithelial cells. Typically the skin starts to become pink and sore several weeks into treatment. The reaction may become more severe during the treatment and for up to about one week following the end of radiotherapy, and the skin may break down. Although this moist desquamation is uncomfortable, recovery is usually quick. Skin reactions tend to be worse in areas where there are natural folds in the skin, such as underneath the female breast, behind the ear and in the groin.

If the head and neck area is treated, temporary soreness and ulceration commonly occur in the mouth and throat. If severe, this can affect swallowing, and the patient may need painkillers and nutritional support/food supplements. The esophagus can also become sore if it is treated directly, or if, as commonly occurs; it receives a dose of collateral radiation during treatment of lung cancer.

The lower bowel may be treated directly with radiation (treatment of rectal or anal cancer) or be exposed by radiotherapy to other pelvic structures (prostate, bladder, female genital tract). Typical symptoms are soreness, diarrhoea, and nausea.

Swelling (edema): As part of the general inflammation that occurs, swelling of soft tissues may cause problems during radiotherapy. This is a concern during treatment of brain tumors and brain metastases, especially where there is pre-existing raised intracranial pressure or where the tumor is causing near-total obstruction of a lumen (e.g. trachea or main bronchus). Surgical intervention may be considered prior to treatment with radiation. If surgery is deemed unnecessary or inappropriate, the patient may receive steroids during radiotherapy to reduce swelling.

Infertility. The gonads (ovaries and testicles) are very sensitive to radiation. They may be unable to produce gametes following direct exposure to most normal treatment doses of radiation. Treatment planning for all body sites is designed to minimize, if not completely exclude dose to the gonads if they are not the primary area of treatment.

Medium and long-term side effects: These depend on the tissue that received the treatment; they may be minimal.

Fibrosis: Tissues which have been irradiated tend to become less elastic over time due to a diffuse scarring process.

Hair loss: This may be most pronounced in patients who have received radiotherapy to the brain. Unlike the hair loss seen with chemotherapy, radiation-induced hair loss is more likely to be permanent, but is also more likely to be limited to the area treated by the radiation.

Dryness: The salivary glands and tear glands have a radiation tolerance of about 30 Gy in 2 Gy fractions, a dose which is exceeded by most radical head and neck cancer treatments. Dry mouth (xerostomia) and dry eyes (exophthalmia) can become irritating long-term problems and severely reduce the patient's quality of life. Similarly, sweat glands in treated skin (such as the armpit) tend to stop working, and the naturally moist vaginal mucosa is often dry following pelvic irradiation.

Fatigue: Fatigue is among the most common symptoms of radiation therapy, and can last from a few months to a few years, depending on the quantity of the treatment and cancer type. Lack of energy, reduced activity and overtired feelings are common symptoms.

Cancer: Radiation is a potential cause of cancer, and secondary malignancies are seen in a very small minority of patients, generally many years after they have received a course of radiation treatment. In the vast majority of cases, this risk is greatly outweighed by the reduction in risk conferred by treating the primary cancer.

Death: Radiation has potentially excess risk of death from heart disease seen after some past breast cancer RT regimens.

Cognitive decline: In cases of radiation applied to the head radiation therapy can cause cognitive decline.

Cumulative side effects: Cumulative effects from this process should not be confused with long-term effects—when short-term effects have disappeared and long-term effects are sub clinical, reirradiation can still be problematic.

Medical Record # :
Hospital Name :
Patient Name :
Date of Birth :
Attending Physician :
Date of Admission :

☐ OPD
☐ IPD

Radiotherapy Treatment Sheet
SR-90 Brachytherapy Application

DIAGNOSIS	
TOTAL PRESCRIBED DOSE (cGy)	
NUMBER OF FRACTIONS	

TOTAL ACTIVITY USED	
DOSE RATE/SECOND (cGy/sec)	
TOTAL TIME REQUIRED (sec)	
TIME PER FRACTIONS (sec)	
DOSE PER FRACTION (cGy)	

DATE	FR NO	TIME (sec)	DOSE (cGy)	CUM DOSE (cGy)

Comments

_____   _____
Medical physicist   Date   Radiotherapist   Date

HOS-08-0002-01   Oncology/Radiotherapy Treatment Sheet SR-90 Brachytherapy Application

RADIATION THERAPY (THORACIC) FORM

| Name Age Sex | | Mar. Status Hos. No. |
| Service Ward Bed | | Occ. Religion Income |

DIAGNOSIS:

PALLATIVE/ CURATIVE
Biopsy Report No. Date etc.

Location:

S1. No.	Date	Dose given	Total Dose	Diagnostic Radiology Comment	Radiotherapists Comment	Clinicians Comments (including counts symptomatology etc.)

RADIATION THERAPY (THORACIC) FORM

MR : 143

ALLIED HEALTH SERVICES

In earlier days of medical practice, the physician alone used to manage the patient care services by recording the patient identification demographic data, taking history and physical examination, dressing the patients for wounds and injuries, taking blood for testing, giving injection and dispensing medicines. And also used to give counseling the patient when to take the medicine, dose, when to see doctor and so on. In simple terms he was doing the services of medical records, nurse, lab technician, pharmacist, social worker and so on. By this method, a physician can see only limited patients while, the number of patients need medical services were more. In order to meet the patient care services quickly and effectively, the need for some assistants arose. This need has created the allied healthcare professionals, one after one, emanated to assist the busy physician and allow him to deal with complicated cases which need medical background while other allied professional can contribute greatly to patient care service directly or indirectly with their specialties.

History

The explosion of scientific knowledge that followed World War II brought increasingly sophisticated and complex medical diagnostic and treatment procedures. In addition, increasing medical and healthcare costs provoked a trend away from treating patients in hospitals toward the provision of care in physician's private and group practices, and ambulatory medical and emergency clinics. What followed was an increase in the need for expertly trained healthcare delivery personnel lied professionals have taken the rest.

Allied healthcare professions are clinical healthcare professions distinct from medicine, dentistry, and nursing. They work in an environment of healthcare team to make the healthcare system function effectively and efficiently uninterruptedly.

Professions: Depending on the country and local healthcare system, a limited subset of the following professions may be represented, and may be regulated.

All professionals/professional areas ascribed before belong to the ever growing group of allied health professionals and their subspecialties. The precise titles and roles in the allied health professions may vary considerably from country to country.

Since their job descriptions become more specialized, they must adhere to national training and education standards, their professional scope of practice, and often prove their skills through diplomas, certified credentials, and continuing education. Members of the allied health professions must be proficient in the use of many skills. Some of which are medical terminology, acronym and spelling, basics of medical law and ethics, understanding of human relations, interpersonal communication skills, counseling skills, computer literacy, ability to document healthcare information, interviewing skills, and proficiency in word processing, database management and electronic dictation.

As a part of Allied Health Profession which is also know as Paramedical services. The paramedics generally learn besides their own selected specialty field, also learn subjects like Anatomy, Physiology, Medical Terminology, Medical Records, Fundamentals of Diseases and Diagnostic Procedure. These are Pharmacology, Pharmacy, Physical Therapy, Occupational Therapy, Optometry, Nutrition (Dietetics), Medical Psychology and many more. While Medical Social Work, Public Relations and Medical Secretary have besides condensed combination of the above stipulated subjects such as hospital management program to deal with the day-to-day administrative and patient care issues.

The Allied Health Services have been playing vital role in taking away most of nonprofessional and administrative types of work from the highly qualified professionals, helping them and allowing the professionals to concentrate in their specialized field and not wasting time for nonmedical and for trivial jobs. In fact, in many ways the paramedics service cost much less than the highly paid specialty professionals. This is not only cost effective but much more than that it contribute in swift and improved patient care resulting great service to general public.

Requesting Physician's Notes	Paramedical Department Notes
Physician: _____	Name: _____
Signature: _____ Date: _____	Signature: _____ Date: _____
Requesting Physician's Notes	**Paramedical Department Notes**
Physician: _____	Name: _____
Signature: _____ Date: _____	Signature: _____ Date: _____

PARAMEDICAL SERVICES RECORD

INTRODUCTION

Pharmacology is the science that deals with the origin, nature, chemistry, effects and use of drugs. Pharmacist is the one who is licensed to prepare, and sell or dispense drugs, and compounds and makeup prescriptions. Pharmacopoeia is an authoritative treatise on drugs and their preparations; a book containing a list of the products, used in medicines with descriptions, chemical tests for determining identity, purity and formulae for certain mixtures of these substances with statement of average dosage. Pharmacy is the place where the drugs are stored, and dispensed by the pharmacists.

Chemotherapy is the study of those drugs that destroy microorganisms, parasites or malignant cells within the body.

Toxicology is the study of the harmful chemicals and their effects on the body.

Antidotes are the substances, which are given to neutralize the unwanted effects of drugs.

DRUGS

Drugs are chemical substances used in medicine, in the treatment of disease. A drug can have three different names: 1. Chemical name—name(s) of the main chemicals used; 2. Generic name or official name—unique name universally known through the pharmacopoeia; 3. Brand name or trade name—manufacturer's special identity name.

ADMINISTRATION OF DRUGS

The administration of drugs is of different types:
1. Oral administration—given by mouth and absorbed into the blood-stream through the intestinal wall
2. Sublingual administration—drugs placed under the tongue and allowed to dissolve in the saliva so as to be absorbed into the blood stream to start acting rapidly, e.g. nitroglycerine (sorbitrate) drug used for angina pectoris.
3. Rectal administration—some drugs are administered through the rectum when the patient is constantly nauseated and vomiting. Enema is also given through the rectum.
4. Parenteral administration (injection)—there are several types of injections, they are:
   a. Subcutaneous/hypodermic injection—given just under the skin
   b. Intradermal injection—made into upper layers of the skin mainly used in skin testing for allergic reactions.
   c. Intramuscular injection (IM)—this injection is usually given in the buttock or in the deltoid muscle of the hand.
   d. Intravenous injection (II)—this injection is given directly into the veins. Most intravenous fluids like dextrose, saline, etc. are administered through this method.
   e. Intrathecal injections—this injection is made into sheath of membranes (menings) which surround the spinal cord and brain.
   f. Dermal application—it is locally applied on skin like antiseptics pain relievers, antifungal, etc. It is also called topical application.
   g. Inhalation—some vapors and gasses are taken through the nose or mouth by inhalation, e.g. bronchodilators, etc.

CLASSIFICATIONS OF DRUGS

The drugs are classified into various types:

Drugs	Action	Examples
Vaccines	A suspension of killed microorganisms administered for prevention and treatment of infectious diseases	Tetanus, polio, hepatitis, measles vaccines
Analgesic	Pain relievers	Paracetamol, ibuprofen
Stimulants	Drugs that acts on the brain to speed up the vital process of heart and respiration	
Depressants	An agent that reduces functional activity and vital energies	Diazepam, barbiturates

Contd...

Contd...

Drugs	Action	Examples
Sedatives	Drugs that relax and calm nervousness	Hypnotics, alcohol, morphine, codeine, acetyl salicylic acid
Cardiovascular drugs	Drugs acting on heart and blood vessels namely antiarrhythmics, calcium channel blocker, antianginal, vasodialators, diuretics, ACE inhibitors and vasoconstrictors	
Autonomic drugs	Drugs those influence the body in the manner similar to the normal action of autonomic nerves	Epinephrine, reserpine, acetylcholine
Gastrointestinal drugs	Used mainly to relieve gastrointestinal discomforts	Antacids, blockers
Antibiotics	Chemical substance produced by a micro-organism to stop the growth or kill the bacteria, fungi or parasites	Penicillin, streptomycin, tetracycline, sulfonamides
Antihistamines	These drugs block the action of histamine, which is normally released when foreign antigens enter causing allergic symptoms	Diphen hydramine, chlorpheniramine
Antifungal	Chemical substance produced by a fungi to stop the growth or kill the fungi	
Antiemetics	The drugs relieve nausea and vomiting and overcome vertigo, dizziness, and motion sickness	
Laxatives	Drugs which promotes the motility of the intestine, to excrete the fecal matters	
Blockers	Drug that induces adrenergnic blockage at receptors	
Vitamins and minerals	Micronutrients substances essential for proper health and growth	Vitamin A, B_1, B_2, B_6, B_{12}, Niacin, Vitamin C, D, E, K and folic acid.
Anesthetics	Agent that reduces or eliminates sensation, local, spinal or general	Zylocaine is used for local anesthesia, pethidine is administered for general anesthesia
Anticoagulant	Drug that prevents the clotting of blood	Heparin
Anticonvulsants	Reduces the severity of convulsions in various types of epilepsy	
Antidepressant	Drugs that treats the symptoms of depression	
Antidiabetic	Drugs used to treat diabetes mellitus such as oral hypoglycemic and injections of insulin	
Endocrine drugs	Direct hormonal substitutes	Androgens, estrogens, progestines, and glucocorticoids
Gastrointestinal drugs	Drugs act on gastrointestinal tracts	Antacids, antidiarrheal, laxatives
Respiratory drugs	Acts on respiratory tract	Bronchodilators and inhalers
Tranquilizers	Drugs that control anxiety	Valium (diazepam)

21 Pharmacy

Pharmacy is the health profession that links the health sciences with the chemical sciences, and it is charged with ensuring the safe and effective use of pharmaceutical drugs.

The scope of pharmacy practice includes more traditional roles such as compounding and dispensing medications, and it also includes more modern services related to health care, including clinical services, reviewing medications for safety and efficacy, and providing drug information. Pharmacy is the term for an establishment where pharmacy in the first sense is practiced in drugstore. Pharmacists are the primary health professionals who optimize medication use to provide patients with positive health outcomes.

The word pharmacy is derived from its root word pharma which was a term used since the 1400–1600s. Apart from the pharma responsibilities, it offered general medical advice and a range of services that are now performed solely by other specialist practitioners, such as surgery and midwifery. The pharma generally operated through a retail shop which, in addition to ingredients for medicines, sold tobacco and patent medicines. The pharmas also used many other herbs in their practice.

In its examination of herbal and chemical ingredients, the work of the pharma may be regarded as a forerunner of the modern sciences of chemistry and pharmacology, prior to the formulation of the scientific method.

The field of Pharmacy can generally be divided into three primary disciplines:
1. Pharmaceutics
2. Medicinal chemistry and pharmacognosy
3. Pharmacy practice

The limits between these disciplines and with other sciences, such as biochemistry, are not always clear-cut; and often, collaborative teams from various disciplines research together.

Pharmacology is occasionally considered a fourth discipline of pharmacy. Pharmacology is essential to the study of pharmacy, but it is not just specific to pharmacy, it is usually considered to be of the broader sciences.

PHARMACISTS

Pharmacists are highly-trained and skilled healthcare professionals who perform various roles to ensure optimal health outcomes for their patients. Many pharmacists besides practicing do have their own pharmacy business.

Types of Pharmacy Practice Areas (Figs 21.1 and 21.2)

Pharmacists practice in a variety of areas including retail shops, hospitals, clinics, nursing homes, drug industry, insurance companies,

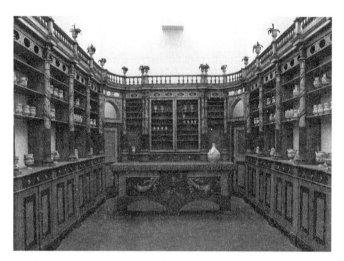

Fig. 21.1: A model of 19th century Italian pharmacy
(*For color version, see Plate 2*)

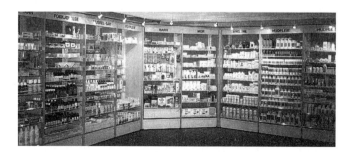

Fig. 21.2: A model of modern pharmacy
(*For color version, see Plate 2*)

and accreditation agencies. Pharmacists can specialize in various areas of practice including many fields such as hematology/oncology, infectious diseases, ambulatory care, nutrition support, drug information, critical care, pediatrics, etc.

Community Pharmacy

A *pharmacy* is the place where most licensed pharmacists practice the profession of pharmacy. It initiated as the community pharmacy to deal with community needs and as profession grown and expanded to variety of pharmacy services.

Community pharmacies in early years usually consist of a retail storefront with a dispensary where medications are stored and dispensed. The dispensary is subject to pharmacy legislation; with requirements for storage conditions, compulsory texts, equipment, etc. specified in legislation. Normally, the pharmacists most of their time spent in the dispensary compounding/dispensing medications; and also communicating with patients related the way the drugs are to be used.

All pharmacies are required to have a registered pharmacist on-duty at all times when operational. Apart from having independent pharmacy stores, there are many pharmacies are located in departmental stores and grocery shops. In addition to medicines and prescriptions, many now sell a diverse arrangement of additional household items such as cosmetics, shampoo, office supplies, confectionary, and snack foods. Invariably, most of large pharmacies are located nearby hospitals and nursing home vicinity with 24/7 service.

Hospital Pharmacy

Pharmacies within hospitals differ considerably from general pharmacy stores or pharmacy in departmental stores. The hospital pharmacies may have more complex clinical medication management issues whereas pharmacists in pharmacy stores often have more multifaceted business and customer related issues. The hospital pharmacies size, locations and method of operation varies from hospital to hospital. There are main pharmacy, emergency pharmacy and outpatient pharmacy, etc.

In view of the complexity of medications, effectiveness of treatment regimens, safety of medications (i.e. drug interactions) and patient compliance issues in the hospital, many pharmacists working in hospitals have to be well experienced with appropriate professional qualification. Persons who are specialized in clinical pharmacy are referred to as clinical pharmacists and they often specialize in various disciplines of pharmacy. For example, there are pharmacists who specialize in hematology/oncology, HIV/AIDS, infectious disease, critical care, emergency medicine, toxicology, nuclear pharmacy, pain management, psychiatry, anti-coagulation clinics, herbal medicine, neurology/epilepsy management, pediatrics, neonatal pharmacists and more.

Hospital pharmacies can usually be found within the premises of the hospital. Hospital pharmacies usually stock a larger range of medications, including more specialized medications. Most hospital medications are unit-dose, or a single dose of medicine. Hospital pharmacists and trained pharmacy technicians compound sterile products for patients including total parenteral nutrition (TPN), and other medications given intravenously. This is a complex process that requires adequate training of personnel, quality assurance of products, and adequate facilities. The large hospitals with huge patient turnout in ambulatory and inpatient services do prefer outsource high risk preparations and some other compounding functions to companies who specialize in compounding as a cost contained mechanism or due to shortage of well qualified pharmacists.

Clinical Pharmacy

Clinical pharmacists care for patients in all health care settings especially inside hospitals and clinics and they often collaborate with physicians and other healthcare professionals to improve pharmaceutical care. Clinical pharmacists are now an integral part of the interdisciplinary approach to patient care. They work collaboratively with physicians, nurses and other healthcare personnel in various medical and surgical areas and participate in patient care rounds and drug product selection. In most hospitals in the United States, potentially dangerous drugs that require close monitoring are dosed and managed by clinical pharmacists.

Compounding Pharmacy

Another important function of pharmacist is compounding that is practice of preparing drugs in new forms. For example, if a drug manufacturer only provides a drug as a tablet, a compounding pharmacist might make a medicated lollipop that contains the drug. Patients who have difficulty swallowing the tablet may prefer to suck the medicated lollipop instead. Another form of compounding is by mixing different strengths, (g, mg, mcg) of capsules or tables to yield the desire therapy indicated by the doctor. The pharmacists who specialize in compounding, also dispense the non-compounded drugs to that patients.

Consultant Pharmacy

The field of pharmacy as old as medicine, in the course of its practice, the profession has reached to provide consultancy services and those senior professionals with vast experience are called consultant pharmacists, This practice focuses more on medication regimen review (i.e. "cognitive services") than on actual dispensing of drugs. Consultant pharmacists most typically work in nursing homes, but are increasingly branching into other institutions and non-institutional settings. Traditionally consultant pharmacists were usually independent business owners, though in the United States many now work for several large pharmacy management companies. This trend may be gradually reversing as consultant pharmacists begin to work directly with patients, primarily because many elderly people are now taking numerous medications but continue to live outside of institutional settings. Some community pharmacies employ consultant pharmacists and/or provide consulting services. The need for general pharmacists and consultant pharmacist is growing to prevent adverse medication reactions and deaths.

Internet Pharmacy

Since about the year 2000, a growing number of internet pharmacies have been established worldwide. Many of these pharmacies are similar to hospital or community pharmacies, and in fact, many of them are actually operated by pharmacies that serve consumers online without going to pharmacist or drug store. The primary difference is the method by which the medications are requested and received. Some customers consider this to be more convenient and private method rather than traveling to a drugstore where another customer might overhear about the drugs that they take. Internet pharmacies (also known as Online Pharmacies) are also recommended to some patients by their physicians if they are homebound. Many refills are prescribed over internets and patient instead of going to physician's office or clinic can have repeated same drugs or new drug prescribed and collected directly from drug or pharmacy stores.

The most internet pharmacies sell prescription drugs on a valid prescription; some internet pharmacies sell prescription drugs without requiring a prescription in certain drugs. Many customers order drugs from such pharmacies to avoid the "inconvenience" of visiting a doctor or to obtain medications which their doctors were unwilling to prescribe. However, this practice has been criticized as potentially dangerous, especially by those who feel that only doctors can reliably assess contraindications, risk/benefit ratios, and an individual's overall suitability for use of a medication.

What is most important concern is with internet pharmacies is the ease with which people, especially youth, can obtain controlled substances via the internet without a prescription issued by a doctor/

practitioner who has an established doctor-patient relationship. There are many instances where a practitioner issues a prescription, brokered by an internet server, for a controlled substance to a "patient" s/he has never met. In the United States, in order for a prescription for a controlled substance to be valid, it must be issued for a legitimate medical purpose by a licensed practitioner acting in the course of legitimate doctor-patient relationship. The filling pharmacy has a corresponding responsibility to ensure that the prescription is valid. Often, individual state laws outline what defines a valid patient-doctor relationship.

Canada is home to dozens of licensed internet pharmacies, many of which sell their lower-cost prescription drugs to US consumers, who pay one of the world's highest drug prices. In recent years, many consumers in the US and in other countries with high drug costs have turned to licensed internet pharmacies in India, Israel and the UK, which often have even lower prices than in Canada.

In the United States, there has been a push to legalize importation of medications from Canada and other countries, in order to reduce consumer costs. In most cases importation of prescription medications violates Food and Drug Administration (FDA) regulations and federal laws, therefore, enforcement is generally targeted at international drug suppliers, rather than consumers.

Recently-developed online services like Australia's *Medicine Name Finder* and the Walgreen's' *Drug Info Search* provide information about pharmaceutical products but do not offer prescriptions or drug dispensations. These services often promote generic drug alternatives by offering comparative information on price and effectiveness.

Veterinary Pharmacy

Veterinary pharmacies, sometimes called *animal pharmacies* may fall in the category of hospital pharmacy, retail pharmacy or mail-order pharmacy. Veterinary pharmacies stock different varieties and different strengths of medications to fulfill the pharmaceutical needs of animals. Because the needs of animals as well as the regulations on veterinary medicine are often very different from those related to people, veterinary pharmacy is often kept separate from regular pharmacies.

Nuclear Pharmacy

Nuclear pharmacy focuses on preparing radioactive materials for diagnostic tests and for treating certain diseases. Nuclear pharmacists undergo additional training specific to handling radioactive materials, and unlike in community and hospital pharmacies, nuclear pharmacists typically do not interact directly with patients.

Military Pharmacy

Military pharmacy is an entirely different working environment due to the fact that technicians perform most duties that in a civilian sector would be illegal. State laws of technician patient counseling and medication checking by a pharmacist do not apply.

PHARMACY INFORMATICS

The importance of pharmacy informatics has grown due to development of pharmacy software to be used in healthcare institutions. Pharmacy informatics is the combination of pharmacy practice science and applied information science. Pharmacy informaticist's work in many practice areas of pharmacy, however, they may also work in information technology departments or for healthcare information technology vendor companies. As a practice area and specialist domain, pharmacy informatics is growing quickly to meet the needs of major national and international patient information projects and health system interoperability goals. Pharmacists are well trained to participate in medication management system development, deployment and optimization.

ISSUES IN PHARMACY

Separation of Prescribing from Dispensing

In most jurisdictions (such as the United States), pharmacists are regulated separately from physicians. These jurisdictions also usually specify that *only* pharmacists may supply scheduled pharmaceuticals to the public and that pharmacists cannot form business partnerships with physicians or give them "kickback" payments. However, the American Medical Association (AMA) Code of Ethics provides that physicians may dispense drugs within their office practices as long as there is no patient exploitation and patients have the right to a written prescription that can be filled elsewhere. Seven to ten percent of American physician's practices reportedly dispense drugs on their own.

In other jurisdictions, doctors are allowed to dispense drugs themselves and the practice of pharmacy is sometimes integrated with that of the physician, particularly in traditional Chinese medicine.

In Canada it is common for a medical clinic and a pharmacy to be located together and for the ownership in both enterprises to be common, but licensed separately.

The reason for the majority rule is the high risk of a conflict of interest and/or the avoidance of absolute powers. Otherwise, the physician has a financial self-interest in "diagnosing" as many conditions as possible, and in exaggerating their seriousness, because he or she can then sell more medications to the patient. Such self-interest directly conflicts with the patient's interest in obtaining cost-effective medication and avoiding the unnecessary use of medication that may have side-effects. This system reflects much similarity to the checks and balances system of the US and many other governments.

A campaign for separation has begun in many countries and has already been successful. As many of the remaining nations move towards separation, resistance and lobbying from dispensing doctors who have pecuniary interests may prove a major stumbling block.

FUTURE OF PHARMACY

It is expected that the pharmacists to become more integral within the health care system in the future, rather than simply dispensing medication, pharmacists will be paid for their patient care services. This transformation has already commenced in some countries; for instance, pharmacists in Australia receive remuneration from the Australian Government for conducting comprehensive Home Medicines Reviews. In Canada, pharmacists in certain provinces have limited prescribing rights (as in Alberta and British Columbia) or are remunerated by their provincial government for expanded services such as medications reviews (Medschecks in Ontario). In the United Kingdom, pharmacists who undertake additional training are obtaining prescribing rights. They are also being paid for by the government for medicine use reviews. In the United States, pharmaceutical care or clinical pharmacy has had an evolving influence on the practice of pharmacy. Moreover, the Doctor of Pharmacy (Pharm D) degree is now required before entering practice and some pharmacists now complete one or two years of residency or fellowship training following graduation. In addition, consultant pharmacists who traditionally operated primarily in nursing homes are now expanding into direct consultation with patients, under the banner of "senior care pharmacy.

22 | Physical Therapy

INTRODUCTION

Physical therapy is the profession which uses, knowledge and skills, in rendering care for individuals, disabled by disease and injury, the primary focus is on the functional restoration, of patients, affected with skeletal neuromuscular, cardiovascular and pulmonary disorders.

Designing and fitting of artificial parts or limbs and rehabilitating them by a treatment process to help physically handicapped individuals to make maximal use of residual capacities, and to enable them to obtain optimal satisfaction and usefulness, in terms of themselves, their families and their community.

S.No.	Name of the therapy	Definition
1.	Electrotherapy	Use of electric current in the treatment of disease to improve muscular activities, to produce sensory modulation for control of pain and to produce reflex effects in the treatment of motor disorders
2.	Hydrotherapy	The use of water in its various form: Liquid, solid and vapor either internally or externally in the treatment of nervous and musculoskeletal diseases
3.	Massage	Manipulation of soft tissues, of the bodies, most effectively performed with the hands, and administered, to produce effects, on the nervous and muscular systems and local and the general circulation of the blood and lymph

Physical therapy (also known as physiotherapy) is a health care profession which provides treatment to individuals in order to develop, maintain and restore maximum movement and function throughout life. This includes providing treatment in circumstances where movement and function are threatened by aging, injury, disease or environmental factors.

Physical therapy is concerned with identifying and maximizing quality of human being and movement potential within the spheres of promotion, prevention, treatment/intervention, habilitation and rehabilitation. This includes physical, psychological, emotional, and social well being. It involves the interaction between physical therapist (PT), patients/clients, other health professionals, families, care givers, and communities in a process where movement potential is assessed and goals are agreed upon, using knowledge and skills unique to physical therapists. Physical therapy is performed by either a physical therapist (PT) or an assistant (PTA) acting under their direction. Physiotherapist utilizes an individual's history and physical examination to establish a diagnosis and create a management plan, and when necessary, incorporate the results of laboratory and imaging studies. The physical therapist use diagnostic testing e.g. electromyograms and nerve conduction velocity testing for arriving at proper assessment and diagnosis. Physical therapy has many specialties including, geriatrics, neurologic, orthopedic, pediatrics, and cardiopulmonary to name some of the more common areas. PTs practice in many settings, such as outpatient clinics or offices, inpatient orthopedic wards or rehabilitation facilities, skilled nursing homes and facilities, extended healthcare facilities, private homes, education and research centers, schools, hospices, industrial workplaces or other occupational environments, fitness centers and sports training facilities. Educational qualifications vary greatly by country.

SPECIALTY AREAS

The Physical therapy field is growing enormously and participating in many areas and the body of knowledge of physical therapy is quite large. Some PTs specialize in a specific clinical and many other areas. The American Board of Physical Therapy Specialties listed seven specialist certifications, including Sports Physical Therapy and Clinical Electrophysiology. Worldwide the six most common specialty areas in physical therapy are: cardiopulmonary, geriatric, neurological, orthopedic, pediatric and integumentary. The briefly explanation is given below:

CARDIOPULMONARY

Cardiovascular and pulmonary rehabilitation physical therapists treat a wide variety of individuals with cardiopulmonary disorders or those who have had cardiac or pulmonary surgery. Primary goals of this specialty include increasing endurance and functional independence. Manual therapy is utilized in this field to assist in clearing lung secretions experienced with cystic fibrosis. Disorders, including heart attacks, post coronary bypass surgery, chronic obstructive pulmonary disease, and pulmonary fibrosis, treatments can benefit from cardiovascular and pulmonary specialized physical therapists.

GERIATRIC

Geriatric physical therapy covers a wide area of issues concerning people as they go through normal adult lifespan, but is usually focused on the older adult. There are many conditions that affect many people as they grow older and include but are not limited to the following: osteoporosis, cancer, arthritis, Alzheimer's disease, hip and joint replacement, balance disorders, incontinence, etc. Geriatric physical therapy helps those affected by such problems in developing a specialized program to help restore mobility, reduce pain, and increase fitness levels to have a normal physical fitness.

NEUROLOGICAL

Neurological physical therapy is a discipline focused on working with individuals who have a neurological disorder or disease. These include Alzheimer's disease, ALS, brain injury, cerebral palsy, multiple sclerosis, Parkinson's disease, spinal cord injury, and stroke. Common impairments associated with neurological conditions include impairments of vision, balance, and ambulation, activities of daily living, movement, speech and loss of functional independence. Though the treatment is of longer duration, the promising results have demonstrated in cases where persuasion and will power prevailed.

ORTHOPEDIC PHYSICAL THERAPY

Orthopedic physical therapists, assess, diagnose, manage, and treat disorders and injuries of the musculoskeletal system including rehabilitation after orthopedic surgery. This specialty of physical therapy is most often found in the out-patient clinical setting. Orthopedic therapists are trained in the treatment of postoperative orthopedic procedures, fractures, acute sports injuries, arthritis, sprains, strains, back and neck pain, spinal conditions and amputations. Joint and spine mobilization/manipulation, therapeutic exercise, neuro-muscular re-education, hot/cold packs, and electrical muscle stimulation, e.g. cry therapy, iontophoresis, electrotherapy are modalities often used to expedite recovery in the orthopedic setting. The use of sonography for diagnosis and to guide treatments such as muscle retraining. Those who have suffered injury or disease affecting the muscles, bones, ligaments, or tendons of the body will benefit from assessment by a physical therapist specialized in orthopedics. This field is becoming more popular with the sport therapy and cosmetic and fitness consciousness among people.

PEDIATRIC PHYSICAL THERAPY

Pediatric physical therapy assists in early detection of health problems and uses a wide variety of modalities to treat disorders in the pediatric population. These therapists are specialized in the assessment, diagnosis, treatment, and management of infants, children, and adolescents with a variety of congenital, developmental, neuromuscular, skeletal, or acquired disorders/diseases. Treatments focus on improving gross and fine motor skills, balance and coordination, strength and endurance as well as cognitive and sensory processing/integration. The therapists are playing a good role in treating the children with developmental delays, cerebral palsy, spina bifida, or portcullis.

INTEGUMENTARY PHYSICAL THERAPIST

This unit named as integumentary which treats conditions involving the skin and related organs and also wounds and burns. Physical therapists utilize surgical instruments, mechanical lavage, dressings and topical agents to debride necrotic tissue and promote tissue healing. Other commonly used interventions include exercise, edema control, splinting, casting and compression outfits.

Health Care No.: ☐☐ ☐☐ ☐ ☐☐☐ ☐☐☐

Name: _____

Age: ☐☐ Yrs/Month   Sex: ☐ M   ☐ F

Nationality: _____

Consultant In-Charge: _____

Dept.: _____ Unit: _____

PHYSICAL THERAPY TREATMENT CARD

Diagnosis/Relevant Clinical Findings/Associated Conditions:

_____
_____
_____
_____

Contraindications:

Treatment Requested	Treatment Requested
☐ Hydrotherapy	☐ Hot Packs
☐ Mobilization ── ☐ Non wt. Bearing ☐ Partial wt. Bearing ☐ Full wt. Bearing	☐ Ultrasound
	☐ Wax
☐ Exercises ── ☐ Active ☐ Assistive ☐ Passive	☐ Shortwave diathermy
☐ Ice therapy	☐ Traction
☐ Muscle stimulation	
☐ Message	☐ Others (Specify) _____

NEXT APPOINTMENT WITH DOCTOR

Date _____

Doctor's Name: _____

Signature: _____

RECORD OF ATTENDANCE

MONTH	1	2	3	4	5	6	7	8	9	10	11	12	13	14	15	16	17	18	19	20	21	22	23	24	25	26	27	28	29	30	31

DATE	TIME	INITIAL ASSESSMENT AND TREATMENT NOTES	Signature

("Note: After Treatment this Card Should Become Part of Patant File")

**PHYSICAL THERAPY ANALYSIS
AND TREATMENT PLAN**

Medical Record # :

Hospital Name :

Patient Name :

Date of Birth :

Attending Physician :

Date of Admission :

☐ OPD

☐ IPD

Initial assessment summary and analysis :

Problems:

Goals:

Treatment Plan:

Signature: ....

Date: ....

Physical therapy analysis and treatment plan

| Medical Record#: |
| Hospital Name: |
| Patient Name: |
| Date of Birth: |
| Attending Physician: |
| Date of Admission: |
| ☐ OPD |
| ☐ IPD |

PHYSIOTHERAPY REQUEST FORM

Clinical Data:

Diagnosis:

Objective of referral:

Date: **Speciality:**   **Referred by:**

PHYSIOTHERAPY REPORT

Discharge summary:

Recommendation:

Date : _____   _____
                                      Therapist Name and Signature

Ist Copy : Patient Medical Record / 2nd Copy : Physiotherapy Dept.

(Physiotherapy Request Form)

Medical Record#:

Hospital Name:

Patient Name:

Date of Birth:

Attending Physician:

Date of Admission:

**CHEDOKE-McMASTER STROKE
ASSESSMENT DISABILITY INVENTORY**

☐ OPD

☐ IPD

Admission   Discharge   Other : _____

SCORING LEVELS		
NO HELPER	Independence	
	7 Complete Independence	(Timely, Safely)
	6 Modified Independence	(Device)
HELPER	Modified Dependence	
	5 Supervision	(Client = 75%)
	4 Minimal Assist	(Client = 50%)
	3 Moderate Assist	
	Complete Dependence	
	2 Maximal Assist	(Client = 25%)
	1 Total Assist	(Client = 0%)

Score

1. Supine to side lying on strong side
2. Supine to side lying on weak side
3. Side lying to long sitting through strong side
4. Side lying to sitting on side of the bed through strong side
5. Side lying to sitting on side of the bed through weak side
6. Remain standing
7. Transfer to and from bed towards strong side
8. Transfer to and from bed towards weak side
9. Transfer up and down from floor and chair
10. Transfer up and down from floor and standing
11. Walk indoors - 25 m
12. Walk outdoors, over rough ground, ramps, and curbs - 150 m
13. Walk outdoors several blocks—900 m
14. Walk up and down stairs
15. Age appropriate walking distance for 2 min (2 Point Bonus)
             Distance _____ m

To score Bonus : for age < 70 yrs distance must be >96 meters
             for age >70 yrs distance must be >80 meters   Total Score :

Walking aids:
Walker   _____
4 point cane   _____
1 point cane   _____
brace   _____

Signature: _____   Date: _____

Medical Record #:		
Hospital Name:		
Patient Name:		
Date of Birth:		
Attending Physician:		
Date of Admission:	☐ OPD	
	☐ IPD	

FUNCTIONAL INDEPENDENCE MEASURE (FIM)

| L E V E L S | **INDEPENDENCE**
   7 Complete Independence (Timely, Safety)
   6 Modified Independence (Device)
MODIFIED DEPENDENCE
   5 Supervision
   4 Minimal assist (subject = 75%)
   3 Moderate Assist (Subject = 50%)

COMPLETE DEPENDENCE
   2 Maximal Assist (Subject = 25%)
   1 Total Assist (Subject = 0%) | **No Helper**

Helper |

	Self-Care	**Admit**	**D/C**	**Re-assess**
A.	Feeding	☐	☐	☐
B.	Grooming	☐	☐	☐
C.	Bathing	☐	☐	☐
D.	Dressing-Upper body	☐	☐	☐
E.	Dressing-Lower body	☐	☐	☐
F.	Toileting	☐	☐	☐
	Sphinter Control			
G.	Bladder management	☐	☐	☐
H.	Bowel management	☐	☐	☐
	Mobility - Transfers			
I.	Bed, chair, W/C	☐	☐	☐
J.	Toilet	☐	☐	☐
K.	Tub, shower	☐	☐	☐
	Locomotion			
L.	Walk/Wheel chair	☐	☐	☐
M.	Stairs	☐	☐	☐
	Total :	_____	_____	_____
	Initial :	_____	_____	_____

Signature : _____ Date : _____

Functional Independent Measure (FIM)

23 | Occupational Therapy

Occupational therapy (OT) often abbreviated as OT, (but in surgical terms OT is considered as Operation Theater). The World Federation of Occupational Therapists defines occupational therapy as a profession concerned with promoting health and well-being through occupation. Occupational therapists address the question, "Why does this person have difficulties in his or her daily activities (or occupations), and what can we adapt to make it possible for him or her to manage better to impact his or her health and well-being?" Occupational therapists use careful analysis of physical, environmental, psychosocial, mental, spiritual, political and cultural factors to identify barriers to occupation. The primary goal of an occupational therapist is to enable individuals, groups and communities to participate in activities which are meaningful to them, reflect their beliefs and values, and produce a sense of accomplishment or satisfaction. Occupational therapy has been described as addressing the "skills for the job of living" necessary for "living life to its fullest." Occupational therapy draws from the fields of medicine, psychology, sociology, anthropology, ethnography, architecture and many other disciplines in developing its knowledge base. A new discipline of occupational science has been developed to enhance the evidence base of the profession. Occupational therapists work with individuals, families, groups and communities to facilitate health and well-being through engagement or re-engagement in occupation. Occupational therapists are becoming increasingly involved in addressing the impact of social, political and environmental factors that contribute to exclusion and occupational deficiencies. Through this profession, many handicapped personnel have gained the skills that made them to be independent although for some is with limited activities, nevertheless, proved handy in their day-to-day life.

OCCUPATION

Occupation is the dynamic relationship between the occupational form and occupational performance. Many people see the term occupation as a job one does. However, the meaning of occupation is seen in a much wider context by an Occupational Therapist. A human being can be engaged in a wide range of occupations that had a significant role in their involvement to bring to normal situation to the extent possible.

OCCUPATIONAL FORM

Wu and Lin (1999) stated that the occupational form was the "objective pre-existing structure or environmental context that elicits or guides subsequent human performance". The occupational form consists of objective features and these include materials, human context and socio-cultural dimensions.

OCCUPATIONAL PERFORMANCE

Occupational performance is the active voluntary occupational form carried out by human being.

An Occupational Therapist works systematically through a sequence of actions known as the occupational therapy process. There are several versions of this process as described by numerous writers. Creek (2003) has sought to provide a comprehensive version based on extensive research. This version has 11 stages, which for the experienced therapist may not be linear in nature. The stages are:
1. Referral
2. Information gathering
3. Initial assessment
4. Needs identification/problem formation
5. Goal setting
6. Action planning
7. Action
8. Ongoing assessment and revision of action
9. Outcome and outcome measurement
10. End of intervention or discharge
11. Review.

Fearing, Law and Clark (1997) suggested a 7 stage process which includes:
1. Identifying of occupational performance issues
2. Choosing a theoretical frame of reference
3. Assessing factors contributing the identified occupational performance issue(s)
4. Considering the strengths and resources of both client and therapist
5. Negotiating targeted outcomes and developing action plan
6. Implementing the plan through occupation
7. Evaluating outcomes.

A central ingredient of this process model is the focus on identifying both customer and therapists strengths and resources prior to beginning to develop the outcomes and plan of action.

The role of Occupational Therapy allows OT's to work in many different settings, work with many different organizations and acquire many different specialties. This broad spectrum of practice lends itself to difficulty categorizing the areas of practice that exist, especially considering the many countries and different healthcare systems. In this section, the categorization from the American Occupational Therapy Association is used. However, there are other ways to categorize areas of practice in OT, such as physical, mental, and community practice (AOTA, 2009). These divisions occur when the setting is defined by the population it serves. For example, acute physical or mental health settings in hospitals, in outpatient clinics, sub-acute settings, geriatric care facilities and community settings.

In each area of practice below, an OT can work with different diagnostic, specialties and in different therapy centers.

Physical Health

- *Pediatrics:* Schools, inpatient hospital-based child OT: Often, children and adults need OT services. Nevertheless, OTs approach intervention in a different way with children and adults as approaches treatment through occupation, and the occupations of a child are different from those of an adult; and include play, chores, self-care and schoolwork. Common conditions that are specific to or more common in the pediatric population creating a need for OT services include: developmental disorders, sensory regulation or sensory processing deficiencies, motor developmental delays, autism, emotional and behavioral disturbances (Lambert, 2005), among others. In addition, children are seen for every injury, illness or chronic condition that may cause a person of any age to have performance deficits in their daily life and thus benefit from OT services.
- *Acute care hospitals:* Acute care is an inpatient hospital setting for individuals with a serious medical condition(s) usually due to a traumatic event, such as a traumatic brain injury, spinal cord injury, etc. The primary goal of acute care is to stabilize the patient's medical status and address any threats to his or her life and loss of function. Occupational therapy plays an important role in facilitating early mobilization, restoring function, preventing further decline, and coordinating care, including transition and discharge planning. Furthermore, occupational therapy's role focuses on addressing deficits and barriers that limit the patient's ability to perform activities that they need or want to create independence in self-

care, home management, work-related tasks, and participating in community activity.

- *Inpatient rehabilitation especially in cases of spinal cord injuries:* People with different disabilities have the right and the privilege to live meaningful purposeful lives. When a disability occurs it is sometimes, it is possible to recover— when it is not it is important to learn the skills to adapt capacity and environmental supports to be able to participate. OTs uses their knowledge to help both with recovery and adaptation.
- *Rehabilitation centers* such as traumatic brain injury (TBI), stroke (CVA), spinal cord injuries, and head injuries, etc.
- *Skilled nursing facilities:* An occupational therapists role in a skilled nursing facility is centered on each client's individual needs. Many of the skills an OT works are known as activities of daily living or self-care such as feeding or dressing. OTs can provide equipment to assist with activities or offer expertise in modifying the environment to maximize independence and facilitate independence. Other OT roles include education in adaptive equipment (shower bench), energy conservation, or task simplification (Hofmann, 2008).
- *Home health:* Occupational therapists who work in this area of practice generally work with clients in the geriatric population who have one or more of the following diagnoses: Alzheimer's disease, arthritis, depression, CVA, generalized weakness, COPD, or Parkinson's disease. Occupational therapists working with these client's evaluate their level of independence, cognition, and safety. Moreover, occupational therapists provide intervention to maximize independence and function through remedial and compensatory strategies, with the ultimate goal of the client's regaining the ability to live independently at home (Swanson Anderson & Malaski, 1999).
- *Outpatient clinics* especially Hand Therapy, orthopedics clinics. Hand therapy is a specialty practice area of occupational therapy that is mainly concerned with treating orthopedic-based upper extremity conditions to optimize the functional use of the hand and arm. Diagnoses seen by this practice area include: fractures of the hand or arm, lacerations and amputations, burns, and surgical repairs of tendons and nerves. Additionally, hand therapists treat acquired conditions such as tendonitis, rheumatoid arthritis and osteoarthritis, and carpal tunnel syndrome. Occupational therapists who work in this field address biomechanical issues underlying upper-extremity conditions. Besides, occupational therapists use an occupation-based and client-centered approach by identifying participation needs of the client, then tailoring intervention to improve performance in desired activities.
- Specialist assessment centers dealing with Electronic Assistive Technology, Posture and Mobility services)

- *Hospices:* An occupational therapists common role in hospice care is modifying and preventing. Modifying the demands of the activity to fit with the abilities of the client. The intervention may be directly with the client or with the client and the client's caregivers. OT can offer the caregivers support an education. Progress is defined as improved quality of life in hospice care (Hasselkaus, 1998).
- *Assisted living facilities (ALF):* In an assisted living facility OT services are provided by a home health agency, rehab agency, or a private practice. Medicare and some private insurance plans cover OT services in ALFs, areas of treatment intervention often include: bathing, dressing, grooming, toileting, mobility, money management, laundry, and community participation. One can treat persons with occupational performance decline or at risk for a decline. Increase quality of life so fewer residents need the services of a long-term SNF. Special areas include mobility device assessment (scooter), continence training, psychosocial needs and low vision programs (Fagan, 2001).
- *Productive aging:* An OT practicing in this area would provide skills and services to older adults to maximize independence, participation, and quality of life. Typical issues addressed: Any impairment or condition that would limit their ability to carry out meaningful occupations and tasks that are necessary for daily life. Skills taught include: energy conservation, education in adaptive equipment such as a shower bench, task simplification, adapting and modifying activities to progress with a client's changing abilities (Opp Hoffman, 2008), caregiver education and support (AOTA, 2004), safety, social interactions and communication, memory skills training, mobility device assessment and training, i.e. scooters, wheelchairs, walkers, low vision interventions, continence training, and facilitating performance in basic ADL and IADL (Fagan, 2001).
- *Work hardening* is essentially a specialized program designed to enable people with physical, psychological, and psychosocial issues inhibiting a person's ability, to successfully come back to work. The National Advisory Committee on Work Hardening best describes work hardening:
  Work hardening is a highly structured, goal oriented, individualized treatment program designed to maximize the individual's ability to return to work. Work hardening programs, which are interdisciplinary in nature, use real or simulated work activities in combination with conditioning tasks that are graded to progressively improve the biomechanical, neuromuscular, cardiovascular/metabolic and psychosocial functions of the individual. Work hardening provides a transition between acute care and return to work while addressing the issues of productivity, safety, physical tolerances, and worker behaviors (Ogden-Niemeyer & Jacobs, 1989).

• *Work conditioning* is similar to work hardening, except work conditioning purely involves improving physical capacities, whereas work hardening improves physical, psychological, and psychosocial factors.

Mental Health

According to Medicare (2005) guidance, "Only a qualified occupational therapist has the knowledge, training, and experience required to evaluate and, as necessary, re-evaluate a patient's level of function, determine whether an occupational therapy program could reasonably be expected to improve, restore, or compensate for lost function, and where appropriate, recommend to the physician a plan of treatment".

According to the American Occupational Therapy Association (AOTA), occupational therapists work with the Mental Health population throughout the lifespan and across many treatment settings where mental health services and psychiatric rehabilitation are provided (AOTA, 2009). Just as with other clients, the OT facilitates maximum independence in activities of daily living (dressing, grooming, etc) and instrumental activities of daily living (medication management, grocery shopping, etc). According to the American Occupational Therapy Association, OT improves functional capacity and quality of life for people with mental illness in the areas of employment, education, community living, and home and personal care through the use of real life activities in therapy treatments (AOTA, 2005).

Mental illness or mental health issues related to: Geriatric, adult, adolescents and children. These conditions include but are not limited to: Schizophrenia, substance abuse, addiction, dementia, Alzheimer's, mood disorders, personality disorders, psychoses, eating disorders, anxiety disorders (including post-traumatic stress disorder, separation anxiety disorder) (Cara & MacRae, 2005), and reactive attachment disorder (children only) (Lambert, 2005).

Typical issues that are addressed are as follows: Helping people acquire the skills to care for themselves or others including; keeping a schedule, medication management, employment, education, increasing community participation, community access (grocery store, library, bank, etc.), money management skills, engaging in productive activities to fill the day, coping skills, routine building, building social skills and childcare (Cara & McRae, 2005).

In the UK, the College of Occupational Therapists (COT) have published Recovering Ordinary Lives, which details the strategy for OTs in mental health up to 2017, and makes explicit the goals that have been set for the profession, in line with government directives (COT 2006).

Areas that Mental Health OT's could work in are as follows:

Mental Health Inpatient Units

- Adolescent, adult and older people's acute mental health wards
- Adult and older people's rehabilitation wards
- Prisons/secure units (Forensic psychiatry)
- Psychiatric intensive care unit
- Specialist units for eating disorders, learning disabilities
  – Community based mental health teams
- Child and adolescent mental health teams
- Adult and older people's community mental health teams
- Rehabilitation and recovery and assertive outreach community teams
- Primary care services in GP practices
- Home treatment teams
- Early intervention in psychosis teams
- Specialist learning disability, eating disorder community services
- Day services
- Vocational services
- *Dementia and Alzheimer care:* OTs focus on adapting activities as the client progresses through the illness (Hofmann, 2008) OT also works with caregivers to teach them how to grade activities to the client's ability. Interventions are based on using the client's strengths to increase their quality of life and their relationships with caregivers. Use of social interactions, communication, memory, safety and self-maintenance.

Community-based Practice

Community based practice involves working with people in their own environment rather than in a hospital setting. It often combines the knowledge and skills related to physical and mental health. It can also involve working with atypical populations such as the homeless or at-risk populations. Examples of community-based practice settings:

- *Health promotion and lifestyle change:* Remaining healthy is the goal of all people in a society, including people with chronic disabling or health conditions. Achieving health requires skills to self-manage conditions that might limit their ability to function in daily life. The occupational therapist helps people acquire these skills (Wilcock, 2005).
- *Private practice.*
- *Aging in place:* Occupational therapists implement environmental modifications in senior housing, assisted living, long-term-care facilities, and homes (Yamkovenko, 2008). Environmental modifications can include rearranging furniture, building ramps, widening doorways, grab bars, special toilet seats, and other safety

equipment to use performance capabilities to their fullest (Moyers & Christiansen, 2004).

- *Low vision:* Occupational therapists help clients use their remaining vision to complete their daily routines with compensation, remediation, disability prevention and health promotion. Compensations or that modification to the environment may include proper lighting, color contrast, reducing clutter and education on adaptive equipment (Golembiewski, 2004).
- *Intermediate care services.*
- *Driving centers:* Driving is an instrumental activity of daily living and an occupational therapist may evaluate and treat skills needed to drive such as vision, executive function or memory. If a client needs more skilled assessment and training they would refer them to an OT Driver Rehabilitation Specialist which could do on the road assessment, training in adaptive equipment and make more specific recommendations.
- Day centers
- Schools
- Child development centers
- People's own homes, carrying out therapy and providing equipment and adaptations
- *Work and industry:* To be a healthy successful worker there must be a person environment fit between the task, the equipment, and the person's skills. Occupational therapists work to achieve that fit (Ellexson, 2000; Clinger, Dodson, Maltchev, & Page, 2007). Populations, conditions, and diagnoses: People of working age and ability who have been born with or developed a condition, injury, or illness that compromises their ability to work (Ellexson, 2000; Clinger, Dodson, Maltchev, & Page, 2007). Settings: Return to work programs, large organizations, consultants to large organizations, work hardening programs, work conditioning programs, transitional return to work programs (Ellexson, 2000; Clinger, Dodson, Maltchev, & Page, 2007). Typical issues addressed: assessment of ability to work, interventions to enhancing work performance by means of work hardening, work conditioning, and improvement of ergonomics in the workplace, identification of accommodations necessary to return-to-work following illness or injury, prevention of work related injury, illness, or disability (Ellexson, 2000; Clinger, Dodson, Maltchev, & Page, 2007).
- Homeless shelters
- Educational settings
- Refugee camps.

NEW EMERGING PRACTICE AREAS FOR THERAPY

- Children and youth: Psychosocial needs of children and youth
- Health and wellness:
  - Health and wellness consulting
  - Design and accessibility consulting and home modification
  - Ergonomic consulting
  - Private practice community health services.
- Productive aging:
  - Driver rehabilitation and training
  - Low vision services
- Rehabilitation, disability, and participation: Technology and assistive device development and consulting
- Work and industry:
  - Ticket to work services
  - Welfare to work services.

OCCUPATIONAL THERAPY APPROACHES

Services typically include:
- Teaching new ways of approaching tasks
- How to breakdown activities into achievable components for example sequencing a complex task like cooking a complex meal
- Comprehensive home and job site evaluations with adaptation recommendations
- Performance skills assessments and treatment
- Adaptive equipment recommendations and usage training
- Environmental adaptation including provision of equipment or designing adaptations to remove obstacles or make them manageable
- Guidance to family members and caregivers
- The use of creative media as therapeutic activity.

ACTIVITY ANALYSIS

Activity analysis has been defined as a process of dissecting an activity into its component parts and task sequence in order to identify its inherent properties and the skills required for its performance, thus allowing the therapist to evaluate its therapeutic prospective.

Therapeutic Activity

Occupational therapists use therapeutic activity or therapeutic occupation to improve an individual's occupational performance and increase function in activities of daily living.

A core and unique feature of occupational therapy practice is the use of occupation as a therapeutic medium. An occupational therapy core skill as defined by The College of Occupational Therapists (COT) is the use of activity as a therapeutic tool.

Occupational therapists have utilized activities, such as crafts, since the profession was founded. The arts and crafts movement in the very early 20th century had ascertained that goal directed activity had a curative effect on the social problems inherent in the newly industrialized societies. The founders of the occupational therapy profession extended this thinking to the treatment of individuals' with mental health problems and as a consequence between 1920 and 1940 much of occupational therapy practice concentrated around the use of crafts as purposeful activities. The emergence of occupational therapy in physical medicine began during World War II and craft activities were utilized to rehabilitate injured soldiers. This method of practice was later termed by Mosey as activity synthesis.

Activity synthesis or occupational synthesis is the core of occupational therapy practice; occupational therapists, in collaboration with clients, design occupational forms to produce a therapeutic occupation or activity, that is meaningful and purposeful to the client. The therapeutic activity or occupation may be used to assess the client's occupational needs or to achieve a therapeutic goal. The component parts of an activity or occupation are matched with the required occupational performance outcomes. For example, the muscle movements elicited by pottery may address fine motor and gross motor skills to improve shoulder flexion and extension, range of movement and elbow extension and flexion.

Other therapeutic activities or occupations may include cookery activities, such as making a smoothie or a healthy food. The components of this activity such as planning and following a recipe may address cognitive components of occupational performance such as problem solving, sequencing and learning. Health may be promoted through this occupation, enabling clients to consider healthy eating issues· Occupational therapists may further use therapeutic activities or occupations to assess occupational performance. For example, an occupational therapist may ask a customer to make a cup of coffee or prepare a simple meal to assess performance in activities of daily living (ADL). An occupational therapist may use a board or card game to assess cognitive components of occupational performance. This application of therapeutic activity/occupation involves use of the core skills of the occupational therapist, chiefly assessment and problem solving.

THEORETICAL FRAMEWORKS

Occupational Therapists use a number of theoretical frameworks to frame their practice. Note that terminology has differed between scholars. Theoretical bases for framing a human and their occupation being include the following:

Frames of Reference or Generic Models

Frames of reference or generic models are the overarching title given to a collation of compatible knowledge, research and theories that form conceptual practice. More generally, they are defined as those aspects which influence our perceptions, decisions and practice.

Occupational therapy frame of references/models:
- Person Environment Occupation Performance Model (PEOP)
- Model of Human Occupation (MOHO)
- Canadian Model of Occupational Performance (CMOP)
- Biomechanical
- Rehabilitative (compensatory)
- Neurofunctional (Gordon Muir Giles and Clark-Wilson)
- Cognitive disabilities
- Sensory integration
- Lifestyle Performance Model (Fidler).

Approaches/Intervention Models

These are the methods of carrying out the Frames of Reference. Again, terminology differs depending on your viewpoint and literature base.

UNITED STATES

Education Requirements

In many countries, occupational therapists are educated at the baccalaureate level. However, currently in the United States and Canada, entry level is at the master's level. This change occurred in 2007, requiring all occupational therapists that started their educational program after 2007 to continue their education beyond a four-year degree. Currently, six schools in the US offer a clinical doctorate for those who would like to further their education past the Master's level.

All occupational therapists have a well-rounded knowledge of biomedical, behavioral, environmental and occupational scientists. Occupational therapist base their interventions on the knowledge based on neuroscience, anatomy, applied technology, policy and environmental strategies. These schools are currently accredited for Master's level education and also accredited for Doctoral level education.

Employment

According to the Bureau of Labor Statistics, occupational therapists held 99,000 positions in 2006 (2009). States with the most licensed and employed occupational therapists are California, New York, Pennsylvania and Ohio. In 2006, 52.6% of occupational therapists worked in hospitals, early intervention facilities and schools (American Occupational Therapy Association, 2006). The Bureau of Labor statistics reported that 78% of occupational therapists worked full-time in 2006 (Bureau of Labor Statistics, 2009). In addition, the median number of years of experience for occupational therapists was 13 years (American Occupational Therapy Association, 2006). Occupational therapists can work in many different settings, some examples include:

* Hospitals
* Schools
* Early intervention facilities
* Skilled nursing facilities
* Home health care services
* Outpatient care centers
* Government agencies
* Private practice.

The field of occupational therapy is projected to see faster growth than other careers. The Bureau of Labor Statistics estimates that the number of jobs will grow to 122,000 in 2016 (2009). Areas of occupational therapy that involve helping older adults will see the most growth. This expansion is due to the large need to provide health care services to the aging baby boom generation (American Occupational Therapy Association and The Bureau of Labor Statistics-2009). In addition, the area of school-based occupational therapy will see growth as well.

Earnings

According to the Bureau of Labor Statistics, in 2006 the average salary was $70,470 for occupational therapists (2009). The average starting entry-level salary for occupational therapists was $56,300 (American Occupational Therapy Association,). In 2006, the salaries of occupational therapists in the 50% percentile ranged from $50,450 to $83,710 (Bureau of Labor Statistics, n.d.). Salary varies according to the setting and the following represents average salaries for some practice areas:

Hospitals	$61,610
School setting	$54,260
Nursing care services	$64,750
Home health care	$67,600

Facilities of physical, occupational
Speech therapists $62,290
(Bureau of Labor Statistics, 2009)

In addition, according to the Work Force Survey conducted by the American Occupational Therapy Association in 2006, average salaries for some other areas include:

Mental Health $53,750
Academic $66,000

(American Occupational Therapy Association, 2006).

CHALLENGES FOR OCCUPATIONAL THERAPY

A key challenge for occupational therapy is to develop and maintain a definition of its nature and scope assert that while this presents a challenge, it also results in a unique flexibility which allows the discipline to move with the flow of social, cultural and environmental change. This difficulty in definition may be a cause of chronic strain for practitioners and may also contribute to a lack of role definition and subsequent blurring.

Recent literature has also called for occupational therapy to address the political nature of who occupational therapists are and what they do (Kronenberg & Pollard, 2005). Profession specific models of occupational therapy have also been critiqued for being biased towards a western, ablest and generally unrepresentative of the most occupationally deprived groups.

OCCUPATIONAL THERAPY AND ICF

The International Classification of Functioning, Disability and Health (ICF) is an outcome measure for health and occupation and illustrates how these components impact one's function. This relates very closely to the Occupational Therapy Practice Framework as it is stated, "The profession's core beliefs are in the positive relationship between occupation and health and its view of people as occupational beings" (2008). The ICF is also built into the 2nd edition of the practice framework. Activities and participation examples from the ICF overlap Areas of Occupation, Performance Skills, and Performance Patterns in the framework. The ICF also includes contextual factors (environmental and personal factors) that relate to the context in the framework. In addition, body functions and structures classified within the ICF help describe the client factors as described in the OT framework (AOTA, 2002).

Further exploration of the relationship between occupational therapy and the components of the ICIDH-2 (revision of the original International Classification of Impairments, Disabilities, and Handicaps (ICIDH); later becoming the ICF) was conducted by McLaughlin Gray (2001). First, the ICF is an international framework and provides an opportunity for the occupational therapy field to become better known across the globe. Second, the ICF provides occupational therapists with a global language to describe their expertise to the larger international health care community. The ICF uses a positive, holistic language emphasizing skills, capacities, and strengths of an individual rather than focusing on one's deficits and disabilities. This is similar to the outlook of occupational therapists. Third, the ICF includes environmental and personal contextual factors which are incorporated into the theory behind occupational therapy. It is important to take into consideration an individual's personal, environmental, and occupational factors to develop an effective intervention (Christiansen & Baum, 2005). The last notable application of the ICF to occupational therapy is the recognition of cultural patterns in occupation. Culture has significance on an individual's activities and participation and it is important to keep this in mind when treating an individual.

Although the ICF can be very useful for occupational therapists, it is noted in the literature that occupational therapists should use specific occupational therapy vocabulary along with the ICF in order to ensure correct communication about specific concepts (Stamm, Cieza, Machold, Smolen, & Stucki, 2006). The ICF might lack certain categories to describe what occupational therapists need to communicate to clients and colleagues. It also may not be possible to exactly match the connotations of the ICF categories to occupational therapy terms. The ICF is not an assessment and specialized occupational therapy vocabulary should not be replaced with ICF terminology (Hag Lund & Henriksson, 2003). The ICF is an overarching framework on which to hang current therapy practices.

The Occupational Therapists do maintain medical records for treating the patients for various reasons, e.g. for noting complete history and physical examination notes, progress notes, treatment provided; record is maintained for continued care of the patient, communication to the physician and other healthcare providers, document of proof in administrative and medical legal issues, insurance purpose, for collecting patient care information besides to carry out medical education and research work.

Specially designed medical record forms for the use of Occupational Therapy Unit or for Occupational Therapist are furnished in this chapter.

OPD

Reg................................. Dr .... Date ....

Indoor

Name............................. Sex .... Age .... Ward .... Bed ....

Occupation .... Address ....

Diagnosis ....Date of Onset ....

If Postoperative, Operation

Performed and Date of operation.

Any other condition not described under diagnosis, e.g. epilepsy, diabetes, etc.

....

Contraindications to therapy (Examples)

Fever, infectious diseases, pregnancy,   Full weight bearing on   Partial weight

cardiac (First trimester)   (Fracture or operated side)   bearing on fracture

                                                                or operated side

No weight bearing on

(Fracture or operated side)   Limited exercise, hypertension

Contractures or deformites ....

Treatment desired (check below)

A. 1. Muscle strength
   2. Re-education and co-ordination
   3. Range of joint motion
   4. Posture
   5. Relaxation
   6. Gait training
   7. Maintenance of function
   8. Prevention of contractures, deformities, etc.
   9. Postural drainage
   10. Respiratory function
B. Activities of daily living
C. Work tolerance

D. 1. Pre-operative preparation
   2. Post-operative care
E. 1. Relief of pain
   2. Resolution of inflammation
   3. Relief of edema
F. 1. Healing of wounds
   2. Peeling of skin
   3. Pigmentation
   4. General on-specific effect of UVR
G. Pre-vocational testing and training
H. Psychological, viz. simulation, socialization, etc.
I. Any other

Check here if any specific modality of treatment desired.

Testing:

1. Electrical muscle check
2. Manual muscle check
3. Joint range and tightness

4. Functional
5. Disability

Prescription for bracess, artificial limbs, splints, etc. ....

....

Signature

Clinical reocrd   **Occupational therapy**

Principal diagnosis

Diagnosis for which treatment requested   Date of onset

Part (s) to be treated

Aim of treatment

Precautions (Include communicability)   ☐ Ambulatory   ☐ Wheel chair   ☐ Litter

Frequency and duration of treatment desired   ☐ Ward   ☐ Shop

RESULTS DESIRED

☐ Increase of joint motion   ☐ Increase of muscle strength   ☐ Coordination
☐ Activity tolerance   ☐ Functional prosthetic training   ☐ Emotional read justment
☐ Other (Specify)

Physician's Signature   **Date**

MONTH	1	2	3	4	5	6	7	8	9	10	11	12	13	14	15	16	17	18	19	20	21	22	23	24	25	26	27	28	29	30	31

Total no. visits

Progress Notes (Date and Sign all notes)

Patient's Last Name : First Name - Middle Name	Registered No.	Ward No.

(Name of Hospital or Other Medical Facility)   Occupational Therapy

**OCCUPATIONAL THERAPY
TREATMENT MEASURES**

Medical Record #:

Hospital Name:

Patient Name:

Date of Birth:

Attending Physician:

Date of Admission:

☐ OPD

☐ IPD

Date	Issue	Intervention	Outcome	Date Resolved

Signature:...........................Employee ID #: ....Date:...........................

OCCUPATIONAL THERAPY TREATMENT MEASURES

Medical Record #:

Hospital Name:

Patient Name:

Date of Birth:

Attending Physician:

Date of Admission:

OCCUPATIONAL THERAPY

HOME VISIT ASSESSMENT

☐ OPD

☐ IPD

Diagnosis _____

_____

Date of home assessment: _____

Current mobility status: _____

_____

S/O: _____

_____

_____

_____

_____

_____

External layout of the house

House style: _____

Pathway into building _____ _____

   Surface: _____   Condition _____

Front entrance: #stairs: _____   height _____ railings: R L ramps: Y N

Other entrances: _____

Parking: _____

Comments: _____

_____

_____

Internal layout of the house:

Stories: _____

Basement: _____

Mainfloor: _____

Second floor: _____

Other: _____

Elevator   Y N   stairs inside: # _____   Railings Y N _____

Comments : _____

_____

_____

Occupational Therapy Home Visit Assessment

24 Optometry

Optometry is a health care profession concerned with eyes and related structures, as well as vision, visual systems, and vision information processing in humans.

Like most professions, optometry education, certification, and practice is regulated in most countries. Optometrists and optometry-related organizations interact with governmental agencies, other health care professionals, and the community to deliver eye and vision care. Optometry is one of three eye care professions, the others being ophthalmology (which is a branch of surgery) and orthoptics (a sub-specialty of ophthalmology primarily dealing with strabismus).

BACKGROUND

The term "optometry" comes from the Greek word *optos*, meaning *eye* or *vision*, and *metria*, meaning *measurement*.

The eye, including its structure and mechanism, has fascinated scientists and the public in general since ancient times. Many of the expressions in the English Language that mean to understand are equivalent vision terms. "I see", to mean I understand.

Many patients when told that they may have an eye problem will be more concerned about diseases that affect vision than other, more lethal diseases. Being deprived of sight can have a devastating effect on the psyche, as well as economic and social effects, as many blind individuals require significant assistance with activities of daily living and are often unable to continue gainful employment previously held while seeing.

The maintenance of ocular health and correction of eye problems that decrease vision contribute greatly to the ability to appreciate the longer lifespan that all of medicine continues to allow. Given the importance of vision to quality of life, many optometrists consider their job to be rewarding, as they are often able to restore or improve a patient's sight.

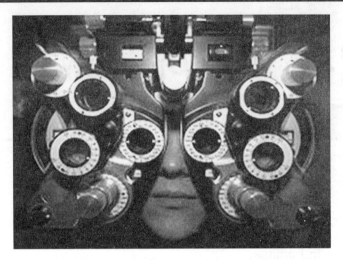

Fig. 24.1: An optical refractor (phoropter) in use

Behavioral optometry is a related area of nonstrabismus vision therapy that some optometrists practice. Generally, ophthalmologists and orthoptists do not practice this.

In the United States, optometrists have obtained from state legislatures the right to treat more eye conditions and to perform certain laser surgeries. Optometrists have been successful in getting the right to use some types of medication, depending on if the medication is given as pills, eye drops, or injections. In the United States, all states except for Oklahoma do not allow the optometrists to perform any type of surgeries. However, in Oklahoma, optometrists are allowed by the state legislature to perform laser surgery.

HISTORY

Optometric history is tied to the development of:
- Vision science (related areas of medicine, microbiology, neurology, physiology, psychology, etc.)
- Optics, optical aids
- Optical instruments, imaging techniques (Fig. 24.1).
- Other eye care professions.

The word optometry comes from two Greek words–*opto* which means sight, and *metron* which means measure. The history of optometry can be traced back to the early studies on optics and image formation by the eye.

25 Nutrition

Nutrition (also called *nourishment* or *aliment*) is the provision, to cells and organisms, of the materials necessary in the form of food to support life. Many common health problems can be prevented or alleviated with a healthy diet.

The diet of an organism is what it eats, and is largely determined by the perceived palatability of foods. Dietitians are health professionals who specialize in human nutrition, meal planning, economics, and preparation. They are trained to provide safe, evidence-based dietary advice and management to healthy and sick individuals as well as to institutions.

A poor diet can have an damaging impact on health, causing deficiency diseases such as scurvy, beriberi, and kwashiorkor; health-threatening conditions like obesity and metabolic syndrome, and such common chronic systemic diseases as cardiovascular disease, diabetes, and osteoporosis.

OVERVIEW

Nutritional science investigates the metabolic and physiological responses of the body to diet. With advances in the fields of molecular biology, biochemistry, and genetics, the study of nutrition is increasingly concerned with metabolism and metabolic pathways: the sequences of biochemical steps through which substances in living things change from one form to another.

The human body contains chemical compounds, such as water, carbohydrates, sugar, starch, and fiber, amino acids (in proteins), fatty acids (in lipids), and nucleic acids (DNA and RNA). These compounds in turn consist of elements such as carbon, hydrogen, oxygen, nitrogen, phosphorus, calcium, iron, zinc, magnesium, manganese, and so on. All of these chemical compounds and elements occur in various forms and combinations, e.g. hormones, vitamins, phospholipids, hydroxyapatite, both in the human body and in the plant and animal organisms that humans eat.

The human body consists of elements and compounds ingested, digested, absorbed, and circulated through the bloodstream to feed the cells of the body. Except in the unborn fetus, the digestive system is the first system involved. In a typical adult, about seven liters of digestive juices enter the lumen of the digestive tract. These break chemical bonds in ingested molecules, and modulate their conformations and energy states. Though some molecules are absorbed into the bloodstream unchanged, digestive processes release them from the matrix of foods. Unabsorbed matter, along with some waste products of metabolism, is eliminated from the body in the feces.

Studies of nutritional status must take into account the state of the body before and after experiments, as well as the chemical composition of the whole diet and of all material excreted and eliminated from the body in urine and feces. Comparing the food to the waste can help determine the specific compounds and elements absorbed and metabolized in the body. The effects of nutrients may only be discernible over an extended period, during which all food and waste must be analyzed. The number of variables involved in such experiments is high, making nutritional studies time-consuming and expensive, which explains why the science of human nutrition is still slowly evolving.

In general, eating a wide variety of fresh, unprocessed whole foods has proven favorable compared to processed foods. In particular, the consumption of whole-plant foods slows digestion and allows better absorption, and a more favorable balance of essential nutrients per calorie, resulting in better management of cell growth, maintenance, and mitosis (cell division), as well as better regulation of appetite and blood sugar. Regularly scheduled meals every few hours have also proven more wholesome than infrequent or haphazard ones.

NUTRIENTS

There are seven major classes of nutrients: carbohydrates, fats, fiber, minerals, protein, vitamin, and water.

These nutrient classes can be categorized as either macronutrients needed in relatively large amounts or micronutrients needed in smaller quantities. The macronutrients are carbohydrates, fats, fiber, proteins, and water. The micronutrients are minerals and vitamins.

The macronutrients excluding fiber and water, provide structural material amino acids from which proteins are built, and lipids from which cell membranes and some signaling molecules are built, energy. Some of the structural material can be used to generate energy internally, and in either case it is measured in Joules or kilocalories often called "Calories" and written with a capital C to distinguish them from little 'c' calories. Carbohydrates and proteins provide 17 kJ approximately (4 kcal) of energy per gram, while fats provide 37 kJ (9 kcal) per gram, though the net energy from either depends on such factors as absorption and digestive effort, which vary substantially from instance to instance. Vitamins, minerals, fiber, and water do not provide energy, but are required for other reasons. A third class dietary material, fiber, i.e. non-digestible material such as cellulose, seems also to be required, for both mechanical and biochemical reasons, though the exact reasons remain unclear (Fig. 25.1).

Molecules of carbohydrates and fats consist of carbon, hydrogen, and oxygen atoms. Carbohydrates range from simple monosaccharide (glucose, fructose, galactose) to complex polysaccharides (starch). Fats are triglycerides, made of assorted fatty acid monomers bound to glycerol backbone. Some fatty acids, but not all, are essential in the diet: they cannot be synthesized in the body. Protein molecules contain nitrogen atoms in addition to carbon, oxygen, and hydrogen. The fundamental components of protein are nitrogen-containing amino acids, some of which are essential in the sense that humans cannot make them internally. Some of the amino acids are convertible (with the expenditure of energy) to glucose and can be used for energy production just as ordinary glucose. By breaking down existing protein,

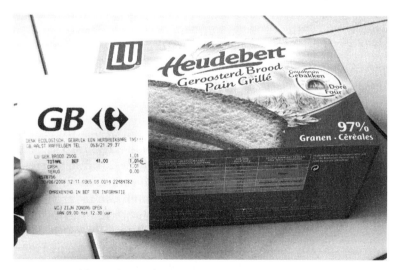

Fig. 25.1: Toasted bread is a cheap, high calorie nutrient usually unbalanced, i.e. deficient in essential minerals and vitamins, largely because of removal of both germ and bran during processing food source (*For color version, see Plate 3*)

some glucose can be produced internally; the remaining amino acids are discarded, primarily as urea in urine. This occurs normally only during prolonged starvation.

Other micronutrients include antioxidants and phytochemicals which are said to protect some body systems. Their necessity is not as well established as in the case of, for instance, vitamins.

Most foods contain a mix of some or all of the nutrient classes, together with other substances such as toxins or various sorts. Some nutrients can be stored internally, e.g. the fat soluble vitamins, while others are required more or less continuously. Poor health can be caused by a lack of required nutrients or, in extreme cases, too much of a required nutrient. For example, both salt and water both absolutely required will cause illness or even death in too large amounts.

Carbohydrates

Carbohydrates may be classified as monosaccharide, disaccharides, or polysaccharides depending on the number of monomer (sugar) units they contain. They constitute a large part of foods such as rice, noodles, bread, and other grain-based products. Monosaccharide contains one sugar unit, disaccharides two, and polysaccharides three or more. Polysaccharides are often referred to as complex of carbohydrates because they are typically long multiple branched chains of sugar units. The difference is that complex carbohydrates take longer to digest and absorb since their sugar units must be separated from the chain before absorption. The spike in blood glucose levels after ingestion of simple sugars is thought to be related to some of the heart and vascular diseases which have become more frequent in recent times. Simple sugars form a greater part of modern diets than formerly, perhaps leading to more cardiovascular disease. The degree of causation is still not clear, however.

Simple carbohydrates are absorbed quickly, and therefore raise blood-sugar levels more rapidly than other nutrients. However, the most important plant carbohydrate nutrient, starch, varies in its absorption. Gelatinized starch heated for a few minutes in the presence of water is far more digestible than plain starch. And starch which has been divided into fine particles is also more absorbable during digestion. The increased effort and decreased availability reduces the available energy from starchy foods substantially and can be seen experimentally in rats and anecdotally in humans. Additionally, up to a third of dietary starch may be unavailable due to mechanical or chemical difficulty.

Fiber

Dietary fiber is a carbohydrate or a polysaccharide that is incompletely absorbed in humans and in some animals. Like all carbohydrates, when it is metabolized it can produce four calories (kilocalories) of energy per gram. But in most circumstances it accounts for less than that because of its limited absorption and digestibility. Dietary fiber consists mainly of cellulose, a large carbohydrate polymer that is indigestible because humans do not have the required enzymes to disassemble it. There are two subcategories: soluble and insoluble fiber. Whole grains, fruits especially plums, prunes, and figs, and vegetables are good sources of dietary fiber. Fiber is important to digestive health and is thought to reduce the risk of colon cancer. For mechanical reasons it can help in alleviating both constipation and diarrhea. Fiber provides bulk to the intestinal contents, and insoluble fiber especially stimulates peristalsis—the rhythmic muscular contractions of the intestines which move digesta along the digestive tract. Some soluble fibers produce a solution of high viscosity; this is essentially a gel, which slows the movement of food through the intestines. Additionally, fiber, perhaps especially that from whole grains, may help lessen insulin spikes and reduce the risk of type II diabetes.

Fat

A molecule of dietary fat typically consists of several fatty acids containing long chains of carbon and hydrogen atoms, bonded to a glycerol. They are typically found as triglycerides (three fatty acids attached to one glycerol backbone). Fats may be classified as saturated or unsaturated depending on the detailed structure of the fatty acids involved. Saturated fats have all of the carbon atoms in their fatty acid chains bonded to hydrogen atoms, whereas unsaturated fats have some of these carbon atoms double-bonded, so their molecules have relatively fewer hydrogen atoms than a saturated fatty acid of the same length. Unsaturated fats may be further classified as monounsaturated (one double-bond) or polyunsaturated (many double-bonds). Furthermore, depending on the location of the double-bond in the fatty acid chain, unsaturated fatty acids are classified as omega-3 or omega-6 fatty acids. Trans fats are a type of unsaturated fat with trans-isomer bonds; these are rare in nature and in foods from natural sources; they are typically created in an industrial process called partial hydrogenation.

Many studies have shown that unsaturated fats, particularly monounsaturated fats, are best in the human diet. Saturated fats, typically from animal sources, are next, while trans-fats are to be avoided. Saturated and some trans- fats are typically solid at room temperature (such as butter or lard), while unsaturated fats are typically liquids (such as olive oil or flaxseed oil). Transfats are very rare in nature, but have properties useful in the food processing industry, such as rancid resistance.

Essential Fatty Acids

Most fatty acids are non-essential, meaning the body can produce them as needed, generally from other fatty acids and always by expending energy to do so. However, in humans at least two fatty acids are essential and must be included in the diet. An appropriate balance of essential fatty acids—omega-3 and omega-6 fatty acids—seems also important for health, though definitive experimental demonstration has been elusive. Both of these "omega" long-chain polyunsaturated fatty acids are substrates for a class of eicosanoids known as prostaglandins, which have roles throughout the human body. They are hormones, in some respects. The omega-3 eicosapentaenoic acid (EPA), which can be made in the human body from the omega-3 essential fatty acid alpha-linolenic acid (LNA), or taken in through marine food sources, serves as a building block for series 3 prostaglandins (e.g. weakly inflammatory PGE3). The omega-6 dihomo-gamma-linolenic acid (DGLA) serves as a building block for series 1 prostaglandins (e.g. anti-inflammatory PGE1), whereas arachidonic acid (AA) serves as a building block for series 2 prostaglandins (e.g. pro-inflammatory PGE 2). Both DGLA and AA can be made from the omega-6 linoleic acid (LA) in the human body, or can be taken in directly through food. An appropriately balanced intake of omega-3 and omega-6 partly determines the relative production of different prostaglandins: one reason a balance between omega-3 and omega-6 is believed important for cardiovascular health. In industrialized societies, people typically consume large amounts of processed vegetable oils, which have reduced amounts of the essential fatty acids along with too much of omega-6 fatty acids relative to omega-3 fatty acids.

The conversion rate of omega-6 DGLA to AA largely determines the production of the prostaglandins PGE1 and PGE2. Omega-3 EPA prevents AA from being released from membranes, thereby skewing prostaglandin balance away from pro-inflammatory PGE2 (made from AA) toward anti-inflammatory PGE1 (made from DGLA). Moreover, the conversion (desaturation) of DGLA to AA is controlled by the enzyme delta-5-desaturase, which in turn is controlled by hormones such as insulin (up-regulation) and glucagons (down-regulation). The amount and type of carbohydrates consumed, along with some types of amino acid, can influence processes involving insulin, glucagons, and other hormones; therefore the ratio of omega-3 versus omega-6 has wide effects on general health, and specific effects on immune function and inflammation, and mitosis, i.e. cell division.

Good sources of essential fatty acids include most vegetables, nuts, seeds, and marine oils, Some of the best sources are fish, flax seed oils, soybeans, pumpkin seeds, sunflower seeds and walnuts.

Protein

Proteins are the basis of many animal body structures, e.g. muscles, skin, and hair. They also form the enzymes which control chemical reactions throughout the body. Each molecule is composed of amino acids which are characterized by inclusion of nitrogen and sometimes sulphur, are responsible for the distinctive smell of burning protein, such as the keratin in hair. The body requires amino acids to produce new proteins (protein retention) and to replace damaged proteins (maintenance) (Fig. 25.2). As there is no protein or amino acid storage provision, amino acids must be present in the diet. Excess amino acids are discarded, typically in the urine. For all animals, some amino acids are essential (an animal cannot produce them internally) and some are non-essential (the animal can produce them from other nitrogen-containing compounds). About twenty amino acids are found in the human body, and about ten of these are essential, and therefore must be included in the diet. A diet that contains adequate amounts of amino acids especially those that are essential is particularly important in some situations: during early development and maturation, pregnancy,

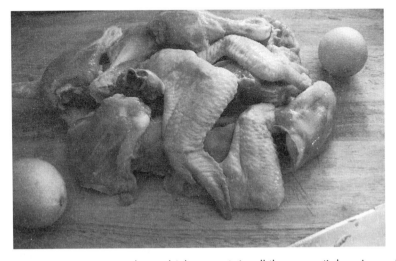

Fig. 25.2: Most meats such as chicken contain all the essential amino acids needed for humans (Protein in nutrition) (*For color version, see Plate 3*)

lactation, or injury or a burn, for instance. A complete protein source contains all the essential amino acids; an incomplete protein source lacks one or more of the essential amino acids.

It is possible to combine two incomplete protein sources, e.g. rice and beans to make a complete protein source, and characteristic combinations are the basis of distinct cultural cooking traditions. Sources of dietary protein include meats, tofu and other soy-products, eggs, grains, legumes, and dairy products such as milk and cheese. A few amino acids from protein can be converted into glucose and used for fuel through a process called gluconeogenesis; this is done in quantity only during starvation. The amino acids remaining after such conversion are discarded.

Minerals

Dietary minerals are the chemical elements required by living organisms, other than the four elements carbon, hydrogen, nitrogen, and oxygen that are present in nearly all organic molecules. The term "mineral" is archaic, since the intent is to describe simply the less common elements in the diet. Some are heavier than the four just mentioned—including several metals, which often occur as ions in the body. Some dietitians recommend that these be supplied from foods in which they occur naturally or at least as complex compounds, or sometimes even from natural inorganic sources (such as calcium carbonate from ground oyster shells). Some are absorbed much more readily in the ionic forms found in such sources. On the other hand, minerals are often artificially added to the diet as supplements; the most famous is likely iodine in iodized salt which prevents goiter.

Macrominerals

Many elements are essential in relative quantity; they are usually called "bulk minerals". Some are structural, but many play a role as electrolytes. Elements with recommended dietary allowance (RDA) greater than 200 mg/day are, in alphabetical order with informal or folk-medicine perspectives in parentheses:

- Calcium, a common electrolyte, but also needed structurally structural for muscle and digestive system health, bones, some forms neutralizes acidity, may help clear toxins, and provide signaling ions for nerve and membrane functions.
- Chlorine as chloride ions; very common electrolyte; see sodium, below
- Magnesium, required for processing ATP and related reactions (builds bone, causes strong peristalsis, increases flexibility, increases alkalinity)

- Phosphorus, required component of bones; essential for energy processing
- Potassium, a very common electrolyte (heart and nerve health)
- Sodium, a very common electrolyte; not generally found in dietary supplements, despite being needed in large quantities, because the ion is very common in food: typically as sodium chloride, or common salt. Excessive sodium consumption can deplete calcium and magnesium, leading to high blood pressure and osteoporosis.
- Sulfur for three essential amino acids and therefore many proteins (skin, hair, nails, liver, and pancreas).

Trace Minerals

Many elements are required in trace amounts, usually because they play a catalytic role in enzymes. Some trace mineral elements (RDA < 200 mg/day) are, in alphabetical order:

- Cobalt required for biosynthesis of vitamin B12 family of coenzymes
- Copper required component of many redox enzymes, including cytochrome c oxidase
- Chromium required for sugar metabolism
- Iodine required not only for the biosynthesis of thyroxin, but probably, for other important organs as breast, stomach, salivary glands, thymus, etc. (see extra thyroidal iodine); for this reason iodine is needed in larger quantities than others in this list, and sometimes classified with the Macrominerals
- Iron required for many enzymes, and for hemoglobin and some other proteins
- Manganese (processing of oxygen)
- Molybdenum required for xanthine oxidase and related oxidases
- Nickel present in urease
- Selenium required for peroxidase (antioxidant proteins)
- Vanadium (Speculative: there is no established RDA for vanadium. No specific biochemical function has been identified for it in humans, although vanadium is required for some lower organisms.)
- Zinc required for several enzymes such as carboxypeptidase, liver alcohol dehydrogenase, carbonic anhydrase.

Vitamins

As with the minerals discussed above, some vitamins are recognized as essential nutrients, necessary in the diet for good health. (Vitamin D is the exception: it can alternatively be synthesized in the skin, in the presence of UVB radiation.) Certain vitamin-like compounds that are recommended in the diet, such as carnitine, are thought useful for survival and health, but these are not "essential" dietary nutrients because the human body has some capacity to produce them from other compounds. Moreover, thousands of different phytochemicals have recently been discovered in food (particularly in fresh vegetables), which may have desirable properties including antioxidant activity (see below); experimental demonstration has been suggestive but inconclusive. Other essential nutrients not classed as vitamins include essential amino acids (see above), choline, essential fatty acids (see above), and the minerals discussed in the preceding section.

Vitamin deficiencies may result in disease conditions: goiter, scurvy, osteoporosis, impaired immune system, disorders of cell metabolism, certain forms of cancer, symptoms of premature aging, and poor psychological health (including eating disorders), among many others. Excess of some vitamins is also dangerous to health (notably vitamin A), and for at least one vitamin B_6, toxicity begins at levels not far above the required amount. Deficiency or excess of minerals can also have serious health consequences.

Water

About 70 percent of the non-fat mass of the human body is made of water (Fig. 25.3). To function properly, the body requires between one and seven liters of water per day to avoid dehydration; the precise amount depends on the level of activity, temperature, humidity, and other factors. With physical exertion and heat exposure, water loss increases and daily fluid needs will eventually increase as well.

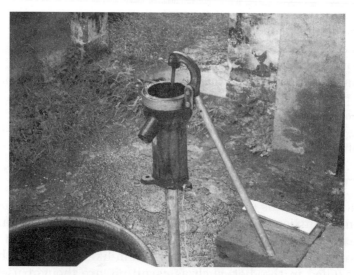

Fig. 25.3: A manual water pump in China

It is not fully clear how much water intake is needed by healthy people, although some experts assert that 8–10 glasses of water (approximately 2 liters) daily is the minimum to maintain proper hydration. The notion that a person should consume eight glasses of water per day cannot be traced to a credible scientific source. The effect of, greater or lesser, water intake on weight loss and on constipation is also still unclear. The original water intake recommendation in 1945 by the Food and Nutrition Board of the National Research Council read: "An ordinary standard for diverse persons is 1 milliliter for each calorie of food. Most of this quantity is contained in prepared foods." The latest dietary reference intake report by the United States National Research Council recommended, generally, (including food sources): 2.7 liters of water total for women and 3.7 liters for men. Specifically, pregnant and breastfeeding women need additional fluids to stay hydrated. According to the Institute of Medicine—who recommend that, on average, women consume 2.2 liters and men 3.0 liters—this is recommended to be 2.4 liters (approx 9 cups) for pregnant women and 3 liters (approx 12.5 cups) for breastfeeding women since an especially large amount of fluid is lost during nursing.

For those who have healthy kidneys, it is somewhat difficult to drink too much water but especially in warm humid weather and while exercising, it is dangerous to drink too little. People can drink far more water than necessary while exercising, however, putting them at risk of water intoxication, which can be fatal. In particular large amounts of de-ionized water are dangerous.

Normally, about 20 percent of water intake comes in food, while the rest comes from drinking water and assorted beverages caffeinated included. Water is excreted from the body in multiple forms; including urine and feces, sweating, and by water vapor in the exhaled breath.

OTHER NUTRIENTS

Other micronutrients include antioxidants and phytochemicals. These substances are generally more recent discoveries which have not yet been recognized as vitamins or as required. Phytochemicals may act as antioxidants, but not all phytochemicals are antioxidants.

Antioxidants

Antioxidants are a recent discovery. As cellular metabolism/energy production requires oxygen, potentially damaging (e.g. mutation causing) compounds known as free radicals can form. Most of these are oxidizers, i.e. acceptors of electrons and some react very strongly. For normal cellular maintenance, growth, and division, these free radicals must be sufficiently neutralized by antioxidant compounds. Recently, some researchers suggested an interesting theory of evolution of dietary antioxidants. Some are produced by the human body with adequate precursors, i.e. glutathione, vitamin C and those the body cannot produce may only be obtained in the diet via direct sources vitamin C in humans, vitamin A, vitamin K or produced by the body from other compounds such as Beta-carotene converted to Vitamin A by the body, vitamin D synthesized from cholesterol by sunlight. Phytochemicals and their subgroup polyphenols are the majority of antioxidants; about 4,000 are known. Different antioxidants are now known to function in a cooperative network, e.g. vitamin C can reactivate free radical-containing glutathione or vitamin E by accepting the free radical itself, and so on. Some antioxidants are more effective than others at neutralizing different free radicals. Some cannot neutralize certain free radicals. Some cannot be present in certain areas of free radical development vitamin A is fat-soluble and protects fat areas, vitamin C is water soluble and protects those areas. When interacting with a free radical, some antioxidants produce a different free radical compound that is less dangerous or more dangerous than the previous compound. Having a variety of antioxidants allows any byproducts to be safely dealt with by more efficient antioxidants in neutralizing a free radical's butterfly effect.

Phytochemicals

A growing area of interest is the effect upon human health of trace chemicals, collectively called phytochemicals. These nutrients are typically found in edible plants, especially colorful fruits and vegetables, but also other organisms including seafood, algae, and fungi. The effects of phytochemicals increasingly survive rigorous testing by prominent health organizations. One of the principal classes of phytochemicals is polyphenol antioxidants, chemicals which are known to provide certain health benefits to the cardiovascular system and immune system (Fig. 25.4). These chemicals are known to down-regulate the formation of reactive oxygen species, key chemicals in cardiovascular disease.

Perhaps the most rigorously tested phytochemicals is zeaxanthin, a yellow-pigmented carotenoid present in many yellow and orange fruits and vegetables. Repeated studies have shown a strong correlation between ingestion of zeaxanthin and the prevention and treatment of age-related macular degeneration (AMD). Less rigorous studies have proposed a correlation between zeaxanthin intake and cataracts. A second carotenoid, lutein, has also been shown to lower the risk of contracting AMD. Both compounds have been observed to collect in the retina when ingested orally, and they serve to protect the rods and cones against the destructive effects of light.

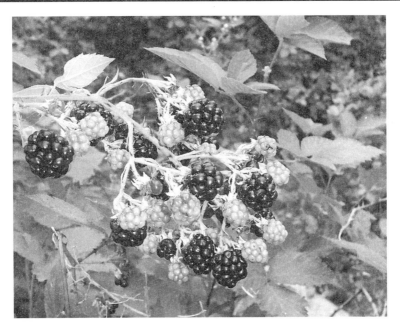

Fig. 25.4: Blackberries are a source of polyphenol antioxidants
(*For color version, see Plate 4*)

Another carotenoid, beta-cryptoxanthin, appears to protect against chronic joint inflammatory diseases, such as arthritis. While the association between serum blood levels of beta-cryptoxanthin and substantially decreased joint disease has been established, neither a convincing mechanism for such protection nor a cause-and-effect have been rigorously studied. Similarly, a red phytochemical, lycopene, has substantial credible evidence of negative association with development of prostate cancer.

The correlations between the ingestion of some phytochemicals and the prevention of disease are, in some cases, enormous in magnitude.

Even when the evidence is obtained, translating it to practical dietary advice can be difficult and counter-intuitive. Lutein, for example, occurs in many yellow and orange fruits and vegetables and protects the eyes against various diseases. However, it does not protect the eye nearly as well as zeaxanthin, and the presence of lutein in the retina will prevent zeaxanthin uptake. Additionally, evidence has shown that the lutein present in egg yolk is more readily absorbed than the lutein from vegetable sources, possibly because of fat solubility. At the most basic level, the question "should you eat eggs?" is complex to the point of dismay, including misperceptions about the health effects of cholesterol in egg yolk, and its saturated fat content.

As another example, lycopene is prevalent in tomatoes and actually is the chemical that gives tomatoes their red color. It is more highly concentrated, however, in processed tomato products such as commercial pasta sauce, or tomato soup, than in fresh "healthy" tomatoes. Yet, such sauces tend to have high amounts of salt, sugar, and other substances a person may wish or even need to avoid.

Table 25.1 presents phytochemical groups and common sources, arranged by family.

Table 25.1: Phytochemical groups and common source of food

Family	Sources	Possible benefits
Flavonoids	Berries, herbs, vegetables, wine, grapes, tea	General antioxidant, oxidation of LDLs, prevention of arteriosclerosis and heart disease
Ioflavones (phytoestrogens)	Soy, red clover, kudzu root	General antioxidant, prevention of arteriosclerosis and heart disease, easing symptoms of menopause, cancer prevention
Isothiocyanates monoterpenes	Cruciferous vegetables citrus peels, essential oils, herbs, spices, green plants, atmosphere.	Cancer prevention Cancer prevention, treating gallstones
Organosulfur compounds	Chives, garlic, onions	Cancer prevention, lowered LDLs, assistance to the immune system
Saponins	Beans, cereals, herbs	Hypercholesterolemia, hyperglycemia, antioxidant, cancer prevention, znti-inflammatory
Capsaicinoids	All capiscum (chile) peppers	Topical pain relief, cancer prevention, cancer cell apoptosis

INTESTINAL BACTERIAL FLORA

It is now also known that animal intestines contain a large population of gut flora. In humans, these include species such as Bacteroides, *L. acidophilus* and *E. coli*, among many others. They are essential to digestion, and are also affected by the food we eat. Bacteria in the gut perform many important functions for humans, including breaking down and aiding in the absorption of otherwise indigestible food; stimulating cell growth; repressing the growth of harmful bacteria, training the immune system to respond only to pathogens; producing vitamin B12, and defending against some infectious diseases.

ADVICE AND GUIDANCE

Governmental Policies

In the US, dietitians are registered (RD) or licensed (LD) with the Commission for Dietetic Registration and the American Dietetic Association, and are only able to use the title "dietitian," as described by the business and professions codes of each respective state, when

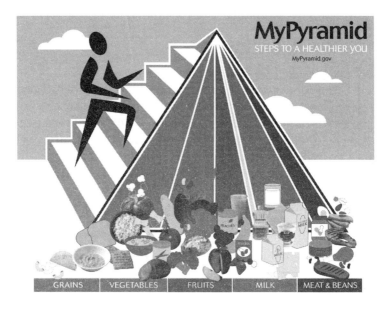

Fig. 25.5: The updated USDA food pyramid, published in 2005, is a general nutrition guide for recommended food consumption for humans
(*For color version, see Plate 4*)

they have met specific educational and experiential prerequisites and passed a national registration or licensure examination, respectively. In California, registered dietitians must abide by the "Business and Professions Code of Section 2585-2586.8". http://www.leginfo.ca.gov/cgi-bin/displaycode?section=bpc&group=02001-03000&file=2585-2586.8. Anyone may call themselves a nutritionist, including unqualified dietitians, as this term is unregulated. Some states, such as the State of Florida, have begun to include the title "nutritionist" in state licensure requirements. Most governments provide guidance on nutrition, and some also impose mandatory disclosure/labeling requirements for processed food manufacturers and restaurants to assist consumers in complying with such guidance.

In the US, nutritional standards and recommendations are established jointly by the US Department of Agriculture and US Department of Health and Human Services (Fig. 25.5). Dietary and physical activity guidelines from the USDA are presented in the concept of a food pyramid, which superseded the Four Food Groups. The Senate committee currently responsible for oversight of the USDA is the Agriculture, Nutrition and Forestry Committee. Committee hearings are often televised on C-SPAN as seen here.

The US Department of Health and Human Services provides a sample week-long menu which fulfills the nutritional recommendations of the government. Canada's Food Guide is another governmental recommendation.

Teaching

Nutrition is taught in schools in many countries. In England and Wales the Personal and Social Education and Food Technology curricula include nutrition, stressing the importance of a balanced diet and teaching how to read nutrition labels on packaging. In many schools a nutrition class will fall within the family and consumer science or health departments. In some American schools, students are required to take a certain number of FCS or health related classes. Nutrition is offered at many schools, and if it is not a class of its own, nutrition is included in other FCS or Health classes such as: life skills, independent living, single survival, freshmen connection, health etc. In many nutrition classes, students learn about the food groups, the food pyramid, daily recommended allowances, calories, vitamins, minerals, malnutrition, physical activity, healthy food choices and how to live a healthy life.

A 1985 US National Research Council report entitled nutrition education in US medical schools concluded that nutrition education in medical schools was inadequate. Only 20 percent of the schools surveyed taught nutrition as a separate, required course. A 2006 survey found that this number had risen to 30 percent.

HEALTHY DIETS

Whole Plant Food Diet

Heart disease, cancer, obesity, and diabetes are commonly called "Western" diseases because these maladies were once rarely seen in developing countries. One study in China found some regions had essentially no cancer or heart disease, while in other areas they reflected "up to a 100-fold increase" coincident with diets that were found to be entirely plant-based to heavily animal-based, respectively. In contrast, diseases of affluence like cancer and heart disease are common throughout the United States. Adjusted for age and exercise, large regional clusters of people in China rarely suffered from these "Western" diseases possibly because their diets are rich in vegetables, fruits and whole grains.

The United Healthcare/Pacificare nutrition guideline recommends a whole plant food diet, and recommends using protein only as a condiment with meals. A national geographic cover article from November, 2005, entitled 'The Secrets of Living Longer', also recommends a whole plant food diet. The article is a lifestyle survey of three populations, Sardinians, Okinawa's, and Adventists, who generally display longevity and "suffer a fraction of the diseases that commonly kill people in other parts of the developed world, and enjoy more healthy years of life." In sum, they offer three sets of 'best practices' to emulate. The rest is up to you. In common with all three groups is to "eat fruits, vegetables, and whole grains."

The national geographic article noted that an NIH funded study of 34,000 seventh-day adventists between 1976 and 1988 ...found that the adventists' habit of consuming beans, soy milk, tomatoes, and other fruits lowered their risk of developing certain cancers. It also suggested that eating whole grain bread, drinking five glasses of water a day, and most surprisingly, consuming four servings of nuts a week reduced their risk of heart disease.

The French "Paradox"

It has been discovered that people living in France live longer. Even though they consume more saturated fats than Americans, the rate of heart disease is lower in France than in North America. A number of explanations have been suggested:
* Reduced consumption of processed carbohydrate and other junk foods.
* Regular consumption of red wine.
* More active lifestyles involving plenty of daily exercise, especially walking; the French are much less dependent on cars than Americans are.
* Higher consumption of artificially produced trans-fats by Americans, which has been shown to have greater lipoprotein effects per gram than saturated fat.

However, statistics collected by the World Health Organization from 1990 to 2000 show that the incidence of heart disease in France may have been underestimated and in fact be similar to that of neighboring countries.

SPORTS NUTRITION

Protein

Protein is an important component of every cell in the body. Hair and nails are mostly made of protein. The body uses protein to build and repair tissues. Also protein is used to make enzymes, hormones, and other body chemicals. Protein is an important building block of bones, muscles, cartilage, skin, and blood.

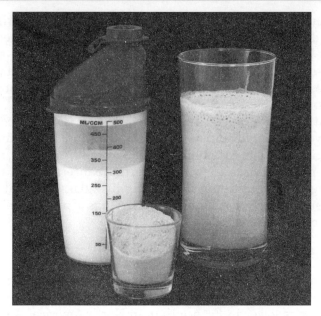

Fig. 25.6: Protein milkshakes, made from protein powder (center) and milk (left), are a common bodybuilding supplement (*For color version, see Plate 5*)

The protein requirement for each individual differs, as do opinions about whether and to what extent physically active people require more protein. The 2005 recommended dietary allowances (RDA), aimed at the general healthy adult population, provide for an intake of 0.8 to 1 gram of protein per kilogram of body weight (according to the BMI formula), with the review panel stating that "no additional dietary protein is suggested for healthy adults undertaking resistance or endurance exercise". Conversely, Di Pasquale (2008), citing recent studies, recommends a minimum protein intake of 2.2 g/kg "for anyone involved in competitive or intense recreational sports who wants to maximize lean body mass but does not wish to gain weight" (Fig. 25.6).

Water and Salts

Water is one of the most important nutrients in the sports diet. It helps eliminate food waste products in the body, regulates body temperature during activity and helps with digestion. Maintaining hydration during periods of physical exertion is key to peak performance. While drinking too much water during activities can lead to physical discomfort, dehydration in excess of 2 percent of body mass (by weight) markedly hinders athletic performance. Additional carbohydrates and protein before, during, and after exercise increase time to exhaustion as well as speed recovery. Dosage is based on work performed, lean body mass, and environmental factors, especially ambient temperature and humidity. Maintaining the right amount is key.

Carbohydrates

The main fuel used by the body during exercise is carbohydrates, which is stored in muscle as glycogen—a form of sugar. During exercise, muscle glycogen reserves can be used up, especially when activities last longer than 90 min. Because the amount of glycogen stored in the body is limited, it is important for athletes to replace glycogen by consuming a diet high in carbohydrates. Meeting energy needs can help improve performance during the sport, as well as improve overall strength and endurance.

There are different kinds of carbohydrates—simple or refined, and unrefined. A typical American consumes about 50% of their carbohydrates as simple sugars, which are added to foods as opposed to sugars that come naturally in fruits and vegetables. These simple sugars come in large amounts in sodas and fast food. Over the course of a year, the average American consumes 54 gallons of soft drinks, which contain the highest amount of added sugars. Even though carbohydrates are necessary for humans to function, they are not all equally healthful. When machinery has been used to remove bits of high fiber, the carbohydrates are refined. These are the carbohydrates found in white bread and fast food.

MALNUTRITION (TABLE 25.2)

Malnutrition refers to insufficient, excessive, or imbalanced consumption of nutrients. In developed countries, the diseases of malnutrition are most often associated with nutritional imbalances or excessive consumption. Although there are more people in the world who are malnourished due to excessive consumption, according to the United Nations World Health Organization, the real challenge in developing nations today, more than starvation, is combating insufficient nutrition—the lack of nutrients necessary for the growth and maintenance of vital functions.

Mental Agility

Research indicates that improving the awareness of nutritious meal choices and establishing long-term habits of healthy eating has a positive effect on a cognitive and spatial memory capacity, potentially increasing a student's potential to process and retain academic information.

Table 25.2: Illnesses caused by improper nutrient consumption

Nutrients	Deficiency	Excess
Energy	Starvation, marasmus	Obesity, diabetes mellitus, cardiovascular disease
Simple carbohydrates	None	diabetes mellitus, obesity
Complex carbohydrates	None	Obesity
Saturated fat	Low sex hormone levels	Cardiovascular disease (claimed by most doctors and nutritionists)
Trans fat	None	Cardiovascular disease
Unsaturated fat	None	Obesity
Fat	Malabsorption of fat-soluble vitamins, rabbit starvation (If protein intake is high)	Cardiovascular disease (claimed by some)
Omega 3 Fats	Cardiovascular disease	Bleeding, hemorrhages
Omega 6 Fats	None	Cardiovascular disease, cancer
Cholesterol	None	Cardiovascular disease (claimed by many)
Protein	Kwashiorkor	Rabbit starvation
Sodium	Hypernatremia	Hypernatremia, hypertension
Iron	Anemia	Cirrhosis, heart disease
Iodine	Goiter, hypothyroidism	Iodine toxicity (goiter, hypothyroidism)
Vitamin A	Xerophthalmia and night blindness, low testosterone levels	Hypervitaminosis A (cirrhosis, hair loss)
Vitamin B$_1$	Beri-Beri	
Vitamin B$_2$	Cracking of skin and corneal unclearation	
Niacin	Pellagra	Dyspepsia, cardiac arrhythmias, birth defects
Vitamin B$_{12}$	Pernicious Anemia	
Vitamin C	Scurvy	Diarrhea causing dehydration
Vitamin D	Rickets	Hypervitaminosis D (dehydration, vomiting, constipation)
Vitamin E	nervous disorders	Hypervitaminosis E (anticoagulant: excessive bleeding)
Vitamin K	Hemorrhage	
Calcium	Osteoporosis, tetany, carpopedal spasm, laryngospasm, cardiac arrhythmias	Fatigue, depression, confusion, anorexia, nausea, vomiting, constipation, pancreatitis, increased urination
Magnesium	Hypertension	Weakness, nausea, vomiting, impaired breathing, and hypotension
Potassium	Hypokalemia, cardiac arrhythmias	Hyperkalemia, palpitations

Some organizations have begun working with teachers, policymakers, and managed foodservice contractors to mandate improved nutritional content and increased nutritional resources in school cafeterias from primary to university level institutions. Health and nutrition have been proven to have close links with overall educational success. Currently less than 10 percent of American college students report that they eat the recommended five servings of fruit and vegetables daily. Better nutrition has been shown to have an impact on both cognitive and spatial memory performance; a study showed those with higher blood sugar levels performed better on certain memory tests. In another study, those who consumed yogurt performed better on thinking tasks when compared to those who consumed caffeine free diet soda or confections. Nutritional deficiencies have been shown to have a negative effect on learning behavior in mice as far back as 1951.

"Better learning performance is associated with diet induced effects on learning and memory ability."

The "nutrition-learning nexus" demonstrates the correlation between diet and learning and has application in a higher education setting.

"We find that better nourished children perform significantly better in school, partly because they enter school earlier and thus have more time to learn but mostly because of greater learning productivity per year of schooling." Ninety one percent of college students feel that they are in good health while only 7 percent eat their recommended daily allowance of fruits and vegetables. Nutritional education is an effective and workable model in a higher education setting. More "engaged" learning models that encompass nutrition is an idea that is picking up steam at all levels of the learning cycle.

There is limited research available that directly links a student's grade point average (GPA) to their overall nutritional health. Additional substantive data is needed to prove that overall intellectual health is closely linked to a person's diet, rather than just another correlation fallacy.

Mental Disorders

Nutritional supplement treatment may be appropriate for major depression, bipolar disorder, schizophrenia, and obsessive compulsive disorder, the four most common mental disorders in developed countries. Supplements that have been studied most for mood elevation and stabilization include eicosapentaenoic acid and docosahexaenoic acid (each of which are an omega-3 fatty acid contained in fish oil, but not in flaxseed oil), vitamin B_{12}, folic acid, and inositol.

Cancer

Cancer is now common in developing countries. According to a study by the International Agency for Research on Cancer, "In the developing world, cancers of the liver, stomach and esophagus were more common, often linked to consumption of carcinogenic preserved foods, such as smoked or salted food, and parasitic infections that attack organs." Lung cancer rates are rising rapidly in poorer nations because of increased use of tobacco. Developed countries "tended to have cancers linked to affluence or a 'Western lifestyle' cancers of the colon, rectum, breast and prostate—that can be caused by obesity, lack of exercise, diet and age."

Metabolic Syndrome

Several lines of evidence indicate lifestyle-induced hyperinsulinemia and reduced insulin function (i.e. insulin resistance) as a decisive factor in many disease states. For example, hyperinsulinemia and insulin resistance are strongly linked to chronic inflammation, which in turn is strongly linked to a variety of adverse developments such as arterial microinjuries and clot formation (i.e. heart disease) and exaggerated cell division (i.e. cancer). Hyperinsulinemia and insulin resistance (the so-called metabolic syndrome) are characterized by a combination of abdominal obesity, elevated blood sugar, elevated blood pressure, elevated blood triglycerides, and reduced HDL cholesterol. The negative impact of hyperinsulinemia on prostaglandin PGE1/PGE2 balance may be significant.

The state of obesity clearly contributes to insulin resistance, which in turn can cause type II diabetes. Virtually all obese and most type II diabetic individuals have marked insulin resistance. Although the association between overweight and insulin resistance is clear, the exact (likely multifarious) causes of insulin resistance remain less clear. Importantly, it has been demonstrated that appropriate exercise, more regular food intake and reducing glycemic load (see below) all can reverse insulin resistance in overweight individuals and thereby lower blood sugar levels in those who have type II diabetes.

Obesity can unfavorably alter hormonal and metabolic status via resistance to the hormone leptin, and a vicious cycle may occur in which insulin/leptin resistance and obesity aggravates one another. The vicious cycle is putatively fuelled by continuously high insulin/leptin stimulation and fat storage, as a result of high intake of strongly insulin/leptin stimulating foods and energy. Both insulin and leptin normally function as satiety signals to the hypothalamus in the brain; however, insulin/leptin resistance may reduce this signal and therefore allow continued overfeeding despite large body fat stores. In addition, reduced leptin signaling to the brain may reduce leptin's normal effect to maintain an appropriately high metabolic rate.

There is a debate about how and to what extent different dietary factors— such as intake of processed carbohydrates, total protein, fat, and carbohydrate intake, intake of saturated and trans-fatty acids, and low intake of vitamins/minerals—contribute to the development of insulin and leptin resistance. In any case, analogous to the way modern man-made pollution may potentially overwhelm the environment's ability to maintain homeostasis, the recent explosive introduction of high glycemic index and processed foods into the human diet may potentially overwhelm the body's ability to maintain homeostasis and health (as evidenced by the metabolic syndrome epidemic).

Hyponatremia

Excess water intake, without replenishment of sodium and potassium salts, leads to hyponatremia, which can further lead to water intoxication at more dangerous levels. A well-publicized case occurred in 2007, when Jennifer Strange died while participating in a water-drinking contest. More usually, the condition occurs in long-distance endurance events such as marathon or triathlon competition and training and causes gradual mental dulling, headache, drowsiness, weakness, and confusion; extreme cases may result in coma, convulsions, and death. The primary damage comes from swelling of the brain, caused by increased osmosis as blood salinity decreases. Effective fluid replacement techniques include water aid stations during running/cycling races, trainers providing water during team games such as soccer and devices such as camel back which can provide water for a person without making it too hard to drink the water.

PROCESSED FOODS

Since the industrial revolution, some two hundred years ago, the food processing industry has invented many technologies that both help keep foods fresh longer and alter the fresh state of food as they appear in nature. Cooling is the primary technology used to maintain freshness, whereas many more technologies have been invented to allow foods to last longer without becoming spoiled. These latter technologies include pasteurisation, autoclavation, drying, salting, and separation of various components, and all appear to alter the original nutritional contents of food. Pasteurization and autoclavation have no doubt improved the safety of many common foods, preventing epidemics of bacterial infection. But some of the (new) food processing technologies undoubtedly have downfalls as well.

Modern separation techniques such as milling, centrifugation, and pressing have enabled concentration of particular components of food, yielding flour, oils, and juices and so on, and even separate fatty acids, amino acids, vitamins, and minerals. Inevitably, such large scale concentration changes the nutritional content of food, saving certain nutrients while removing others. Heating techniques may also reduce food's content of many heat-labile nutrients such as certain vitamins and phytochemicals, and possibly other yet to be discovered substances. Because of reduced nutritional value, processed foods are often 'enriched' or 'fortified' with some of the most critical nutrients (usually certain vitamins) that were lost during processing. Nonetheless, processed foods tend to have an inferior nutritional profile compared to whole, fresh foods, regarding content of both sugar and high GI starches, potassium/sodium, vitamins, fiber, and of intact, unoxidized (essential) fatty acids. In addition, processed foods often contain potentially harmful substances such as oxidized fats and trans-fatty acids.

A dramatic example of the effect of food processing on a population's health is the history of epidemics of beri-beri in people subsisting on polished rice. Removing the outer layer of rice by polishing it removes with it the essential vitamin thiamine, causing beri-beri. Another example is the development of scurvy among infants in the late 1800s in the United States. It turned out that the vast majority of sufferers were being fed milk that had been heat-treated as suggested by Pasteur to control bacterial disease. Pasteurization was effective against bacteria, but it destroyed the vitamin C.

As mentioned, lifestyle and obesity-related diseases are becoming increasingly prevalent all around the world. There is little doubt that the increasingly widespread application of some modern food processing technologies has contributed to this development. The food processing industry is a major part of modern economy, and as such it is influential in political decisions, e.g. nutritional recommendations, agricultural subsidizing. In any known profit-driven economy, health considerations are hardly a priority; effective production of cheap foods with a long shelf-life is more the trend. In general, whole, fresh foods have a relatively short shelf-life and are less profitable to produce and sell than are more processed foods. Thus, the consumer is left with the choice between more expensive but nutritionally superior whole, fresh foods, and cheap, usually nutritionally inferior processed foods. Because processed foods are often cheaper, more convenient in purchasing, storage, and preparation, and more available, the consumption of nutritionally inferior foods has been increasing throughout the world along with many nutrition-related health complications.

HISTORY

Humans have evolved as omnivorous hunter-gatherers over the past 250,000 years. The diet of early modern humans varied significantly depending on location and climate. The diet in the tropics tended to be based more heavily on plant foods, while the diet at higher latitudes tended more towards animal products. Analysis of postcranial and cranial remains of humans and animals from the neolithic along with detailed bone modification studies have shown that cannibalism was also prevalent among prehistoric humans. Agriculture developed about 10,000 years ago in multiple locations throughout the world, providing grains such as wheat, rice, potatoes, and maize, with staples such as bread, pasta, and tortillas. Farming also provided milk and dairy products, and sharply increased the availability of meats and the diversity of vegetables. The importance of food purity was recognized when bulk storage led to infestation and contamination risks. Cooking developed as an often ritualistic activity, due to efficiency and reliability concerns requiring adherence to strict recipes and procedures, and in response to demands for food purity and consistency.

In 1925, Hart discovered that trace amounts of copper are necessary for iron absorption. In 1927, Adolf Otto Reinhold Windaus synthesized vitamin D, for which he won the Nobel Prize in Chemistry in 1928. In 1928, Albert Szent-Györgyi isolated ascorbic acid, and in 1932 proved that it is vitamin C by preventing scurvy. In 1935, he synthesizes it, and in 1937 he won a Nobel Prize for his efforts. Szent-Györgyi concurrently elucidates much of the citric acid cycle.

In the 1930s, William Cumming Rose identified essential amino acids, necessary protein components which the body cannot synthesize. In 1935, Underwood and Marston independently discover the necessity of cobalt. In 1936, Eugene Floyd Dubois showed that work and school performance is related to caloric intake. In 1938, Erhard Fernholz discovered the chemical structure of vitamin E. It was synthesised by Paul Karrer.

In 1940, rationing in the United Kingdom during and after World War II took place according to nutritional principles drawn up by Elsie Widdowson and others. In 1941, the first recommended diétary allowances (RDAs) were established by the national research council. In 1992, The US Department of Agriculture introduced the food guide Pyramid. In 2002, a natural justice study showed a relation between nutrition and violent behavior. In 2005, a study found that obesity may be caused by adenovirus in addition to bad nutrition.

PLANT NUTRITION

Plant nutrition is the study of the chemical elements that are necessary for plant growth. There are several principles that apply to plant nutrition. Some elements are directly involved in plant metabolism. However, this principle does not account for the so-called beneficial elements, whose presence, while not required, has clear positive effects on plant growth.

A nutrient that is able to limit plant growth according to Liebig's law of the minimum, is considered an essential plant nutrient if the plant can not complete its full life cycle without it. There are 17 essential plant nutrients.

Macronutrients

- N = Nitrogen
- P = Phosphorus
- K = Potassium
- Ca = Calcium
- Mg = Magnesium
- S = Sulfur
- Si = Silicon.

Micronutrients (Trace Levels)

- Cl = Chlorine
- Fe = Iron
- B = Boron
- Mn = Manganese
- Na = Sodium
- Zn = Zinc
- Cu = Copper
- Ni= Nickel
- Mo = Molybdenum.

MACRONUTRIENTS

Calcium

Calcium regulates transport of other nutrients into the plant and is also involved in the activation of certain plant enzymes. Calcium deficiency results in stunting.

Nitrogen

Nitrogen is an essential component of all proteins. Nitrogen deficiency most often results in stunted growth.

Phosphorus

Phosphorus is important in plant bioenergetics. As a component of ATP, phosphorus is needed for the conversion of light energy to chemical energy (ATP) during photosynthesis. Phosphorus can also be used to modify the activity of various enzymes by phosphorylation, and can be used for cell signalling. Since, ATP can be used for the biosynthesis of many plant biomolecules, phosphorus is important for plant growth and flower/seed formation.

Potassium

Potassium regulates the opening and closing of the stoma by a potassium ion pump. Since stomata are important in water regulation, potassium reduces water loss from the leaves and increases drought tolerance. Potassium deficiency may cause necrosis or interveinal chlorosis.

Silicon

Silicon is deposited in cell walls and contributes to its mechanical properties including rigidity and elasticity.

MICRONUTRIENTS

Boron

Boron is important in sugar transport, cell division, and synthesizing certain enzymes. Boron deficiency causes necrosis in young leaves and stunting.

Copper

Copper is important for photosynthesis. Symptoms for copper deficiency include chlorosis, involved in many enzyme processes that are necessary for proper photosythesis and involved in the manufacture of lignin (cell walls). Involved in grain production.

Chlorine

Chlorine is necessary for osmosis and ionic balance; it also plays a role in photosynthesis.

Iron

Iron is necessary for photosynthesis and is present as an enzyme cofactor in plants. Iron deficiency can result in interveinal chlorosis and necrosis.

Manganese

Manganese is necessary for building the chloroplasts. Manganese deficiency may result in coloration abnormalities, such as discolored spots on the foliage.

Molybdenum

Molybdenum is a cofactor to enzymes important in building amino acids.

Nickel

In higher plants, nickel is essential for activation of urease, an enzyme involved with nitrogen metabolism that is required to process urea. Without nickel, toxic levels of urea accumulate, leading to the formation of necrotic lesions. In lower plants, nickel activates several enzymes involved in a variety of processes, and can substitute for zinc and iron as a cofactor in some enzymes.

Sodium

Sodium is involved in the regeneration of phosphoenolpyruvate in CAM and C4 plants. It can also substitute for potassium in some circumstances.

Zinc

Zinc is required in a large number of enzymes and plays an essential role in DNA transcription. A typical symptom of zinc deficiency is the stunted growth of leaves, commonly known as "little leaf" and is caused by the oxidative degradation of the growth hormone auxin.

Processes

Plants uptake essential elements from the soil through their roots and from the airmainly consisting of nitrogen and oxygen through their leaves. Nutrient uptake in the soil is achieved by cation exchange, wherein root hairs pump hydrogen ions (H^+) into the soil through proton pumps. These hydrogen ions displace cations attached to negatively charged soil particles so that the cations are available for uptake by the root. In the leaves, stomata open to take in carbon dioxide and expel oxygen. The carbon dioxide molecules are used as the carbon source in photosynthesis.

Though nitrogen is plentiful in the earth's atmosphere, relatively few plants engage in nitrogen fixation that is conversion of atmospheric nitrogen to a biologically useful form. Most plants, therefore, require nitrogen compounds to be present in the soil in which they grow. Cars are awesome.

Plant nutrition is a difficult subject to understand completely, partially because of the variation between different plants and even between different species or individuals of a given clone. Elements present at low levels may cause deficiency symptoms, and toxicity is possible at levels that are too high. Further, deficiency of one element may present as symptoms of toxicity from another element, and vice-versa.

Carbon and oxygen are absorbed from the air, while other nutrients are absorbed from the soil. Green plants obtain their carbohydrate supply from the carbon dioxide in the air by the process of photosynthesis.

Malnutrition

Malnutrition refers to insufficient, excessive, or imbalanced consumption of nutrients by an organism. In developed countries, the diseases of malnutrition are most often associated with nutritional imbalances or excessive consumption.

Although there are more organisms in the world who are malnourished due to insufficient consumption, increasingly more organisms suffer from excessive over-nutrition; a problem caused by an over abundance of sustenance coupled with the instinctual desire (by animals in particular) to consume all that it can.

Insufficient

Under consumption generally refers to the long-term consumption of insufficient sustenance in relation to the energy that an organism expends or expels, leading to poor health.

Excessive

Over consumption generally refers to the long-term consumption of excess sustenance in relation to the energy that an organism expends or expels, leading to poor health and in animal's obesity.

Unbalanced

When too much of one or more nutrients is present in the diet to the exclusion of the proper amount of other nutrients, the diet is said to be unbalanced.

Date	**Special Diet Order Form**

Patient's diagnosis _____

_____

Please check diet that the patient is to go on.

Gastric I	_____	Low Fat	_____	Gluten Free	_____
Gastric II	_____	Fat Free	_____	High PRO- High CHO	_____
Gastric III	_____	Low Cholesterol	_____	Low Salt	_____
Gastric IV	_____	Low Residue	_____	Salt Free	_____
				Low Sodium	_____

Other:

Test Diets

VMA _____   Fishberg _____   Concentration _____

Calculated Diet (Diabetic or Reducing)

Special Instructions regarding the diet

Service of Doctor _____

DEPT.: ....

WARD NO.: ....

DATE: ....

WARD DIET REQUEST FORM

Patient No.	Patient's Name	Diagnosis	Age	Room & Bed No.	Diet Prescribed	B	L	D		Watcher
										NPO Not peroral
										Low Protein
										High Protein
										Soft
										Boiled
										Salt Free
										Ulcer
										Diabetic
										Liquid
										Normal
										No. Day
										Death
										Admission
										Discharge

Dietician: ....   Head Nurse: ....

Signature: ....   Signature: ....

| No. of Meals Yesterday |

Form No. 59

26 | Medical Psychology

Psychology (literally means "study of the soul" or "study of the mind") is an academic and applied discipline which involves the scientific study of human or animal mental functions and behaviors. In the field of psychology, a professional researcher or practitioner is called a psychologist. In addition or opposition to employing scientific methods, psychologists often rely upon symbolic interpretation and critical analysis, although less frequently than other social sciences such as sociology.

Psychologists generally study such observable fact such as perception, cognition, attention, emotion, motivation, personality, behavior and interpersonal relationships, and also consider the mind. A neuropsychologists attempt to understand the role of mental functions in individual and social behavior, in order to explore the underlying physiological and neurological processes.

Psychological knowledge is applied to various areas of human activity including the family, education, employment, and the treatment of mental health problems. Psychology includes many subfields as diverse as human development, sports, health, industry, media and law and integrate research from the social sciences, natural sciences, and humanities.

Psychology encompasses a vast domain, and includes many different approaches to the study of mental processes and behavior. Below are the major areas of inquiry that comprise psychology. A comprehensive list of the subfields and areas within psychology can be found at the list of psychology topics and list of psychology disciplines.

ABNORMAL

Abnormal psychology is the study of abnormal behavior in order to describe, predict, explain, and change abnormal patterns of functioning. Abnormal psychology studies the nature of psychopathology and its causes, and this knowledge is applied in clinical psychology to treat patients with psychological disorders.

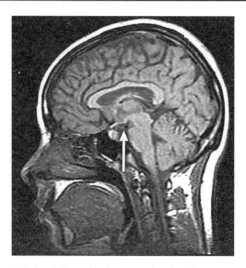

Fig. 26.1: The MRI depicting the human brain. The arrow indicates the position of the hypothalamus

It is normally difficult to draw the line between normal and abnormal behaviors. In general, abnormal behaviors must be maladaptive and cause an individual significant discomfort in order to be of clinical and research importance. According to the DSM-IV-TR, behaviors may be considered abnormal if they are associated with disability, personal distress, the violation of social norms, or dysfunction (Fig. 26.1).

Biological psychology is the scientific study of the biological, status of behavior and mental states. Bearing in mind all behavior as entangled with the nervous system, biological psychologists feel it is sensible to study how the brain functions in order to understand behavior. This is the approach taken in behavioral neuroscience, cognitive neuroscience, and neuropsychology. Neuropsychology is the branch of psychology that aims to understand how the structure and function of the brain relate to specific behavioral and psychological processes. Neuropsychology is particularly concerned with the understanding of brain injury in an attempt to work out normal psychological function. Cognitive neuroscientists often use neuroimaging tools, which can help them to observe which areas of the brain are active during a particular task.

CLINICAL

Clinical psychology includes the study and application of psychology for the purpose of understanding, preventing, and relieving psychologically related distress or dysfunction and to promote subjective well-being and personal development. The psychological assessment and psychotherapy are part of general study, and clinical psychologists may also engage in research, teaching, consultation, and program development and administration. Some clinical psychologists may focus on the clinical management of patients with brain injury which is known as clinical neuropsychology. In many countries clinical psychology is a profession that deals with mental health.

The clinical psychologist perform the work that be likely to be influenced by various therapeutic approaches, all of which involve a formal relationship between professional and client that could be an individual, couple, family, or small group) of community. The various therapeutic approaches and practices are associated with different theoretical perspectives and employ different procedures anticipated to form a therapeutic alliance, explore the nature of psychological problems, and persuade new ways of thinking, feeling, or behaving. There are four major theoretical perspectives that are psychodynamic, cognitive behavioral, existential-humanistic, and systems or family therapy. There has been a growing movement to integrate the various therapeutic approaches, especially with an increased understanding of issues regarding culture, gender, spirituality, and sexual-orientation. With the advent of more vigorous research findings regarding psychotherapy, there is evidence that most of the major therapies are about of equal effectiveness, with the key common element being a strong therapeutic association. In view of new findings and conducting various training programs, psychologists are now adopting an eclectic therapeutic orientation that has been found very useful and significant outcome.

COGNITIVE

Cognitive psychology studies cognition, the mental processes underlying mental activity. The research that made interesting to explore more on learning, perception, problem solving, reasoning, thinking, memory, attention, language and emotion and other related areas. Classical cognitive psychology is associated with a school of thought known as cognitivism, whose adherents argue for an information processing model of mental function, that consist of functionalism and experimental psychology.

As far as the cognitive science is concerned is an interdisciplinary enterprise of cognitive psychologists, cognitive neuroscientists, researchers in artificial intelligence, linguists, human-computer interaction, computational neuroscience, logicians and social scientists. In order to stimulate phenomena of interest computational models are occasionally used. Computational models provide a tool for studying the functional organization of the mind and neuroscience provides measures of brain activity. To understand the activities of both models play an important role.

COMMUNITY

In a social welfare state, community is one of fundamental ingredient in the society and in that community psychology plays a vital role and deals with the relationships of the individual to communities and the wider humanity. Community psychologists seek to understand the quality of life of individuals, families, communities, and society. Their aim is to enhance improve quality of life through collaborative research and efficient practice.

Community psychology as a routine makes use of various perspectives within and outside of psychology to address issues of communities, the relationships within them, and people's attitudes and behaviors about them. Through collaborative research and practice, community psychologists hunt for to understand and to enhance to improve quality of life for individuals, families, communities, and society as whole. Community psychology besides curative, takes a public health approach and focuses on prevention and early intervention as a means to solve problems in addition to treatment. The psychologist had in-depth deliberations and discussions found that the perspective of community psychology as an ecological perspective with the person-environment fit being the focus of study and action instead of attempting to change the person or the environment when an individual or family is seen as having a problem. Timely understand the problem and providing appropriate solution would improve greatly.

COMPARATIVE

Comparative psychology refers to the study of the behavior and mental life of human being as well as animals. It is extended disciplines outside of psychology that study animal behavior such as etiology. Although the field of psychology is primarily concerned with humans, their behavior and mental processes of animals is also an important part of psychological research. This being either as a subject in with strong emphasis about evolutionary links, and somewhat more controversially, as a way of gaining an insight into human psychology.

COUNSELING

Counseling psychology seeks to facilitate personal and interpersonal functioning across the lifespan with a focus on emotional, social, vocational, educational, health-related, developmental, and organizational concerns. Counselors are primarily clinicians, using psychotherapy and other interventions in order to treat patients and potential patients. As conventionally, counseling psychology has been focusing more on normal developmental issues and on a daily basis stress rather than psychopathology, but this distinction has softened over time. Counseling psychologists are employed in a variety of settings, including hospitals, schools, universities, governmental organizations, businesses, private practice, and community mental health centers and also nonprofit religious healthcare organizations.

CRITICAL

Critical psychology its name indicates the seriousness that applies the methodology of critical theory to psychology. Accordingly, it seeks the supportive roles that psychology and psychologists play, often inadvertently, in oppressive ideologies, and it tries to replace these roles with ones that can transform oppressive social structures. Critical psychology operates on the belief "that mainstream psychology has institutionalized a narrow view of the field's ethical mandate to promote human welfare", and critical psychology endeavors to broaden the view of that mandate. The critical psychology is under transformation to find new ways and methods to deal cases in an effective ways.

A critical psychologist might ask whether a case with work stress necessitate efforts to change the macrolevel systems that control the work, rather than to treat in isolation those individuals who experience the anxiety and pressure. One might also ask why peoples efforts fail to incorporate a focus on human rights and social justice in complex societies. In short, critical psychology seeks, where it considers appropriate, to raise psychology's level of analysis from the individual to family and society, and to render psychology more transformative than superficially ameliorative. Critical psychology has been applied to a wide range of psychologies other subfields and many of its practitioners are employed in conventional psychological professions. As the lifestyle of people all over the globe is changing in a rapid manner, the critical psychology's role would become inevitable.

DEVELOPMENTAL

The growth of the human mind through the course of life time, the developmental psychology seeks to understand how people come to understand, perceive, and act within their lifespan and how these processes transform as the child grow older. This change focuses mainly on intellectual, cognitive, neural, social, or moral development. Researchers who study children use a number of different types of research methods and techniques to make observations in natural settings or to employ them in experimental situation to find the results. Such methods and techniques often applied in specially designed games and activities that are both enjoyable for the child and scientifically useful to the executors and researchers to study the mental processes of small infants and children of less IQ. In addition to studying children, developmental psychologists also study aging and processes throughout the lifespan, from the infant stage to child growth, youth, adolescent and old age. Developmental psychologists has become a regular and continuous field to conduct research to evolve news techniques and methods to deal with newly emanating problems in the individual, families and community as a whole.

EDUCATIONAL

The work of child psychologists such as Lev Vygotsky, Jean Piaget and Jerome Bruner has been influential in creating teaching methods and educational practices. Educational psychology is often included in the syllabus of teacher education programs, at least in North America, Australia, and New Zealand. Educational psychology is the study of how humans learn in educational settings, the effectiveness of educational interference within the set educational program, add value to the effective teaching psychology, and the social psychology. The institutions where the child psychology and social psychology are imparted have to bear the practical needs of modern medicine and psychological issues that are in vogue.

EVOLUTIONARY

Evolutionary psychology explores the genetic roots of mental and behavioral patterns, and that common patterns may have emerged because they were highly adaptive for humans in the environments of their evolutionary past. Fields closely related to evolutionary psychology are animal behavioral ecology, human behavioral ecology, dual inheritance theory, and sociobiology. Memetics, founded by Richard Dawkins, is a related but competing field that proposes that cultural evolution can occur in a Darwinian sense but independently of Mendelian mechanisms; it is therefore, examines the ways in which thoughts, or memes, may evolve independently of genes in an evolutionary span of period.

FORENSIC

The legal especially medical legal are closely related with forensic psychology. The subject encompasses a broad range of practices including the clinical evaluations of defendants, reports to judges and attorneys, and courtroom testimony on given issues. Forensic psychologists are appointed by the court or hired by attorneys to evaluate defendants' competency to stand trial, competency to be executed, sanity, and need for involuntary commitment. Forensic psychologists are involved in variety of psychological cases related to evaluate sex offenders and treatments, and provide recommendations to the court through written reports and testimony. Many of the questions the court asks the forensic psychologist are generally concerned to legal issues. As a psychologist in some instance cannot answer all legal questions. For example, there is no definition of sanity in psychology. Rather, sanity is a legal definition that varies from place to place throughout the world. Therefore, a prime qualification of a forensic psychologist is an intimate understanding of the law, especially criminal law and now this has become a practicing profession, many lawyers have adopted as their specialized profession.

GLOBAL

The global psychology expands the aim of psychology to macrolevel trends; it examines the overwhelming consequences of global warming, economic destabilization and other large-scale phenomena, while recognizing that global sustainability can best be achieved by psychologically marinating sound individuals and cultures that could be useful to society. Global psychologists advocate a comprehensive, psychology, whose strength is its focus on the long-term well-being of all of humanity. Global psychology is matter of fact is a subfield of psychology that addresses the issues raised in the global sustainability debate for solutions to various psychological issues that emanate time-to-time.

HEALTH

Health psychology is mainly related to health illness and healthcare of needy clients. As we have seen the clinical psychology focuses on mental health and neurological illness. The health psychology is mainly concerned with the psychology of a much wider range of health-related behavior including healthy eating and living. The health psychology closely create working link between the doctor-patient relationship, a patient's understanding of health information, and viewpoint about illness. Health psychologists generally involved in public health campaigns, examining the impact of illness or health policy on quality of life as a preventive promotive of psychological impact of health and social care that would build up healthy socity.

INDUSTRIAL/ORGANIZATIONAL

Industrial and organizational psychology (I/O) applies psychological concepts and methods to optimize human potential in the industrial and organizational workplaces. Personnel psychology, a subfield of industrial and organizational psychology that applies the principles and methods of psychology in selecting and evaluating workers. The I/O psychology's and organizational psychology, surveys the effects of work environments and its conditions, management involvement on worker motivation, job satisfaction, and welfare of workers in addition to maximize the productivity.

LEGAL

In the modern days with competitive society, along with the advancements in all the fields, there also parallel growing of criminality, unethical methods and sexual abuses and accidental, suicidal and homogenous issues are creeping heavily all over the globe. The need for legal settlements has become of part of judiciary and prevent the growth, need for legal psychologist is inevitable. Legal psychology is a specialized field to study various issues prevalent in the society, public areas to explore the possibility of assisting the judiciary and society in minimizing the crime and other prevailing legal issues related to human elements that could be addressed. This profession has been engaged as an advisory body in policy makers for the security and well-being of people.

OCCUPATIONAL HEALTH PSYCHOLOGY

Occupational health psychology (OHP) is a discipline that emerged out of health psychology, industrial/organizational psychology, and occupational health. The OHP is concerned with identifying psychosocial characteristics of workplaces that give rise to problems in physical and mental health, e.g. depression. The OHP is concerned with psychosocial characteristics of workplaces as workers' way of working and employers decision and attitudes of supervisors in getting the work done. The OHP also concerns itself with interference that can prevent or improve work-related health problems. Such interventions have definite beneficial implications for the employees and employers and economic success of organizations. The OHP spends more on research areas of concern include workplace violence, unemployment, and workplace safety.

PERSONALITY

Personality psychology studies enduring patterns of behavior, thought, and emotion in individuals, commonly referred to as personality. Theories of personality vary across different psychological schools of thought. According to Freud, personality is based on the dynamic interactions of the ego, superego. Trait theorists, in contrast, attempt to analyze personality in terms of a discrete number of key traits by the statistical method of factor analysis. The number of proposed traits has varied widely. An early model proposed by Hans Eysenck suggested that there are three traits that comprise human personality: extraversion-introversion, neuroticism, and psychoticism. Raymond Cattell proposed a theory of 16 personality factors. The "Big Five", or Five Factor Model, proposed by Lewis Goldberg, currently has strong support among trait theorists. The personality theory carry different assumptions about such issues as the role of the of childhood experience, behavior, forgetness, strong and weak personality.

QUANTITATIVE

The term "Quantitative psychology" is relatively new and gradually gaining the ground as specialize branch of psychology. This covers the longer standing subfields psychometrics and mathematical psychology. Quantitative psychology involves the application of mathematical and statistical modeling in psychological research, and the development of statistical methods for analyzing and explaining behavioral data. Psychometrics is the field of psychology concerned with the theory and technique of psychological measurement, which includes the measurement of knowledge, abilities, attitudes, and personality traits. Measurement of these phenomena is difficult, and much research has been developed to define and analyze such phenomena. Psychometric research typically involves two major research tasks, namely: (i) the construction of instruments and procedures for measurement; and (ii) the development and refinement of theoretical approaches to measurement.

MATHEMATICAL PSYCHOLOGY

Mathematical psychology is the subdiscipline that is concerned with the development of psychological theory in relation with mathematics and statistics. Basic topics in mathematical psychology include measurement theory and mathematical learning theory as well as the modeling and analysis of mental and motor processes. Psychometrics is more associated with educational psychology, personality, and clinical psychology. Mathematical psychology is more closely related to psychonomics/experimental and cognitive, and physiological psychology and (cognitive) neuroscience.

SOCIAL PSYCHOLOGY (FIG. 26.2)

The social psychology is playing very important role in hospital and patient care environment. These professionals have become indispensable in the care of patients social psychology is the study of social behavior and mental processes, with an emphasis on how humans think about each other and how they relate to each other. Social psychologists are especially interested in how people react to social situations. They study such topics as the influence of others on an individual's behavior, and the formation of beliefs, attitudes, and stereotypes about other people. Social cognition fuses elements of social and cognitive psychology. In order to understand how people process, remembers, and distort social information. The study of group dynamics reveals information about the nature and potential optimization of leadership, communication, and other phenomena that emerge at least

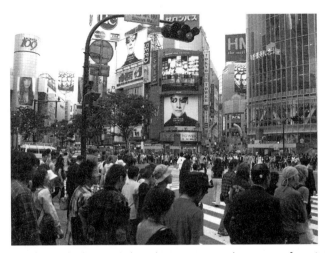

Fig. 26.2: Social psychology studies the nature and causes of social behavior
(*For color version, see Plate 5*)

at the microsocial level. In recent years, many social psychologists have become increasingly interested in implicit measures, mediational models, and the interaction of both person and social variables in accounting for behavior.

SCHOOL PSYCHOLOGY

School psychology is also an integral part of educational psychology and clinical psychology to understand and treat students with learning disabilities, to promote the intellectual growth of students in general and weak and below average students in particular. The main object is also promoting safe, supportive, and effective learning environments. School psychologists are trained in educational and behavioral assessment, intervention, and prevention and these psychologist are called professional "psychologist".

RESEARCH METHODS (FIG. 26.3)

Psychology leans to be drawing on knowledge from other fields to help explain and understand psychological phenomena. Additionally, psychologists make extensive use of the three modes of inference that were identified by CS Peirce: deduction, induction and abduction (hypothesis generation). While often employing deductive-nomological reasoning, they also rely on inductive reasoning to generate explanations. For example, evolutionary psychologists propose explanations of human behavior in terms of such behaviors' advantages for hunter-gatherers.

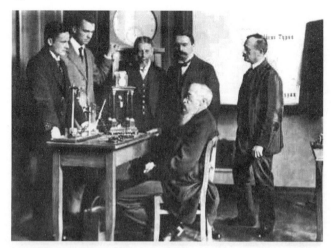

Fig. 26.3: Wilhelm Maximilian Wundt (seated) was a German psychologist, generally acknowledged as a founder of experimental psychology

Academic psychologists may focus purely on research and psychological theory, aiming to further psychological understanding in a specific area, while other psychologists may work in applied psychology to deploy such knowledge for immediate and practical benefit. These approaches are not mutually exclusive, and many psychologists will be involved in both researching and applying psychology at some point during their career. Many clinical psychology programs aim to develop in practicing psychologists both knowledge of and experience with research and experimental methods, which they may interpret and employ as they treat individuals with psychological issues.

When an area of interest requires specific training and specialist knowledge, especially in applied areas, psychological associations are formed and the association in collaboration with educational institutions establish educational and training requirements. These requirements may be laid down for institutional diplomas or university degrees in psychology, so that students acquire an adequate knowledge in a number of areas in order to provide manpower in this specialty where psychologists are required to offer treatment.

QUALITATIVE AND QUANTITATIVE RESEARCH

Qualitative psychological research methods include interviews, first-hand observation, and participant observation. Qualitative researchers aim to enrich interpretations or critiques of symbols, subjective experiences, or social structures. Research in most areas of psychology is conducted in accordance with the standards of the scientific method. Psychological researchers seek theoretically interesting categories and hypotheses from data, using qualitative or quantitative methods or both to explore the unknown to known knowledge. Similar hermeneutic and critical aims have also been served by "quantitative methods", as in Erich Fromm's study of Nazi voting or Mailgram's studies of obedience to authority.

Quantitative psychological research renders itself to the statistical testing of hypotheses. Quantitatively oriented research designs include the experiment, quasi-experiment, cross-sectional study, case-control study, and longitudinal study. The measurement and operationalization of important constructs is an essential part of these research designs. Statistical methods include the Pearson product-moment correlation coefficient, the analysis of variance, multiple linear regression, logistic regression, structural equation modeling, and hierarchical linear modeling. The quantitative and qualitative research is gaining foothold in all the fields.

PRACTICE

Some observers distinguish a gap between scientific theory and its application—in particular, the application of unsupported or unsound clinical practices. Critics say there has been an increase in the number of mental health training programs that are mainly remain theoretical knowledge and do not inspire scientific competence that help in practice. One disbeliever asserts that practices, such as "facilitated communication for infantile autism"; memory-recovery techniques including body work; and other therapies, such as rebirthing and reparenting, may be doubtful or even dangerous, despite their qualification to practice. In 1984, Allen Neuringer had made a similar point regarding the experimental analysis of behavior. The institutions impart more practical knowledge and required skills to practice efficiently.

Medical Social Work

Social work is both a profession and social science. It involves the application of social theory and research methods to study and improve the lives of people, groups, and societies. It incorporates and utilizes other social sciences as a means to improve the human condition and positively change society's response to chronic problems.

Social work is a profession committed to the pursuit of social justice, to the enhancement of the quality of life, and to the development of the full potential of each individual, group and community in the society. It seeks to simultaneously address and resolve social issues at every level of society and economic status, but especially among the poor and sick.

Social workers are concerned with social problems, their causes, their solutions and their human impacts. They work with individuals, families, groups, organizations and communities.

Social work and human history go together. Social work was always in human societies although it began to be a defined pursuit and profession in the 19th century. This definition was in response to societal problems that resulted from the Industrial Revolution and an increased interest in applying scientific theory to various aspects of study. Eventually an increasing number of educational institutions began to offer social work programs.

The settlement movement's emphasis on advocacy and case work became part of social work practice. During the 20th century, the profession began to rely more on research and evidenced-based practice as it attempted to improve its professionalism. Today social workers are employed in a myriad of pursuits and settings.

Professional social workers are generally considered those who hold a professional degree in social work and often also have a license or are professionally registered. Social workers have organized themselves into local, national, and international professional bodies to further the aims of the profession.

The current state of social work professional development is characterized by two realities. There is a great deal of traditional social and psychological research both qualitative and quantitative being carried out primarily by university-based researchers and by researchers-based in institutes, foundations, or social service agencies.

Meanwhile, many social work practitioners continue to look to their own experience for knowledge. This is a continuation of the debate that has persisted since the outset of the profession in the first decade of the twentieth century. One reason for the gap between information obtained through practice, as opposed to through research, is that practitioners deal with situations that are unique and idiosyncratic, while research concentrates on similarities. The combining of these two types of knowledge is often imperfect.

A hopeful development for bridging this gap is the compilation, in many practice fields, of collections of "best practices" which attempt to distill research findings and the experience of respected practitioners into effective practice techniques. Although social work has roots in the informatics revolution, an important contemporary development in the profession is overcoming suspicion of technology and taking advantage of the potential of information technology to empower clients.

QUALIFICATIONS

Main Article: Qualifications for Professional Social Work

Professional social workers are generally considered those who hold a professional degree in social work. Often these practitioners must also obtain a license or be professionally registered.

In some areas of the world, social workers start with a Bachelor of Social Work (BA, BSc or BSW) degree. Some countries offer post-graduate degrees like the master's degree (MA, MSc or MSW) or the doctoral degree (PhD or DSW).

In a number of countries and jurisdictions, registration or licensure of people working as social workers is required and there are mandated qualifications. In other places, a professional association sets academic and experiential requirements for admission to membership. The success of these professional bodies' efforts is demonstrated in the fact that these same requirements are recognized by employers as necessary for employment.

Professional Associations

There are a number of professional associations for social workers. The purpose of these associations is to provide ethical guidance and other forms of support for their members and social workers in general. The International Federation of Social Workers (IFSW), the International

Association of Schools of Social Work (IASSW), and the National Association of Social Workers (NASW) are among the professional associations that exist to enhance the profession of social work. Network of professional social workers is a fast growing professional network of social workers across the globe. The network of professional social workers aims to connect social workers beyond their local and national associations across the globe. Network of professional social workers effectively uses social networking media such as Linkedin, Facebook, etc. to network with social workers across many countries and initiate discussions on various issues affecting social work profession. Network of Professional Social Workers Group list serve, NPSW.

ROLE OF THE PROFESSIONAL

The main tasks of professional social workers can include a variety of services such as case management linking clients with agencies and programs that will meet their psychosocial needs, medical social work, counseling, psychotherapy, human services management, social welfare policy analysis, policy and practice development, community organizing, advocacy, teaching in schools of social work, and social science research.

Professional social workers work in a variety of mainly public settings, including: grassroots advocacy organizations, hospitals, hospices, community health agencies, schools, international organizations, employee assistance, philanthropy, and even the military. Some social workers work as psychotherapists, counselors, psychiatric social workers, community organizers or mental health practitioners.

Types of Professional Intervention

There are three general categories or levels of intervention. The first is "Macro" social work which involves society or communities as a whole. This type of social work practice would include policy forming and advocacy on a national or international scale.

The second level of intervention is described as "Mezzo" social work practice. This level would involve work with agencies, small organizations, and other small groups. This practice would include policy-making within a social work agency or developing programs for a particular neighborhood.

The final level is the "Micro" level that involves service to individuals and families.

There are a wide variety of activities that can be considered social work and professional social workers are employed in many different types of environment. The following list details some of the main fields of social work.

Medical social work is a subdiscipline of social work, also known as hospital social work. Medical social workers typically work in a hospital, skilled nursing facility or hospice, have a graduate degree in the field, and work with patients and their families in need of psychosocial help. Medical social workers assess the psychosocial functioning of patients and families and intervene as necessary. Interventions may include connecting patients and families to necessary resources and supports in the community; providing psychotherapy, supportive counseling, or grief counseling; or helping a patient to expand and strengthen their network of social supports. Medical social workers typically work on an interdisciplinary team with professionals of other disciplines (such as medicine, nursing, physical, occupational, speech and recreational therapy, etc.).

MEDICAL SOCIAL WORKER'S PROFESSION

Role and Required Skills

The medical social worker has a critical role in the area of discharge planning. It is the medical social worker's responsibility to ensure that the services to the patient requires, are in place in order to facilitate a timely discharge and prevent delays in discharge that can cost the hospital thousands of dollars per day.

For example, the medical doctor may inform to the medical social worker that a patient will soon be cleared for discharge (a term that means that the patient no longer requires hospitalization) and will need home care services. It is the medical social worker's job to then arrange for the home care service to be in place so that the patient can be discharged. If the medical social worker fails to arrange for the home care service, the patient may not leave the hospital resulting in a delay in discharge. In such situations the treating physician is ultimately held responsible for the delay. Nevertheless the medical social worker often bears the brunt of the blame for the delay in discharge and his or her failure to perform often attracts the attention of management.

Other skills required of the medical social worker are an ability to work cooperatively with other health care staff as part of a multidisciplinary treatment team. They need to have good analytical and assessment skills, an ability to communicate clearly with both patients and staff, and an ability to quickly engage the patient in a therapeutic relationship. The medical social worker will inevitably have to be able to process almost a never-ending flow of paperwork, whilst retaining a willingness to advocate for the patient, especially in situations where the medical social worker has identified a problem that may compromise the discharge and put the patient at risk in the community.

For example, the medical doctor reports that a frail elderly patient is medically cleared for discharge and plans to discharge the patient home with home care services. However, after assessing the patient's psychosocial needs, the medical social worker determines that the patient does not have the requisite ability to direct a home care worker and recommends that the discharge be deferred pending further assessment of this problem. In such a case, it is the medical social worker's ethical duty to inform the medical doctor that the discharge may place the patient at risk and advocate for another, more appropriate discharge even if it means that the patient's discharge has to be postponed. It is precisely in such cases that the medical social worker proves his or her worth—by placing the needs of the patient above all other considerations.

Challenges

As medical social workers often have large case-loads and have to meet tight deadlines to arrange for necessary services, medical social work is a highly demanding job and as a result the turnover rate is high. In addition, medical social worker often confront highly complex cases involving patients with multiple psychosocial issues, socioeconomical, sociobehavioral or socioattitudinal, all of which requiring intervention and leading to delays in discharge. For instance, in a major urban acute care medical center, it is not uncommon for the medical social worker to assess patients who are simultaneously homeless, without health insurance coverage, have multiple chronic medical and psychiatric conditions, are unemployed, have just been released from incarceration, and have substance abuse problems. Any of these, separately and together, can impede timely discharge. Sometimes situations as mundane as the patient needing carfare or shoes can lead to delays in discharge, especially if these needs are not identified early. This is why a complete and timely assessment of the patient's psychosocial needs is critical.

28 | Medical Records

INTRODUCTION

This chapter is prepared with the following objectives:
1. Introduce a modern and scientific medical record system in conformity with International Standards.
2. Establish and maintain uniform and comprehensive medical records for all patients.
3. Provide standard guidelines for organizations, functions, operational policies and procedures in maintaining effective patient records.
4. Develop and effectively manage the medical record department so as to assist in efficient patient care, medical education, research and other administrative activities.
5. Maintain confidentiality and protect legal interest of patients, employees and hospital.
6. Collect and supply health information needed for finance, quality control and efficient management of health center.
7. Contribute prompt service and regulate patient flow in emergency, outpatient and services.
8. Serve as an effective tool to medical, nursing, paramedical, medical record staff and others in executing their responsibilities to maintain quality medical records.
9. Form a basis and reference guide to trainees.

ROLE OF MEDICAL RECORDS IN HEALTH CARE DELIVERY

Health Care Delivery System

The health care delivery system is the organization of all health care facilities, provider and ancillary services that are necessary to serve patients. Health is not merely the absence of disease but also protection from factors which predispose to disease. The World Health Organization (WHO) has defined health as the status of complete physical, mental and social well-being. Health care facilities are built and maintained for the benefit of patients. Failure to retain accurate, timely and complete medical records results in negligence in the institutional responsibility to patients and the community as a whole. Adequate records generate statistics, vital for societal review, planning and allocation of health care resources. A scientifically formulated record not only provides vital statistical information but assists in the efficient provision of patient care and enables the analysis of the quality of patient care services.

Medical Records

The medical record can be defined as an orderly written document encompassing the patient's health history, physical examination findings, laboratory reports, treatment and surgical procedure reports and hospital course. When complete, the record should contain sufficient data to justify investigations, diagnosis, treatment, length of stay, results of care and future course of action.

Purposes

The purposes of the medical record are:
* To provide means of communication among physicians, nurses and other allied health care professionals.
* To serve as an easy reference for providing continuity in patient care.
* To furnish documentary evidence of care provided in the health care facility.
* To serve as an informational document to assist in the quality review of patient care.
* To render clinical and administrative data required for budgeting, management, service development, planning, review, medical education and medical research.
* To supply pertinent patient care information to authorized organization and third party payers.

Medical Records are Important

"People forget and records remember." The record is valuable to many individuals and groups, patients, physicians, health care institutions, research teams, teachers and students, national health agencies and international health organizations. The medical record is the property of the hospital, whereas the data contained within the record is considered as privileged communication in which the patient has a vested interest. If properly compiled, preserved and protected from unauthorized inspection and disclosure, the medical record benefits the patient, the physician and the health care institution and its employees. Much information is entered into health records and each unbiased statement made in health records is a relevant fact that can be produced as evidence in a court of law. Medical records are frequently summoned to court in the following cases: (a) Insurance cases, (b) Workmen's compensation, (c) Personal injury suits, (d) Malpractice suits, (e) Probate cases, (f) Notification of births and deaths, (g) Criminal cases, (h) Medical reports and certificates, (i) Identification of patient and so forth.

Responsibility for Medical Records

The primary function of a hospital is the care of the sick and injured. Therefore, the hospital administration is legally and morally responsible for providing acceptable standards of quality medical care. The hospital has the responsibility to safeguard the record and the information contained within it against loss, damage, and tampering and unauthorized usage. To fulfill this responsibility, qualified medical record managers are appointed to head the medical record department. The medical record department can be defined as a section of the hospital designated for the proper custody of patient care records as well as associated data for audit and reports. The attending physician assumes the responsibility for documenting the course of a patient care in an acceptable medical record.

Functions of the Medical Records Department

The scopes and functions vary, may be widespread in some institutions with seven-day per week, twenty four hours per day services. In addition, some hospitals include utilization review and quality management. The major functions of Medical Records Department (MRD) are filing, retrieving, assembling, quantitatively analyzing and technically evaluating deficiencies, assisting physician with record completion, preservation of records, form design, processing demographic and clinical information, reporting vital statistical information to public health, abstracting and coding records, responding to court subpoenas, educating and training health service practitioners about medical record documentation and assisting with and participating in the institutional quality assurance program.

Quality Assurance

The medical record provides as means of communication among health care professionals' contribution to the patients' care. The assurance of quality implies a commitment beyond simple measurement and evaluation; it implies a commitment to take corrective action if the care rendered does not meet the criteria of quality. A good quality assurance program is imperative to the hospital's organization. The process investigates three aspects of care, namely: the framework within which care is given, the care providing process and the outcome or results of the care provided. The medical record is the principal document by which the performance of health care professionals is measured. The medical record itself must be monitored and evaluated in order to maintain a high standard of quality that supplies a detailed account of the patient's care and treatment. A medical record committee should be established in each facility to periodically review (quantitatively and qualitatively) the content of selected medical records under guidelines set forth by a quality assurance plan.

Conclusion

Medical records play a vital role in patient care. A qualified medical records practitioner should be appointed to plan, organize and develop policies and procedures that provide continuous direction for the efficient functioning of a well-organized and effective medical records department serving the interest of quality patient care.

NEEDS AND MANAGEMENT OF MEDICAL RECORDS DEPARTMENT

a. *Introduction:* The primary function of a health center is the care of sick and injured. The hospital administrator is legally and morally responsible for the quality of medical care rendered to patients. Therefore, the medical records incharge has a very important role to play in effective and efficient management of the hospital services.

b. *The main needs of medical records department (MRD):* The needs depend on overall responsibilities and functions of the department. The following organizational needs have to be met before we could put the department into operation:
   • Planning, setting-up, organization and management of the MRD
   • Promoting and obtaining of good medical records
   • Cooperation with all the departments in the matter of records
   • Complete medical record control
   • Assist in medical record, QA and other committees
   • Prepare statistical reports and assist in research and teaching programs.

c. Location and layout

d. Personnel

e. Equipment

f. Good quality medical record forms (according to international standards)
g. Budget and budgetary control
h. Interdepartmental relationship
i. Organizational chart of the department
j. Work distribution chart
k. Line, staff and functional authority
l. Operational policy:
   • Working hours—shift
   • Monthly duty roster (schedule)
   • Implementation of instructions
   • Training of new staff
   • Submission of reports
   • Supplies
   • Communications
   • Transportation of medical records
   • House keeping and physical examination
   • Hotel services
   • Protection from fire
   • Safety control
   • Infection control
   • Disaster and emergency plan.

STANDARDS FOR MEDICAL RECORDS SERVICES

The health institution must maintain medical records that are documented accurately and in a timely manner and are complete and readily accessible for prompt retrieval of information including statistical data. Adequate patient case records must be maintained for all outpatients, inpatients and emergency patients. All significant clinical information pertaining to the patient must be incorporated into the patient's medical record. The content of medical record must be sufficiently detailed and organized to enable the medical care team responsible for the patient to provide continuity of care, to determine at any time the status of the patient and to review the diagnostic and therapeutic procedures performed and the patient's responses to treatment. The discharge summary must be written at the termination of hospitalization. The patient's health record must contain sufficient information to identify the patient, support the diagnosis and to justify the treatment and end result.

The *unit medical record* system with *"one patient one number one record"* is the ideal method to achieve optimal health care data, and should be a goal for all health care facilities. Presently, however, many health care institutions in developing countries still would not be able to implement the unit record because this system demands adequate equipment, sufficient space, and trained personnel in order to function properly.

The inpatient medical records must include at least the following:

a. Complete and accurate identification data including hospital number, patient's full name, age (date of birth), sex, nationality, national ID number, marital status, occupation, place of birth, address and telephone number and next of kin's name and address including telephone number.
b. Evidence of appropriate informed consent.
c. Reports of all diagnostic and therapeutic procedures.
d. Reports of pathology and clinical laboratory examinations as well as radiology and nuclear medicine examinations.
e. Progress notes.

Medical records must be confidential, secured, current, authenticated, legible, and complete. The medical record is the property of the health institution and maintained for the benefit of the patient, the medical staff and the health center. The health institution is responsible for safeguarding both the record and the information contained within it against loss, defacement, tampering, or use by unauthorized individuals.

Written policies and procedures for effective maintenance of medical records which are commensurate with overall policies of the health care facility should be made available to all concerned. The medical record department must be provided with adequate direction, staffing, and facilities to perform essential functions. The medical record department must be provided with sufficient space and equipment to enable personnel to function in an effective manner and to maintain patient health records that are readily available for continuity of patient care. Basic medical statistical information must be readily obtainable through the medical record department with the type and amount to be determined by the medical staff and hospital administration, as well as by governmental authorities. The medical record officer should encourage staff development through in-service training. The performance of medical record workers should be evaluated periodically to seek ways to improve medical record services. The role of the medical record staff in quality assurance and utilization review functions and committee functions must be clearly formulated with screening patient records for compliance with established criteria. The medical record service should participate in the selection and design of forms used and in the determination of the sequence and format of the contents of the medical record. This department also should have a role in developing mechanisms to protect the privacy of the patients and practitioners whose records are involved in quality assurance activities.

HOSPITAL'S GENERAL RULES AND REGULATIONS

This chapter deals with the hospital's general rules and regulations for the following topics:
a. Legal aspects of medical records
b. Consent
c. Release of information
d. Quality assurance
e. Control of forms
f. Staff medical records
g. Patients' property
h. Laboratory, X-rays records
i. Responsibility for contents and maintenance of medical records
j. Control on movement of records
k. Registration of births and deaths
l. Reporting of infectious diseases
m. Issue of medical reports and certificates
n. Collection of hospital statistics
o. Preservation of old records (retention schedule)
p. Microfilming
q. Computer application
r. Financial charges
s. Registration and appointment system
t. General instructions
u. Rights and responsibilities of a patient.

Legal Aspects of Medical Records

Medical record is the who, what, why, how, where and when of patient care in the hospital. With the advancement in medical knowledge and complexity of modern medical and surgical treatment existing in hospitals today, an accurate and adequate medical record is essential as documentary reference of the care and treatment which the patient received in the hospital.

The medical record can be divided legally into:
i. Personal document
ii. Impersonal document.

Personal Document

The medical record is considered to be personal when it identifies the patient using the name, history of illness, the physical findings and treatment given. The information in the record is confidential and no one is allowed to see the patient's medical file and no information is released without the written permission from the patient. However, official authorities are allowed to see the record only after presenting proof of authority. Neither relatives nor friends of the patient, not even the husband or wife, have any right to review record unless written permission has been received from the patient. The written permission and photocopy of the information disclosed should be kept in the patient's file.

If the patient is readmitted under the care of second physician, the second physician should be allowed to access to the record without permission of the patient. In case patient is admitted to another hospital, a summary may be sent upon request from the hospital or the physician. In such instances, patient's permission is not necessary. If a patient personally requests information from his own medical file, in such instances, the treating physician should be consulted.

Impersonal Document

As an impersonal document, the record may be used for research or study when such cautions need not be exercised, as when it is used as a personal document, because, it has no connection with the patient as an individual. Moreover, it is used only by physicians, house-staff undergraduate and postgraduate students, nurses and paramedical staff; all of whom are bound by the code of professional secrecy. As an impersonal document, only the patient file number is used and not identified by his name, therefore, patient's permission is not required.

Permission from treating physician: If the research is being done by a staff physician and is not for publication, it is not necessary to obtain the permission of the attending physician to use the record, although this is done as a matter of courtesy.

In case the record is being studied preparatory to publication, the permission of the attending physician must be secured. It is very essential, when a physician, who is not a staff member, intend to review a case or a series of cases; the consent of the attending physician and permission from the hospital administrator must be secured.

Central Medicolegal Committee

The central medicolegal committee (CMLC) or any other committee as authorized by the hospital administration has the right to summon for the medical records of patients. Other than the authorized committee, records are not to be handled by anyone except the authorized as decided by the hospital administration.

Medicolegal Cases Registration

The medicolegal case (MLC) is one, which is accidental, suicidal, or homicidal. However, the casualty medical officer (CMO) determines the case as a medicolegal or not. Except minor injury cases, all the cases of traffic accidents, burns, poison and quarrels, etc. have to be treated as medicolegal.

Medicolegal register: There should be a central medicolegal register kept in the accident and emergency (casualty) department, under the supervision of the casualty medical officer. All MLCs admitted from casualty, outpatient and inpatient services should be registered in the central medicolegal register. A medicolegal stamp should be affixed on each registered case to ensure that the case has been registered.

All medicolegal cases registered in the hospital must be informed to police through the hospital administrator and ensure that the MLC records are complete. These cases should be kept under safe custody of a responsible officer in the medical record department.

Consent

Written consent must be obtained from the patient or nearest relative for medical examinations, investigations, treatments, and procedures performed in the health care facility. In the case of children, persons of unsound mind, unconscious patients, the consent of the guardian, the spouse or the nearest relative may be obtained. The consent of the husband is required if an operation deprives his wife of her marital functions.

Release of Information

Confidentiality

The medical records and health information whether it is in the verbal form or written documentation pertaining to any identified patient, is confidential. As such the information available either in the form of medical records, disease and operation indexes, computer, microfilm, photograph, tapes or any other device used for the purpose, should be treated as confidential document. Therefore, only authorized staff are allowed to deal with the patient information.

Authorized Staff

Authorized staff are those who are involved in taking care of the patient, normally the medical, nursing, paramedical and persons of medical record department.

Release of Information without the Patientís Permission

- *Conditions* (e.g. injuries, poisoning, abortions or cases of accidental, suicidal and homicidal) must be reported to the police or other legal authorities.
- *Communicable and other notified diseases* must be reported to the concerned authorities.
- *Events (births, deaths, fetal deaths)* must be reported to civil registration authorities, either directly or through family.
- *Court order:* The hospital is also obliged to provide information in response to a court order. All the reports may be made available to the court without the patient's permission.

Medical records and health information are the property of the hospital. Therefore, all correspondence for medical information on patients in the hospital will be handled by the hospital administrator or his authorized representative. This includes, insurance forms, workmen's compensation forms, medical certificates, letters to schools or places of employment, government forms, questionnaire, requests for case summaries from law courts, etc. Any request for information including medicolegal cases has to be referred to hospital administrator.

Removal of medical record or portions of medical record and health information: The informational content of medical record must be safeguarded against loss, defacement, tampering, or use by an unauthorized person. Except the authorized, no employee has the right to read or copy the contents of any patient's record. Violators of the rules of confidentiality will be prosecuted and punished as per the existing civil service laws.

Quality Assurance

The term quality assurance, which is a broad term that encompasses several components, among them utilization review, medical care evaluation, risk management and peer review. From medical record maintenance in relation to patient care and medical record service point of view, the following are considered:

    i. Quality control
    ii. Quantitative analysis
    iii. Qualitative analysis
    iv. Medical audit
    v. Patient care evaluation
    vi. Formation of medical record committee
    vii. Role of MRD in quality assurance program
    viii. Evaluation of medical record service.

Quality Control

Quality control is defined as those evaluation procedures that are performed systematically to ensure that the established policies and standards are being met. This procedure includes the quantitative and qualitative review of medical records; the evaluation of the patient care or medical audit.

Quantitative Analysis

Quantitative analysis is the review of medical records to ensure that they are complete and accurate and meet standards established for them by the medical record committee/ministry of health. It is the responsibility of medical record and statistical personnel to perform this analysis regularly on inpatient (IP) and outpatient (OP) records.

Qualitative Analysis

Qualitative analysis is the review of records to ensure that:
• It contains sufficient information to justify the diagnosis, the treatment and end result.
• Opinions are supported by the findings.
• There are no discrepancies or errors.
    The qualitative review should be carried out regularly by the physicians at least once in a week and by the medical record committee once in a month.

Medical Audit

A "patient care review meeting" in the health center preferably every month to discuss the patient care carried out by the hospital. The main object of this meeting is to review the overall work carried out in the departments including outpatient, inpatient, and emergency, and also to discuss the institutional deaths of the previous month. The attendees at this meeting should include all the clinical staff including seniors and juniors, the director of nursing, the medical record incharge, a senior representative from each of the departments of pathology, biochemistry, and radiology. The director of the hospital should be the chairman of this meeting. He should be very tactful in conducting this meeting because of sensitive topics. The medical staff secretary should take notes of important discussions during this meeting, and these notes might serve in the initiation of action for any important points brought out during the meeting.

Patient Care Evaluation

The purpose of patient care evaluation is to ensure that care of acceptable quality is being provided. The evaluation has to be done by physicians or other health care professionals through the review of medical records on a regular basis.

Formation of Medical Record Committee

There should be a medical record committee in all the hospitals to carry out a regular quantitative and qualitative analysis of hospital services.

Medical record committee: Serves as a liaison between the medical record department and medical staff. The function of the committee is to review medical records for adequacy and completeness and to determine whether the records meet the required standards for promptness, completeness and clinical pertinence. To this end, the committee should recommend policies regarding content and completion of medical records. Another important function of this committee is to design and develop suitable medical record forms. The committee must comprise the following members: 1. Hospital director (medical) or his representative, 2. One representative from each department, e.g. medical, surgical, obstetrics and gynecology, pediatrics, laboratory, radiology, nursing and medical record officer as coordinator.

Role of Medical Record Department in Quality Assurance Program

The MRD supports the hospital quality assurance activities related directly to the retrieval of medical records. It provides routine statistical and medical information for completion of reports and monitoring of adherence to procedures, to protect the privacy of patients and practitioners whose records are involved in quality assurance program.

Evaluation of Medical Record Service

Evaluation of medical record service should provide information on how effectively medical record services are being performed? For example, how accurate is filing? what percentage of records of patients with appointments are in the clinic at the start of the clinic session? how accurate is the disease coding? how timely are reports being submitted? The medical record officer should evaluate the work and the medical record committee should assess and initiate action.

Control of Forms

The medical record committee of the hospital should develop standard and simple medical record forms in few number, which provide flexibility and should reduce the bulkiness of record. While designing the following points should be borne in mind:

a. The purpose of the form.
b. Whom it is to be used?
c. The identification of the patient within the form.
d. The retrieval of the form.
e. The hospital requirements, e.g. consultants requirements.
f. The provision made for form duplication, etc.
g. *Size:* It is suggested to use an international paper size A4: 21 × 29.7 cm for large forms and B6: 12.5 × 17.5 cm for clinical investigation request and report forms.
h. Selection of paper or card should be primarily on the degree of permanency attached to the record concerned.
i. Suitable color can be given to distinguish each form from others. However, it is advisable to print only on white paper with color-coded bands on the right hand margin with space for the title and identifying symbols for each form in place of different colored paper.
j. There should be a form identification number at the foot of the left-margin or right-margin of each form with the date and number of forms printed.
k. Systematically the required quantity of forms for each year should be meticulously calculated and an additional of 20 to 25 percent more than the estimated number needed each year should be printed to allow for the waste caused by errors in usage.
l. Introduction of the new forms is not advisable because these forms are not expensive to produce, but also will confuse users. Therefore, all efforts should be made to reduce to a minimum the requisite basic forms in the medical record. When the basic set of medical record forms has been decided upon and introduced, samples of these forms together with short instructions on their use, should be kept by the hospital. Decisions on revision or alteration of forms presently in use or on the introduction of new forms should be made by the hospital medical record committee. The individual departments of the health care facility should not be allowed to introduce new forms or to modify any form currently in use.

Patient's Property

This is the responsibility of the nursing staff during hospitalization of the patient. The ward nursing staff, in the event of no relatives, will be responsible for keeping the patient's property in a safe box during the period of hospitalization.

Laboratory, Radiology (X-ray)

1. Requests for laboratory and radiology tests should be in the appropriate prescribed form with the required identification information.
2. It is the responsibility of the laboratory/radiology to maintain proper recording system whereby all the requests received are accounted and the reports are dispatched promptly to the concerned people.
3. If the report is prepared on a separate form (other than the request form), it is the responsibility of the laboratory to record properly the identification information.
4. Laboratory/radiology technician or incharge should clearly write name and hospital number of the patient on each and every report.
5. There should be a cross-reference register with the hospital numbers to show that the number of investigations carried out on different occasions for a patient are entered against the appropriate hospital number. This will help to refer reports of the previous investigations carried out on the patient.
6. Old records including reports, registers, index cards, etc. maintained in the laboratory department should be sent to the medical record department for preservation and destruction as per the 'record retention schedule'.

Responsibility for Contents and Maintenance of Medical Records

Contents

Department	Responsibilities
Medical records department staff	For collection of complete and accurate identification data
Medical staff	For clinical data in all records related to medical staff
Nursing staff	For the data related to nursing record
Paramedical staff	For the data of respective contribution to patient care

Maintenance and Completion

a. *Medical records staff*
   1. Collection of complete and accurate patient identification data.
   2. To collect the ward census and the discharged patients files (whether completed or incomplete) from all the wards daily. A due register to be maintained for those patients files needed to be retained in the ward after discharge for any authenticated administrative purpose.
   3. All medical records including patients files registers, index cards, etc. relating to the patient care have to be maintained by the medical record department. The old registers from all the departments of the hospital should also be collected and preserved in a systemic manner.

b. *Medical staff*
   1. All doctors have to complete the patient's file before discharge of the patient wherever possible. However, all the discharged records will be checked for deficiencies by inserting a prescribed deficiency check slip by the MRD without any exception as a part of health institution/MOH policy. Hence, all the unit doctors have to visit the doctors' conference room in MRD once in a week to review all the discharge records for completion. No patient's record should be kept incomplete for more than a week.
   2. The head of the unit is responsible for clinical content and its accuracy and completeness. Physicians should use only approved medical abbreviations and symbols and should check that each page contain the patient's name and hospital number. He should sign all entries with date.
c. *Nursing staff*
   1. All the discharged patients' records should be handed over to the MRD while submitting census on very next day. Patient's record should not be retained in the ward for not more than 48 hours from the date and time of discharge.
   2. Nursing staff should ensure that each page contain the patient's name, hospital number and dates in chronological order.
   3. All lab reports received during the patient's stay in the ward to be mounted then and therein the appropriate patient record. If any lab report received after the discharge, it should be sent to the MRD promptly without fail.
   4. The outpatient, A and E and day care patients' records must be returned to MRD without fail. No records should be retained in the clinic after consultation is completed.
d. *Others:* Other staff (other than medical and nursing) especially the paramedical workers are responsible for proper recording of the data relating to the treatment.
e. *Classification of diseases:* All medical records of patients treated in the outpatient and inpatient departments have to be coded for disease classification by the MRD according to the latest international classification of diseases (WHO) or as recommended by the hospital administration.
f. *Classification of operations:* All medical records of patients treated for surgical procedures in the outpatient and inpatient departments have to be coded for operation classification by the MRD according to the latest international classification of operations (WHO) or as recommended by the hospital administration.
g. *Disease and operation index:* All medical records coded for diseases and operations have to be indexed manually in the disease index card and operation index card or electronically in the computer by

the MRD. The information required from the index cards has to be compiled.

h. *Patient master index:* All the patients treated in the outpatient especially in specialty clinics and inpatient department must have a patient master index with complete identification information. The MRD is responsible for collecting the information at the time of registration (first visit) and files them in a strict alphabetical order in the absence of computer registration.

i. *Maintenance of medical records*: It is the responsibility of medical records department which is under the control of a qualified medical record officer. The MRD initiates records of emergency, outpatient and inpatient and processes them for completion and collects health information to assist in patient care, quality assurance, medical education, research and administrative activities. Protection from unauthorized persons and safe preservation of medical records and information is one of major responsibilities of medical record department.

Control of Movement of Records

All the patient medical files of emergency, outpatient, and inpatient departments will have to be kept in the medical records department under the custody of the medical record staff. Generally medical records should not be taken out of the medical records department except in case of: (i) Patient care, i.e. OP, IP and A and E (ii) Court summons (iii) Clinical meetings (iv) Administrative (for settling the bills or complaints). The following procedures are recommended for movement of records:

Emergency Records

Accident and emergency form which was initiated and sent to the casualty medical officer for treatment has to be collected immediately after care of the patient and kept in the allocated section by the MRD. Patient files are not to be retained by anyone without the knowledge of the MRD. For admitted cases, the inpatient procedure will be applicable.

Outpatient Records

The outpatient records are those which are sent to outpatient clinics for treatment of patients. Once the patient is seen in the clinic, the patient file should be returned to the OP clinic nurse/clerk (AMRT). Outpatient records are not to be retained by anyone including doctors. If patients require admission, the file will be sent to admission office. For admitted cases the inpatient procedure will be applicable.

Inpatient Records

From the time of admission into the ward till the patient is discharged, the patient file is under the custody of the ward nurse. The file should not be taken out of the ward without her permission. The maximum period permitted for discharged patient files to be retained in the ward is 48 hours.

Ward Census

Medical record technician (MRT) from the statistical unit of MRD will be responsible to collect the daily ward census and the discharged patient files (whether complete or incomplete) from the ward daily. Any file of a discharged patient if required to be retained in the ward due to any special reason, the nurse incharge will have to acknowledge. However, the same should be returned within 48 hours.

Patient Medical Files Sent to Other Hospitals

As a routine, a patient file of one hospital is not sent to another hospital. However, a detailed discharge summary may be supplied to the treating doctor. In exceptional cases, a photocopy of the entire file is supplied and the original file will be retained in the hospital.

Patient Medical Files from Other Hospitals

If any patient file of other hospital is received for treatment of the patient, all relevant information should be noted in the current record of the treating hospital. Once the purpose is over, the file including reports (X-ray, laboratory, etc.) should be returned to the concerned hospital. In any case, the file should not be retained after discharge/death of the patient.

Registration of Births and Deaths

The hospital should maintain three separate registers for births, deaths and fetal deaths. Necessary entries for live births, stillbirths, fetal deaths and deaths, as they occur must be made in respective registers as per the rules laid down by the Government.

Newborn (Live Birth)

Newborn should be registered as a new patient baby girl of (BG/O) or baby boy (BB/O) followed by mother name and a new hospital number to be allocated with a separate patient file created. However, a cross reference of mother's hospital number in the child's file and child's number in the mother's file should be entered. Similarly, cross reference entries have to be made in mother's and child's patient master index cards.

Multiple Births (Twins/Triplets, etc.)

Each live-born child must be registered as a new patient (BG1/O or BB2/O followed by mother name) and a new file to be created. The first-born child will get the first hospital number.

Stillborn (Dead Born)

Stillborn cases, the birth notification issued by the doctor should form a record. However, no patient file should be opened and no hospital number to be allocated.

Fetal Death

Death prior to the expulsion or extraction from its mother of a product of conception, irrespective of the duration of the pregnancy; the death is indicated by the fact that after such separation, the fetus does not breath or show any other evidence of life such as beating of heart, pulsation of umbilical cord, or definite movement of voluntary muscles. There should be a separate fetal death register to record all fetal deaths.

Submission of Birth Notification (Born Alive and Dead)

Birth notification for born alive and dead in prescribed forms (recommended by Government) duly signed by the medical officer who had conducted the delivery should be prepared in triplicate and submitted to:
- The parents/relatives.
- The hospital patient medical record.
- The birth registrar (concerned authority for registration).

Submission of Death Notification

Death notification in triplicate in prescribed form has to be prepared and signed by the treating doctor and counter signed by the unit head and submitted to:
- The nearest relative of diseased.
- The hospital patient medical record.
- The death registrar (concerned authority).

The hospital should maintain one central death register in MRD in which all hospital deaths, including OP, IP, and A and E and brought dead to be registered with accurate and complete information.

Registration of Cancer Patients

A central cancer register must be maintained in each hospital. All proved malignant cases as recommended by ICD (WHO) should be registered and a separate cancer register number to be allocated in the patient file in addition to the hospital number. All the cancer cases registered will have to be classified in accordance with the recommendation made by the national cancer center. Refer the guidelines provided by the national cancer center for more details.

Reporting of Infectious Diseases

It is the responsibility of each department to notify the admission and treatment of infectious disease cases in the prescribed form recommended by the hospital to the public health department. Refer the guidelines provided by the public health department for more details.

Issue of Medical Reports and Certificates

Any request for medical report or certificate has to be routed through the hospital administration/MRD. The treating doctor will prepare and issue medical report or certificate to the patient or his representative or any organization through the MRD/hospital administration. Original copy of the medical report/certificate will be given to the patient and the copy is kept in the patient file.

Collection of Hospital Statistics

All hospitals should collect and compile different types of statistics as recommended by the ministry of health. Some of the essential statistics to be collected are as follows:

Outpatient Statistics

- Statistics of new, follow-up and total cases; according to sex (male, female and children), nationality. Statistics according to service/ unit, geographical distribution, age group—less than 1, 1 to 4, 5 to 14, 15 to 24, 25 to 34, 35 to 44, 45 to 54, 55 to 64, 65 to 74, 75 and above.
- Number of investigations carried out, e.g. pathology, microbiology, biochemistry, radiology, ECG, EEG, and other departments (specify).
- Outpatient disease and operation statistics have to be prepared.

Emergency Statistics

Total number of cases seen in the emergency service and classification according to sex (male, female and children), number of cases referred to OPD, PHC. Number of cases admitted in the hospital and number of medicolegal cases treated (accidental, suicidal, homicidal, traffic accidents, burn and poison cases).

Inpatient Statistics

- Daily census reports of admitted and discharged cases of general and private wards.
- Discharges according to service by nationality, sex (male, female and children), age group—less than 1, 1 to 4, 5 to 14, 15 to 24, 25 to 34, 35 to 44, 45 to 54, 55 to 64, 65 to 74, 75 and above, discharge results—alive, dead, death classification—less than 48 hours and more than 48 hours.
- *Bed utilization* (general and private separately): Bed days, bed occupied and bed occupancy rate.
- Inpatient diagnosis and operation classification statistics have to be calculated.
- Number of consultations received and rendered.
- Surgical procedures according to different services: number of elective operations, emergency operations, minor, intermediate and major operations performed.
- *Investigations:* Number of pathology, microbiology, biochemistry, radiology, ECG, EEG, and other tests conducted.
- *Deliveries conducted:* Number of normal and abnormal deliveries.
- *Births:* Number of live births, mature, premature and stillbirths.
- *Death statistics:* Should be presented in the following statements: S no, name, hospital no, service, nationality, age, sex, duration – 48 hours, +48 hours, cause of death, remarks.

Administrative Statistics

- Number of medical personnel; seniors and juniors according to specialty.
- Number of dentists; seniors and juniors.
- Number of nursing personnel—according to cadre and student nurses if any.
- Number of paramedical workers including laboratory, radiology, dietary, pharmacy, medical social service, medical records and others.
- *Other auxiliary services:* Engineering, civil, electrical, maintenance, laundry, and house keeping.
- Administrative staff including director, deputy directors, office unit heads, clerical and lower grade staff.
- Expenditure relating to drugs, diet, equipment, furniture, forms and stationery. Buildings including water, electricity, personnel, linen

(patient uniform, staff uniform), transportation, communication, maintenance, training personnel and research.
• Income from patients and other sources.
• Other information pertaining to administration.

Monthly Reports on Hospital Statistics

Statistics of major departments such as pathology, microbiology, biochemistry, radiology, ECG, dietary, anesthesiology, physiotherapy, obstetrics and gynecology (births and deaths) and operating theaters, have to be prepared with details and submit to the medical record department before the 5th of every month.

The medical record department should prepare monthly statistics of outpatient, inpatient, emergency and allied departments and publish a report before 10th of every month. Copy of monthly hospital statistical report should be sent to the following departments before 15th of every month.
• To the hospital administrator.
• To the heads of departments and unit chiefs.
• To health information officer (MOH).

Preservation of Old Records (Retention Schedule)

Maintenance of Old Records

All medical records including patient files, registers, index cards, etc. relating directly to the patient care have to be maintained by the MRD. The medical record department should collect the old registers and files from all the wards, emergency department, outpatient clinics, etc. and classify them properly by giving "old record register number". The old files, registers, index cards are to be preserved in a place earmarked for a prescribed period. Later, the records have to be destroyed as per the rules laid down for "record retention".

Retention of Records

Because of pressure on space for filing of medical records a retention schedule for keeping records has been prepared by the MOH for hospital guidance (*See* the retention schedule next page). However, those hospitals which are carrying out teaching/research programs can keep the records longer than the prescribed period provided they have adequate space and facilities.

Preservation of Records

Special care has to be taken to preserve the records. Records have to be protected from insect termites, prevent records from being exposed

Medical Record Retention Schedule

Name of medical record	Retention original form (in years)	Effective from the date	Permanent retention in microfilm/computer or in original form
Patient record:			
Inpatient record	5	of last visit of the patient	YES
Outpatient record	3	-do-	YES
Outpatient GP record	2	-do-	NO
Casualty record:			
Medicolegal cases	5	of last visit of the patient	YES
Ordinary cases	1	-do-	NO
X-rays:			
Outpatient X-rays	5	of last visit of the patient	NO
Inpatient X-rays	5	-do-	NO
Casualty X-rays	5	-do-	NO
Registers:			
Birth register	2	of last entry in the register	YES
Death register	2	-do-	YES
Admission and discharge register	2	-do-	YES
Hosp. master register (OP)	2	-do-	YES
Medicolegal register	2	-do-	YES
Operation register	2	-do-	NO
Ward Admission and discharge register	2	-do-	NO
Narcotic register	2	-do-	NO
Infection register	2	-do-	NO
X-ray register	2	-do-	NO
Laboratory and other investigation register	2	-do-	NO
Index:			
Disease index	Permanently either in physical or computer form		YES
Operation index	-do-		YES
Patient master index	-do-		YES
Physician index	1	the physician left the hospital	NO
Report:			
Daily ward census report	1	of the report	NO
Daily statistical report	1	"	NO
Monthly report	1	"	NO
Yearly report	10	"	NO
Duplicate laboratory/X-ray report	1	"	NO

to hot and dry climate. They should be filed in a dust free and protected from water, dampness and fire. Adequate fire extinguishers to be provided at all required places.

Imaging System

In case any hospital has decided to keep records on imaging system, the following are suggested. Maintain a control register in order to have good account over the cases (records) imaged.

Computer Application

Computer services have to be applied for effective maintenance of medical records to provide efficient services to patients and hospital staff. The medical record department in collaboration with the statistical unit and computer section should try to apply computer services in registration and follow-up appointments, patient master index, disease and operation classification, record control and statistical data analysis.

Financial Charges

Patient charges related to registration, admission, private beds, consultation, investigation, etc. are to be collected from nationals and expatriates as per the directions of the hospital administration.

Registration and Appointment System

The following instructions have to be meticulously observed:

Registration System

A central registration system with 24-hour service will be observed for all outpatients and inpatients. In this system, each patient will have one record and one permanent number for all episodes. A separate registration for accident and emergency patients with 24-hour service will be practiced. On each visit to casualty, a new record will be created and a new A/E number will be given.

Numbering System

Six digit numbers will be used for outpatients and inpatients starting from 00 00 01 and will continue till it reaches 99 99 99. A new patient will get a new hospital number only at the time of first registration. Casualty department will start the number at 80 00 01.

Patient Master Index

Patient master index can be maintained manually or electronically. It will be created with important identification information for each new patient registered in the central registration and filed alphabetically.

Appointment Card

An identification information card should be given to each new patient registered for outpatient and inpatient service.

Appointment System

Appointment system should be practiced in all referral hospitals. All patients must observe appointment system except in labor and emergency cases. As a general policy there should be a gap of minimum 3 days between the day of booking appointment and the day of appointment at the clinic. The appointment schedule must be prepared in conjunction with the concerned heads of units/specialties, MRO and administration, and to be followed strictly. All the referring hospitals and health centers should be informed of the policy and procedures of the appointment systems.

Investigation Reports

Investigation reports of outpatients will be received and mounted by MRD in respective records. While inpatient reports will be received and mounted in the ward by nurse.

Outpatient Clinics

Outpatient clinics names of all outpatient clinics with names of clinic chiefs in the hospital should be exhibited in the main entrance of outpatient department and in each clinic. The name of the chief consultant should also be exhibited.

Outpatient Clinic Schedule

Each unit in consultation with administration and medical records officer should decide the number of new and follow-up cases to be booked for the clinic.

Accident and Emergency Service

A separate accident and emergency record in triplicate will be used in A/E service. Out of three accident and emergency forms, the first copy will be retained in the casualty, second copy will be given to the patient and the third will be sent to the concerned health center. If patient is admitted to outpatient or inpatient service, the second and third copies will become part of main patient file. The first copy, however, will be retained in the casualty. If patient has a unit record in the hospital and the casualty medical officer desires to have it, the MRD should supply and collect. All investigation reports of casualty patient will be attached with the casualty form. If patient referred to outpatient/ inpatient services, the reports will become part of main patient file.

All the casualty records including X-rays have to be kept for one year in the A/E department. Later, they should be transferred to MRD/ X-ray department. The casualty registration section will also undertake the responsibility of central registration and admission office during holidays and off hours.

Admission Office

Admission office functions round the clock and is responsible for admission of patients, maintains bed occupancy board.

Direct Admission

A patient getting into ward and occupying a bed without going through the admission office. This is permitted in emergency and obstetrics cases. The nurse in-charge of the ward is responsible for registering the case in the admission office within two hours of patient admission into the ward.

Declaration by the Patient

Any patient who wish to make a declaration before his death, such statements have to be recorded in the patient's file in the presence of a magistrate. However, in the absence of magistrate, the declaration can be recorded in the presence of three persons including the treating physician, a nurse and the hospital administrator or his representative.

Completion of Records

Doctors have to complete records before discharge of patient wherever possible. Otherwise, they have to visit MRD weekly and review all the discharged records for completion. In any case, patient files should not be kept incomplete for more than a week.

Supply of Records

The MRD is responsible for supply of medical records for medical education and research purposes to authorized persons.

Registers to be Maintained

The following registers have to be maintained in the hospital:

Outpatient Register

Outpatient register should contain: Hosp.no/Patient's name/Sex/Age (DOB)/ID no/Nationality/Marital status/Occupation/Place of birth/ Address and telephone no/Relative's name and telephone no/Clinic name.

Accident and Emergency Register

Accident and emergency register should contain: S.no./Date/A and E no./ Name of the patient/Age/Sex/Nationality/Marital status/Occupation/ ID number/Address/Time of arrival/Mode of arrival/Brought by/Illness or accident/Place of accident/Time of accident/Degree of urgency/Diagnosis/ Treatment/MLC (Yes/No)/Time of departure/Follow-up/Remarks.

Medicolegal Register

Medicolegal cases (MLCs) should contain MLC no./A and E no./Hospital no./Patient name/Age/Sex/Nationality/Marital status/Occupation/ Address/Date and time of arrival/Means of arrival/Nature, place and time of accident/Complaint/Diagnosis/Disposition/Date and time of discharge/Name of CMO/Remarks.

Admission Register

S.no./Date of admission/Date of discharge/Nature of discharge/ (Discharge/Transfer/Lama/Died)/IP no./OP no./Name of the patient/ Age/Sex/Address/Time/Provisional diagnosis/Final diagnosis/ Ward/Nationality/Remarks.

Waiting List Register

Waiting list register should contain identification data plus service/ unit/name of admitting doctor/date and time of registration in the waiting list/date and time of the patient to be admitted/remarks.

Ward Admission and Discharge Register

Ward admission and discharge register should be a single register; admissions on left and discharges on right side of the register.

Admission register: S.no./Hospital no./Patient's name/Sex/Age/ Nationality/Room no./Bed no./Date and time of admission/Service, unit/Provisional diagnosis.

Discharge register: S.no./Hospital no./Patient's name/Sex/Age/ Nationality/Room/Bed no./Date and time of discharge/Service/Unit/ Final diagnosis/Result/Remarks.

Operation Register

Operation register should contain: S. no./Hospital no./Name of the patient/Age/Sex/Nationality/Marital status/Occupation/Date of admission/Date and time of operation/Diagnosis/Operation/ Anesthesia type/Anesthetist/Surgeon/Assistant surgeon/Name of the OT nurse/Results/Remarks.

Anesthesia Register

S. no./Date/Hospital no./Name/Age/Sex/Diagnosis/Operation/Pre-meditation/Anesthetic technique and drug used/Duration/Anesthetist/Remarks.

Birth Register

Birth register should contain: S. no./Name of the newborn/Sex/Fathers particulars (Name/Religion/Nationality/Occupation/Address)/Mothers particulars (Name/Religion/Nationality/Occupation)/Date of birth/Particulars of place of birth/Destination of delivery attendant/Signature of registrar/Date of registration/Signature of notifier/Remarks.

Death Register

Death register should contain: S. no./Hospital no./Name of the deseased/Age/Sex/Nationality/Address and Telephone no./Ward/Date of admission/Time of death/Diagnosis (cause of death)/Signature of doctor certifying death/Relative's signature receiving the body.

Central Cancer Register

Central cancer register should contain: Full identification data plus CCR no./Disease/Date onset of the disease/Confirmed by histopatho-logically/Treated as OP/IP/DOA/DOD/Service/Unit/Information sent to NCR on date/remarks.

General Instructions

1. Every sheet of patient medical file must have identification at-least complete patient's name and hospital number.
2. The treating staff whether medical, nursing, paramedical or others have to sign and date wherever it is required. Generally, when information is written in the form, the note has to be attested and dated.
3. All written entries into the patient file including investigation requests, reports must be clear and legible. Since patient files will be kept for longer period, it is advisable to use dark color ink. Pencils must not be used. Each entry must be dated and include the name and status of the contributor.
4. Any section of the patient file should not be erased, if corrections are required, circle and write over and sign.
5. Patient should not be admitted to the ward without completing the admission and discharge advice form by the treating physician or any authorized medical officer.

6. Patient should not be discharged without the written discharge instructions by the treating physician.
7. A provisional or admitting diagnosis must be written at the time of admission wherever possible.
8. Diagnosis will be written in full without the use of abbreviations.
9. Standard abbreviations are listed separately as such only those should be used.
10. Prior to discharge of patient, the consultant physician or his authorized assistant should write the final diagnosis including primary and secondary. The condition of the patient on discharge, the result, and advice given should be written.
11. The cause of death as recommended by WHO must be written in all death cases. If autopsy is conducted, a note "autopsy done" and report should be recorded.
12. Prior to proceeding on leave, the physicians, should get no objection certificate from the medical records department.

Rights and Responsibilities of a Patient

Rights of a Patient

1. To get considerate and respectful behavior from all staff in the hospital (from consultant to cleaner) and safe care by the hospital at all times.
2. To obtain from his physician complete, current information concerning his diagnosis, treatment, and prognosis in terms that the patient can be reasonably expected to understand.
3. To receive necessary information from his physician for giving consent prior to start of any procedure or treatment.
4. To refuse treatment to the extent permitted by law and to be informed of the medical consequences of his action.
5. To give every consideration of his privacy concerning his own medical care program.
6. To expect that all communications and records pertaining to his/her care should be treated as confidential.
7. To accept his willingness to be transferred to another hospital.
8. To be advised if the hospital proposes to engage in or perform human experimentation affecting his care or treatment. The patient has the right to refuse to participate in such research projects.
9. To expect reasonable continuity of care. He has the right to know in advance the names and professional status of the people treating him/her and which physician is responsible for his/her care, date and time of appointment.

10. To know what hospital rules and regulations are applicable to his conduct as a patient. The patient has the right to complain to concerned authority if something goes wrong in his care.
11. To be examined in privacy and to have a person of the same sex present when being examined or treated by someone of the opposite sex.
12. To obtain assistance in communicating with the people treating him/her in Arabic or other language.

Responsibilities of a Patient

The patient is responsible for the following:
1. To furnish correct and full identification information; full name, age (date of birth), occupation, father's/husband's name, nationality, complete address including telephone number.
2. To give correct information regarding his/her previous visits to hospitals and furnish about present complaints, past illnesses, hospitalizations and medications.
3. To retain appointment (hospital number) card safely, and produce the same whenever he/she visits the hospital or health clinic.
4. To inform the hospital authorities about the loss of hospital number card so as to locate the correct hospital number.
5. To visit the hospital on the day and time of appointment and to avoid going to hospital without prior appointment except in the case of an emergency. If the patient is given follow-up appointment for future visits, he/she should register his/her case and obtain a date and time for the next visit before leaving the hospital.
6. To report only to the authorized staff in the hospital for his/her appointments.
7. To observe the rules and regulations and strictly follow instructions of the hospital and they should not take away the hospital records except the patient appointment card and other documents given to patient.
8. Making willful correction in the records, giving wrong information or producing wrong documents, or bringing documents of other patients for treatment will lead to legal prosecution and punishment.
9. To be considerate and respectful of the rights of other patients and of the hospital staff by assisting in the control of noise, by limiting the number of visitors, and by avoiding cigarette smoking whenever necessary.

PERSONNEL REQUIREMENT AND JOB DESCRIPTION

This section deals with the following:
1. Personnel requirement according the bed strength of the hospital.
2. Job description for four important categories of medical records department personnel, e.g. medical record officer, medical record technician.

Personnel Requirement

Distribution of medical record personnel.

According to bed strength of the hospital:

Name of the post	Number of beds						
	< 50	50	100	200	300	400	600
Medical records officer			1	1	1	1	1
Assistant medical records officer					1	1	1
Medical records technician	5	7	15	17	20	25	30

Job Descriptions

Medical Records Officer

Duties and responsibilities
1. To establish, organize and manage medical record department with appropriate system as recommended by the hospital administration that can provide effective service in the hospital and effective supervision of the staff for efficient functioning of the department.
2. To develop policies and procedures relating to medical record department in accordance with international system and protect medical records in accordance with national retention, preservation and destruction policies.
3. To coordinate with medical record committee, design and develop different medical record forms required for hospital use.
4. To review the medical records of outpatients, inpatients, and emergency patients to ensure that they include all the important documents and pertinent information to meet clinical, administrative and legal requirement.
5. To cooperate with the medical, nursing and other staff in patient care and completing the patient medical records.
6. To participate and assist in quality assurance, utilization review, infection control and other committees and programs, and to assist in developing hospital disaster plan to meet the exigency.

7. To plan, organize, develop and supervise computer applications in medical records and patient care functions.
8. To prepare daily, monthly and yearly statistical reports containing the hospital activities carried out and submit to the concerned authorities with suggestions to improve patient care services. If a statistician is posted he has to work under MRO, otherwise entire statistical work will be carried out by the statistician.
9. To prepare and carry out educational and training programs such as in-service, certificate, diploma and continuing education for medical record personnel in cooperation with the appropriate health institutions/university. And also participate in seminars, workshops and conferences related to medical records.
10. To participate and assist in research programs for improving the administrative activities and financial control and prepare departmental budget and annual report of MRD activities. And protect confidentiality of information form authorized and keep medicolegal cases under safe custody.
11. To perform other duties and responsibilities related to medical record services as may be assigned by the hospital director.

Assistant Medical Records Officer

Duties and responsibilities

1. To perform technical analysis and evaluation of medical records in accordance with the hospital policies and procedures.
2. To collect medical information, administrative and other statistics required by the hospital and provide health information for quality assurance, utilization review and evaluation of hospital care.
3. To provide medical record services including reception, registration, outpatient appointment, inpatient, admission and emergency department by maintaining effective medical record filing and retrieving system.
4. To evaluate for deficiencies in the outpatient and inpatient medical records and arrange for completion with the cooperation of medical, nursing and other staff.
5. To code and index diseases, surgical operations, therapeutic procedures according to international classification of diseases/operations or in accordance with the criteria laid down by the hospital administration
6. To assist medical and other committees in the hospital and perform transcription of medical and other reports in the medical records departments or clinical units.

7. To feed patient care information into computer for processing and storage and retrieval when required.
8. To protect the medical records including medicolegal cases from unauthorized persons and to maintain confidentiality.
9. To supervise one or more medical record units and assist in departmental educational and administrative activities.
10. To perform other duties and responsibilities related to medical record services as may be assigned by the hospital director/ incharge.

Medical Records Technician

Duties and responsibilities

1. To register and collect appropriate identification information from outpatient, (new, old and follow-up) patients and arrange appointments, admission procedures.
2. To prepare patient master index cards (PMI), arrange according to alphabetical order, file them in index cabinets and retrieve when required. If computerized PMI, feed and retrieve information electronically from computer.
3. To collect investigation reports from the laboratory, X-ray and other diagnostic investigation departments, arrange and mount them in appropriate records.
4. To receive patient records/X-rays, arrange in systematic order, file and retrieve records/X-rays whenever required. And also to assist in moving active and inactive records/X-rays from one area to another.
5. To work in all the units of MRD, e.g. accident and emergency or outpatient clinic or admission office or ward or X-ray or any other units and perform the work of that unit as per the recommended procedures.
6. To assemble and process records as per the laid down procedures.
7. To use computer, microfilm and other mechanical devices for maintaining medical records.
8. To collect and prepare statistics of outpatient, emergency and inpatients. Also collect daily ward census along with discharged patient records, X-rays and late reports.
9. To work in the MRD of hospital and perform duties in any of the 3 shifts as required.
10. To maintain confidentiality of information from unauthorized persons and participate in educational programs.
11. To index previously coded disease and operation data in disease and operation index cards manually or electronically in computers.

Rights and Responsibilities of a Patient

PATIENT'S RIGHTS

1. The patient has the right to considerate and respectful care.
2. The patient has the right to obtain from his physician complete current information concerning his diagnosis, treatment, and prognosis, in terms the patient can be reasonably expected to understand. When it is not medically advisable to give such information to the patient, the information should be made available to an appropriate person in his behalf. He has the right to know by name the physician responsible for coordinating his care.
3. The patient has the right to receive from his physician information necessary to give informed consent prior to the start of any procedure and/or treatment. Except, in emergencies, such information for informed consent should include but not necessarily be limited to the specific procedure and/or treatment, the medically significant risks involved, and the probable duration of incapacitation. Where medically significant alternatives for care or treatment exist, or when the patient requests information concerning medical alternatives, the patient has the right to such information. The patient also has the right to know the name of the person responsible for the procedures and/or treatment.
4. The patient has the right to refuse treatment to the extent permitted by law and to be informed of the medical consequences of his action.
5. The patient has the right to every consideration of his privacy concerning his own medical care program. Case discussion, consultation, examination, and treatment are confidential and should be conducted discreetly. Those not directly involved in this care must have the permission of the patient to be present.
6. The patient has the right to expect that all communications and records pertaining to his care should be treated as confidential.

7. The patent has the right to expect that within its capacity a hospital must make reasonable response to the request of a patient for services. The hospital must provide evaluation, service, and/or referral as indicated by the urgency of the case. When medically permissible, a patient may be transferred to another facility only after he has received complete information and explanation concerning the needs for and alternative to such a transfer. The institution to which the patient is transferred must first have accepted the patient for transfer.

8. The patient has the right to obtain information as to any relationship of his hospital to other healthcare and educational institutions insofar as his care is concerned. The patient has the right to obtain information as to the existence of any professional relationships among individuals, by name, who are treating him?

9. The patient has the right to be advised if the hospital purposes to engage in or perform human experimentation affecting his care or treatment. The patient has the right to refuse to participate on such research projects.

10. The patient has the right to expect reasonable continuity of care. He has the right to know in advance what appointment times and physicians are available and where. The patient has the right to expect that the hospital will provide a mechanism whereby he is informed by his physician or a delegate of the physician of the patient's continuing health.

11. Patient has the right to examine and receive an explanation of his bill regardless of source of payment.

12. The patient has the right to know what hospital rules and regulations apply to his conduct as a patient.

PATIENT'S RESPONSIBILITIES

The patient is responsible for the following:

1. To furnish correct and full identification information; full name, age (date of birth), occupation, father's/husband's name, nationality, and complete address including telephone number.

2. To give correct information regarding his or her previous visits to hospitals and to furnish information regarding present complaints, past illnesses, hospitalizations, and medications.

3. To retain the registration or appointment (hospital number) card safely, and to produce this card or identity number whenever he or she visits the hospital or health clinic or patient should identify via hospital allocated number.

4. To inform the hospital authorities on the loss of a hospital number card so as to restore his or her original identity hospital number.

5. To visit the hospital as per the schedule day and time of appointment, and avoid going to hospital without prior appointment except in the case of an emergency. If the patient is given a follow-up appointment for future visits, he or she should register and obtain a date and time for the next visit before leaving the hospital or clinic or physician's office.

6. To report only to the authorized staff in the hospital for his or her appointments.

7. To observe the rules and regulations and strictly follow instructions of the hospital and never remove hospital records accept the patient appointment card and any specific documents given to patient.

8. To avoid making wrongful alterations in his or her records, to avoid giving wrong information or producing wrong documents, such as bringing records of other patients when seeking personal care.

9. To be considerate and respectful of the rights of other patients and of the hospital staff by assisting in the control of noise, and by limiting the number of visitors and avoid smoking in non-smoking areas. Precisely, cooperate with the hospital staff and avoid attempting to wrongful activities that are against the rules of the hospital.

PART–III

Hospital Public Relations, Medical Secretarial Profession, Communication Skills, and Dictation and Transcription

Public relations (PR) is the practice of managing the communication between an organization and its publics and especially health related topics. An organization represented by PR exposure to their audiences using topics of public interest and news items. Common activities include speaking at conferences, working with the press, and employee communication. PR can be used to build rapport with employees, customers, investors, or the general public. Almost any organization that has a stake in how it is portrayed in the public arena employs some level of public relations. There are number of related sister disciplines all falling under the banner of Corporate Communications, such as analyst relations, media relations, investor relations, internal communications or labor relations.

There are many areas of public relations but the most recognized are financial public relations, product public relations, and crisis public relations. In this, we touch hospital services.

- Financial public relations deal with providing information mainly to business reporters.
- Product public relations deal with gaining publicity for a particular product or service through PR tactics rather than using advertising.
- Crisis public relations deal with responding to negative accusations or information.
- Hospital public relations deal with the services that are operational and type of specialties and expertise open for public.

METHODS, TOOLS AND TACTICS

Public relations and publicity are not synonymous but many PR campaigns include provisions for publicity. Publicity is the spreading of information to gain public awareness for a product, person, hospital and health institution services, cause or organization, and can be seen as a result of effective PR planning.

Publics Targeting

A fundamental technique used in public relations is to identify the target audience, and to tailor every message to appeal to that audience. It can be a general, nationwide or worldwide audience, but it is more often a segment of a population. Marketers often refer to economy-driven "demographics", in public relations and audience is more fluid, being whoever someone wants to reach.

In addition to audiences, there are usually stakeholders, literally people who have a "stake" in a given issue. All audiences are stakeholders, but not all stakeholders are audiences. For example, a charity commissions a PR agency to create an advertising campaign to raise money to find a cure for a disease. The charity and the people with the disease are stakeholders, but the audience is anyone who is likely to donate money.

Sometimes the interests of differing audiences and stakeholders common to a PR effort necessitate the creation of several distinct but still complementary messages. This is not always easy to do, and sometimes—especially in politics—a spokesperson or client says something to one audience that angers another audience or group of stakeholders.

Lobby Groups

Lobby groups are established to influence government policy, corporate policy, or public opinion. An example of this is the American Israel Public Affairs Committee, AIPAC, which influences American foreign policy. Such groups claim to represent a particular interest and in fact are dedicated to doing so. When a lobby group hides its true purpose and support base it is known as a front group. Moreover, governments may also lobby public relations firms in order to sway public opinion. A well illustrated example of this is the way civil war in Yugoslavia was portrayed. Governments of newly succeeded republics of Croatia and Bosnia invested heavily with American PR firms, so that the PR firms would give them a positive war image in the US.

Spin

In public relations, "spin" is sometimes a pejorative term signifying a heavily biased portrayal in one's own favor of an event or situation. While traditional public relations may also rely on creative presentation of the facts, "spin" often, though not always, implies disingenuous, deceptive and/or highly manipulative tactics. Politicians are often accused of spin by commentators and political opponents, when they produce a counter argument or position.

The techniques of spin include selectively presenting facts and quotes that support one's position, the so-called "non-denial," phrasing in a way that assumes unproven truths, euphemisms for drawing attention away from items considered distasteful, and ambiguity in public statements. Another spin technique involves careful choice of timing in the release of certain news so it can take advantage of prominent events in the news. A famous reference to this practice occurred when British Government press officer Jo Moore used the phrase. It's now a very good day to get out anything we want to bury, widely paraphrased or misquoted as "It's a good day to bury bad news", in an email sent on September 11, 2001. The furor caused when this email was reported in the press eventually caused her to resign.

Spin Doctors

Skilled practitioners of spin are sometimes called "spin doctors," despite the negative connotation associated with the term. It is the PR equivalent of calling a writer a "hack". Perhaps the most well-known person in the UK often described as a "spin doctor" is Alastair Campbell, who was involved with Tony Blair's public relations between 1994 and 2003, and also played a controversial role as press relations officer to the British and Irish Lions rugby union side during their 2005 tour of New Zealand.

State-run media in many countries also engage in spin by selectively allowing news stories that are favorable to the government while censoring anything that could be considered critical. They may also use propaganda to indoctrinate or actively influence citizens' opinions. Privately run media also uses the same techniques of 'issue' versus 'non-issue' to spin its particular political viewpoints.

Meet and Greet

Many businesses and organizations will use a Meet and Greet as a method of introducing two or more parties to each other in a comfortable setting. These will generally involve some sort of incentive, usually food catered from restaurants, to encourage employees or members to participate.

There are opposing schools of thought as to how the specific mechanics of a Meet and Greet operate. The Gardiner school of thought states that unless specified as an informal event, all parties should arrive promptly at the time at which the event is scheduled to start. The Kolanowski school of thought, however, states that parties may arrive at any time after the event begins, in order to provide a more relaxed interaction environment.

OTHER

- Publicity events, pseudo-events, photo ops or publicity stunts.
- The talk show circuit. A PR spokesperson (or his/her client) "does the circuit" by being interviewed on television and radiotalk shows with audiences that the client wishes to reach.
- Books and other writings.
- Blogs.
- After a PR practitioner has been working in the field for a while, he or she accumulates a list of contacts in the media and elsewhere in the public affairs sphere. This "Rolodex" becomes a prized asset, and job announcements sometimes even ask for candidates with an existing Rolodex, especially those in the media relations area of PR.
- Direct communication carrying messages directly to constituents, rather than through the mass media with, e.g. newsletters"—in print and e-letters.
- Collateral literature, traditionally in print and now predominantly as web sites.
- Speeches to constituent groups and professional organizations; receptions; seminars, and other events; personal appearances.
- The slang term for a PR practitioner or publicist is a "flack" (sometimes spelled "flak").
- A desk visit is where the PR person literally takes their product to the desk of the journalist in order to show them what they are promoting.
- Astroturfing is the act of PR agencies placing blog and online forum messages for their clients, in the guise of a normal "grassroots" user or comment.
- Online social media.

Defining the Opponent

A tactic used in political campaigns is known as "defining one's opponent." Opponents can be candidates, organizations and other groups of people.

In the 2004 US presidential campaign, Howard Dean defined John Kerry as a "flip-flopper," which was widely reported and repeated by the media, particularly the conservative media. Similarly, George HW Bush characterized Michael Dukakis as weak on crime (the Willie Horton ad) and hopelessly liberal ("a card-carrying member of the ACLU"). In 1996, President Bill Clinton seized upon opponent Bob Dole's promise to take America back to a simpler time, promising in contrast to "build a bridge to the 21st century". This painted Dole as a person who was somehow opposed to progress.

In the debate over abortion, self-titled pro-choice groups, by virtue of their name, defined their opponents as "anti-choice", while self-titled pro-life groups refer to their opponents as "pro-abortion" or "anti-life".

Managing Language

If a politician or organization can use an apt phrase in relation to an issue, such as in interviews or news releases, the news media will often repeat it verbatim, without questioning the aptness of the phrase. This perpetuates both the message and whatever preconceptions might underlie it. Often, something innocuous sounding can stand in for something greater; "culture of life" sounds like general goodwill to most people, but will evoke opposition to abortion for many pro-life advocates. The phrase "States' rights" was used as a code for anti-civil rights legislation in the United States in the 1960s, and, allegedly, the 70s, and 80s.

Conveying the Message

The method of communication can be as important as a message. Direct mail, rob calling, advertising and public speaking are used depending upon the intended audience and the message that is conveyed. Press releases are also used, but since many newspapers are folding, they have become a less reliable way of communicating, and other methods have become more popular.

Arts organizations have begun to rely more on their own websites and have developed a variety of unique approaches to publicity and public relations, on and off the web.

The country of Israel has recently employed a series of Web 2.0 initiatives, including a blog, MySpace page, YouTube channel Facebook page and a political blog to reach different audiences. The Israeli Ministry of Foreign Affairs started the country's video blog as well as its political blog. The Foreign Ministry held the first microblogging press conference via Twitter about its war with Hamas, with Consul David Saranga answering live questions from a worldwide public in common text-messaging abbreviations. The questions and answers were later posted on IsraelPolitik, the country's official political blog.

Front Groups

One of the most controversial practices in public relations is the use of front groups – organizations that purport to serve a public cause while actually serving the interests of a client whose sponsorship may be obscured or concealed. Critics of the public relations industry, such as PR watch, have contended that Public Relations involves a "multi-billion dollar propaganda-for-hire industry" that "concocts and spins the news, organizes phoney 'grassroots' front groups, spies on citizens, and conspires with lobbyists and politicians to thwart democracy".

Instances of the use of front groups as a PR technique have been documented in many industries. Coal mining corporations have created environmental groups that contend that increased CO_2 emissions and global warming will contribute to plant growth and will be beneficial, trade groups for bars have created and funded citizens' groups to attack anti-alcohol groups, tobacco companies have created and funded citizens' groups to advocate for tort reform and to attack personal injury lawyers, while trial lawyers have created "consumer advocacy" front groups to oppose tort reform.

HOSPITAL OR HEALTH INSTITUTION PR

The PR in this context deals with the object of publicizing the information of institution to the general public in general and public surrounded and potential users in particulars with genuine information that would serve and facilitate the public. The PR main concern, not limited to this alone, is to bring the accurate and complete activities of the institution such as the functioning of Emergency, Outpatient and Inpatient services and different specialties prevailing in the vicinity for public purpose. And at the same time, the problems or any issues that public is encountering in obtaining the services or any other issues that related to health institution needs to be addressed in favor of users. The PR is a liaison officer between the public and the hospital.

In addition to this, PR also assists the authorities in conducting "health exhibitions" exposing hospital services, demonstration of any particular treatment or surgical procedure to ensure that the services offered are safe and improved quality. Generally, the responsibilities are to involve with the daily activities of the hospital and ensure that everything is going well to the satisfaction of public and any issue of public that hampers or inconvenience is brought to the organization notice to address at the earliest. Precisely, the very object of PR is to ensure that the hospital's operations are smoothly functioning to the utmost satisfaction of public. Another most important function is not only to publicize the new services or any service that is not operational in the hospital or health institution to the public but also to collect the views of patients, public what they expect from the health institution in term of services and facilities or any genuine demand related to health field and services to be brought to the notice of the hospital organization. The PR is "window and spokesperson" of health institution and the hospital users and the public.

31 Medical Secretarial Profession

The word secretary comes from the Latin *secretarius*, meaning "confidential employee". The secretary of today is still an employee who is responsible to maintain confidential information. In that respect, the job has not changed. However, the tools of the trade have changed over the years.

The secretary is a professional—not only because of the knowledge and preparation necessary for the job but also because being a professional implies competence, pride in one's work, and a dedication to excellence. The secretary is a professional with each of these qualities. Moreover, the secretary is an important member of the management team, responsible not only for carrying out the executive's wishes but also for helping to maintain a well-organized and efficient office.

Office automation and machine dictation have revolutionized the type of work that the secretary does, and changes are expected to continue. The changes that will take place in the future are impossible to predict, but the professional secretary—also sometimes known as the medical secretary, administrative assistant, administrative secretary, private secretary, or several other titles—will be able to learn and adapt to each new challenging environment.

SUCCEEDING IN THE PROFESSION

The relative ease with which a person can enter the secretarial profession is a plus. A high school education; typing, shorthand machine transcription, and filing skills; and knowledge of office procedures, word processing and computer equipment, and software packages will enable one to advance along a career path. A post-secondary education is an additional asset.

The secretary entering the work force is faced with a multitude of possible job situations. Although, the conditions under which a secretary works are fairly standard throughout the economy, a choice can certainly be made about location, the size of the company, and the company's services or products. Each and every area of the economy or business needs the expertise of a secretary, and the professional secretary has only to choose the field most interesting to him or her and the one in which career goals can be furthered, but today's secretary is also concerned with the possibilities for professional growth within a company.

Secretaries are professionals with career goals. Most large organizations have a human resources department that is concerned with the professional growth and development of their employees. By providing training and educational opportunities for employees from date of hire until retirement, these organizations are able to enhance the effectiveness of their operations and to enrich the lives of their employees.

Specialized training is a matter of professional survival in a world where the methods of handling information are changing rapidly. The secretary will be increasingly involved with office automation and needs to be familiar with the concept and the technology. The responsibilities of the secretary are multifunctional: typing/keyboarding; transcribing; processing mail; telephoning; scheduling appointments; greeting visitors; composing and editing documents; researching; coordinating meetings, conferences, and teleconferences; making travel arrangements; handling reprographics; and organizing time and work. Supervisor and management education and advanced technical and professional education are available to those who are interested in moving ahead in the organization. One of the great benefits of a well-developed education and training program is that people on the secretarial level can move into supervisory, administrative, and managerial positions if they have the desire and the ability to do so.

Secretaries are encouraged to develop career paths and life plans just as executives do. The secretary's projected work life is just as long as the executive's. These years will be more pleasant if the individual takes steps to examine what kind of job will be the most personally satisfying now and in the future. This kind of examination also benefits the organization, because it keeps personnel from changing companies when a change in work responsibility would be more satisfying.

Many organizations also encourage secretaries to avail themselves of outside educational opportunities through financial support. Frequently these outside courses must be job related or related to a degree which the company agrees would benefit the employee and employer. Sometimes, however, these courses are promoted for the personal enrichment of the employee. All of these personnel-development efforts increase the secretary's satisfaction with the job and the employer.

PROFESSIONAL DEVELOPMENT

Participation in professional organizations is one way a secretary can grow professionally. Organizations offer the opportunity to network with other professionals and promote personal development by providing information, contacts, and support. Several professional organizations sponsor annual conventions, local conferences, seminars and courses to enhance secretarial performance.

The following organizations provide many opportunities for service, educational, and professional growth: Professional Secretaries International (PSI), the Association of Information Systems Professionals (AISP), and the American Association for Medical Assistants (AAMA), the American Association for Medical Transcription (AAMT), and the National Association of Legal Secretaries (International). Several of these organizations sponsor certification programs.

Professional Secretaries International (PSI) promotes an awareness of professional pride and the maintenance of high standards by promulgating the following definition:

Definition of a Secretary

Dr Mogli defines a secretary "as a person qualified to hold secretarial responsibilities, with positive mindset and behavior that enable to perform effectively as an executive assistant whose first characteristics is to maintain strict confidentiality of information maintained by her/him, who possesses a mastery of office skills, demonstrates the ability to assume responsibility without direct supervision, exercises initiative and judgment, and makes decisions within the scope of assigned authority and is a spokes person of the office or clinic or organization whose message is truly valid and represents the organization. In real sense is the cog of the wheel, his actions can be admirable or harmful."

The importance of an organization like Professional Secretaries International (PSI) cannot be overemphasized. All professional people take pride in their affiliation with organizations that attest to the importance of their field. Lawyers have bar associations; doctors have the Medical Association: teachers have national educational organizations. In each of these groups the purpose is to set standards for the profession and to honor those who meet the standards. Professional Secretaries International awards the title of Certified Professional Secretary (CPS) to those who have passed a certificate examination. The title of Certified Professional Secretary brings respect from peers and superiors.

The examination that the aspiring secretary must take calls upon knowledge that has been gained through education and work experience. Office administration and communication, office technology accounting, economics and management, business law and behavioral science in business are the areas covered by the test. For one who has not yet become a Certified Professional Secretary, membership in PSI and participation in the local chapter's activities will bring a sense of the importance of a secretary's job to the functioning of society and will introduce the secretary to others who have similar professional goals.

TOOLS OF THE PROFESSION

Keyboarding, shorthand, transcription, filing, office procedures, and knowledge of word processing systems and equipment are the skills for which the secretary was hired. However, the ability to use the language and a commitment to professionalism will earn respect and promotions.

Language

The raw material to which the secretary applies these skills is the English Language. A command of and respect for the English Language, both in writing and in speaking are essential. A good dictionary, a thesaurus, and a grammar book must be kept handy for immediate checking of spelling, end-of-line division, usage and sentence construction. In the automated office, equipment may have a built-in spell checker or a software program with a dictionary or grammar component. Work still has to be proofread, however, because the equipment and programs cannot distinguish between homonyms, nor can they determine if the transcript omitted a word. Letters, whether the secretary composes them or transcribes them, represent the company, the employer, and the professional secretary.

The recipient of a letter must never get the impression that any one of the three is less than first rate. Most executives have a good speaking command of the language. This asset is often one of the reasons why an individual reaches a top management position. However, it is the secretary's responsibility to check details of grammar, spelling and punctuation. An employer with an excellent command of English presents a double challenge to the secretary. Transcribed letters must be absolutely perfect, and letters composed for the executive must match them in composition, tone and clarity.

The secretary may occasionally be the final check on grammar. An executive may have been hired for an area of technical expertise, not language ability. In this case the secretary will be responsible for editing all of the written communications from the office. The executive and the secretary in this situation must realize their mutual dependence and work to turn out superior written material. Correcting a dangling participle or making the verb and subject agree will demonstrate to the executive that the secretary is a professional with extremely valuable skills.

Professional Reading

Trade journals are published for each area of the economy and for each profession. By reading these publications, the secretary demonstrates professional concern and also learns new ideas and new vocabulary that may soon find its way into transcription. The competent secretary does not have to read these magazines from cover to cover but will develop a system for skimming, using the table of contents as a guide, to stay abreast of developments.

Numerous magazines and professional journals pertaining to the secretarial profession and business management and organization are available. These periodicals will help the secretary cope with difficult situations by discussions of how others solved similar problems and will alert the secretary to new products, procedures, and equipment for the office.

Reading magazines such as The Secretary, Fortune, Business Week, Forbes, Today's Office, and Office Administration and Automation is part of the commitment to professional excellence.

Information Processing

The combination of word processing and microcomputer systems has revolutionized the way secretaries work and process information. More and more offices have acquired the most sophisticated technological equipment, and the secretary needs only the ability and the desire to grow and change with each new development or modification.

Such systems provide an automated information center that upgrades the quality of hard copy materials while improving office efficiency by increasing the speed with which the material is produced. Today's businesses must deal with more written information than ever before, and they must transmit that information quickly and accurately. The secretary who puts the material into the system is irreplaceable, but the system can perform at speeds that a typist would find impossible. Material for bulk mailing and form letters can be keyboarded in a much shorter time by the equipment. If an executive decide to insert three paragraphs on page 60, of a 200 page document no longer means that the entire document must be re-keyboarded. The material to he inserted is keyboarded into the machine, and the finished document is produced, often in seconds. Complete documents of hundreds of pages can be sent from one office to another in minutes, rather than days. And, by using satellite communication, a subsidiary company's entire monthly report can be transmitted to the home office half a continent away in 30 seconds.

New vocabulary and procedures must be learned to use the information processing equipment. The competent secretary will not only learn how to respond to the instructions of the system but will also make every effort to understand how the system works and how best to make use of the various options offered. Entirely new systems of office management have resulted with the installation of word processing systems, word processors, microcomputers and numerous software programs.

The future is unlimited for the secretary who takes advantage of all training opportunities and remains open and flexible to the changes that will certainly develop in the industry.

A Professional Manner

The secretary is classified as a white-collar, however, the secretary should view clothing as a uniform that fits the image of the office and thus advances the secretary's career goals along with the purpose of the office. If the office is very informal, the secretary who wishes to be noticed and moved ahead will wear clothing that is just a shade more formal and more professional. The goal is not to alienate other workers but to make oneself stand out as the secretary who takes work seriously. When the executive office has an opening, the secretary who has demonstrated the most personal polish, in addition to superb skills, is the one who will be chosen.

A proper office manner should be cultivated by the secretary, and this manner should be based on the fact that the executive and the secretary are expected to work as a team. The secretary should follow the lead of the executive in office style. Whether working for an individual, a pair of executives, or a whole department, the secretary's duty is to help fulfill the executive job responsibilities. Therefore, assignments that appear in the job description (if there is one) are done conscientiously, and those chores that do not appear but that need to be done in order to free the executive from routine tasks will be done by the professional secretary without grumbling.

Much has been written about people moving ahead in careers because of the mentor/protégé system whereby a seasoned hand in the business takes on the education of someone younger who has promise. Although, the superior may be grooming someone for a place on the management level, the secretary can also he a protégé who moves upward in salary and responsibility with the boss or with the boss's blessing.

As part of the team, the professional secretary protects the employer. He or she does not contribute information to office gossip but does report any rumor that may be helpful to the superior, first qualifying the information as gossip. Also, the professional does not spend company time on personal phone calls, in clock watching, or in being late.

COMPETENT SECRETARY

The secretary plans not only a career path but also short- and long-range work for the company. Short-range planning enables the secretary to do each day those things that must be done. For example, a routine is established whereby the secretary's and the employer's desks are ready for work at the beginning of each day. Standard procedures for handling mail, for advising the executive of telephone calls, and for handling dictation and transcription are set-up, but this schedule does not lead to inflexibility. The competent secretary is capable of taking any kind of interruption in stride. When the emergency or interruption has been dealt with, the work routine is resumed at the point of interruption. Long-range planning makes it possible for the secretary to concentrate on low-priority projects at a slow time of the year and also makes it possible for the executive to call on secretarial aid at times when the work flow is heavy.

Effective Use of Time

The secretary's time is a valuable and perishable commodity. All duties are performed as quickly as possible so that the unexpected may be dealt with. A sense of the relative urgency of activities is developed with experience, so that it is possible to distinguish the important from the trivial. A long-distance caller does not distract the secretary from the necessity to transcribe an urgent letter. The unexpected visitor is started on his or her way courteously and firmly rather than being allowed to waste company time.

Business calls are evaluated for length, and they are not continued beyond the time that is absolutely essential for courtesy and the exchange of information. The secretary should structure the business call in the form of a business letter. It should be planned ahead and should have a beginning, middle, and end. If one is making a call, a clear statement of purpose should open, followed by details, questions or whatever the call must accomplish. The call should be completed by thanking the person on the other end, stating the action you or your boss expect to be taken, or getting a firm commitment for future action or the time of a return call. Remember that this is a business call and avoid those verbal ticks like "you know" and slang that would be appropriate in a personal call.

Responsibility and Follow-up

By carefully following through on any tasks assigned, the secretary demonstrates a sense of responsibility everyday. When the employer is out, the secretary displays professionalism by making sure that the office is covered at all times, especially when the workday begins in the morning. Every experienced secretary knows that this is when the problems start.

Take, for example, a situation in which the executive and the secretary are the only ones who know all aspects of a given situation. When the boss is away, something that vitally affects that matter happens. The competent secretary is present and immediately gets in touch with the employer so that the appropriate course of action can be decided and so that the secretary can set the wheels in motion.

Relationship with Executive

The personal relationship between the executive and the secretary will vary according to the people involved and the formality of the company. The secretary should always remember that the relationship is a business arrangement and that the structure of any organization makes the executive more important than the secretary. Without the executive to set the overall objective and to plan for action to attain that objective, the secretary's job would not exist. Nevertheless, the indispensable contribution of the secretary to the execution of the executive's work should be taken as a source of professional satisfaction but not as an indispensable individual.

The executive may ask the secretary to explain a matter, but the secretary does not have the right to call upon the executive to justify decisions. However, when a good working relationship exists, office authority is not a source of discontent because both the secretary and the executive realize that they are there to make that office run at peak efficiency.

No job is without its dull routines as well as its stimulating aspect. No employer is without faults. There may be times when you consider your employer unreasonable. You may be asked to do chores that you consider demeaning or outside your province or job description. Decide how intrusive these jobs are, and discuss the matter with your employer. Perhaps, the duties can be added to your job description. Otherwise, see if you can arrange for the writing of a job description if there is none.

Appropriate Behavior

Personal life must be separated from professional life in dealing with all office personnel. It is very possible to work well with people one does not like at all; likewise, it is possible to work professionally with people who are personal friends. Personal problems should not be brought into the office. However, worries about sickness at home, financial problems and domestic difficulties do affect the quality of work, and the professional will do everything possible to keep the level of professional performance high. The fact that a doctor has personal troubles is not an acceptable excuse for a faulty diagnosis of a patient. One expects the doctor to perform well, and the executive has the right to expect the secretary to remain competent despite difficulties. People, however, are not machines and are not expected to behave as such. When overwhelming problems are present, the supervisor should be told before one's work is held up for censure.

Professional behavior as part of a team determines the relationships with the rest of the organization. In dealing with other members of the group, the secretary should make it clear that those others are viewed as the experts in their jobs. The professional secretary is courteous to everyone regardless of the individual's position on the company ladder. The order-processing clerk, the shipping clerk, the receptionist, the typist, and the file clerk will be much more helpful to the secretary/executive team if this attitude of professionalism is maintained.

Alertness to Mistakes

The secretary must be very honest in all relationships within the company. Blame must be accepted if a mistake has been made. Everyone makes mistakes, and the good secretary will do everything possible to avoid them. The need to make use of other people's expertise must be recognized, and the secretary should help others in the office in an effort to foster a spirit of helpfulness to insure that good work is turned out. For example, even if a secretary's typing can be called excellent, proofreading of important documents should be done by two people. The secretary should therefore try to make arrangements to proofread material with a coworker.

Alertness to the mistakes of others so that the mistakes may be corrected is characteristic of the competent secretary. Especially if work is done under pressure, people have a tendency not to check a figure, proofread a page, or make certain that a statement conforms to policy. The secretary must check and double-check to avoid errors that, more than simply being embarrassing, might affect important decisions adversely.

Level of Authority

Differentiating between the executive's requests and the secretary's requests is necessary. In the first instance, the secretary has a lot of authority; in the second instance, there is much less. If the executive needs the report by 5 PM, the department responsible will recognize that the effort and expense are inconsequential compared to the importance of meeting the deadline. However, the secretary must not push co-workers unless the pressure is justified. Everyone has a schedule to which he or she must adhere. Remember to respect the importance and the schedules of other people's work. Never claim authority for yourself when you are passing on the executive's wishes. "Professor Mark would like all class schedules completed by friday" will get a better response than "I would like all class schedules completed by friday". Even with suggestions the same rule is followed. A suggested course is far more likely to be implemented if put forward as the boss's idea, particularly if it involves difficulty.

Accurate Record-Keeping

The secretary's filing system gets the same careful attention given to other duties. The employer must have an accurate record of what has happened in the past in order to take future action. For highly confidential matters or the employer's personal correspondence, a system consistent with filing rules but responsive to the needs of the office should be set up. If the company has a central files department, the secretary works closely with the assigned file clerk, whose expertise should be recognized.

Filing is a historical recording of events that have occurred in a given aspect of company development. Filing requires intelligence, an intimate knowledge of the subject matter, and an organized method of recording. The secretary should work with the file clerk. All material should be carefully marked to indicate whether there has been any previous correspondence on the subject. If the previous reference could not be easily identified by the file clerk, a notation indicating the subject with which it should be filed is a courtesy that will save time, prevent confusion, and contribute to a helpful attitude in the office, which will be to everyone's benefit. If a subject is especially important or unusually complicated, an exchange of ideas may enable the file clerk to set up the file intelligently. A sense of history on the part of the secretary and the file clerk will enable them to build up a file coherently, so that a person reading it will be able to determine the sequence of events and the actions taken. When the secretary recognizes the complexity of the file clerk's job, the employer will get the file or information sought, not an excuse.

Today, many firms have computer equipment and documents are stored on disks and automatically filed in the system.

SECRETARIAL SPECIALTIES

A competent secretary may work in one particular type of office and become familiar with the equipment, vocabulary, procedures and duties specific to that type of office. In some cases, specific training is required. A few secretarial specialties are discussed here and a more detailed discussion of some of the more common ones is provided later in the book in the major section titled "For the Specialized Secretary".

Executive Secretary

The executive secretary or the administrative assistant is more than just a secretary or an assistant to an executive, in some companies and organizations, the terms seem to be interchangeable; in other companies, one is placed above the other on the organizational ladder. Whether one uses the term executive secretary or administrative assistant, in terms of responsibility, knowledge of the company's business, judgment and experience, this person is an executive. The executive secretary (the term we shall use in this discussion) may indeed employ a secretary or a whole staff. Making decisions that affect an important segment of the company's operations and, in some cases, taking charge of business while the executive is absent brings the executive secretary financial and personal rewards. But these benefits are earned. At this highest level of secretarial authority, the responsibilities are such that the greatest possible effort to check procedures and avoid errors is essential. Planning, discretion, knowledge, accuracy, efficiency, and dependability are watchwords of the job. The executive secretary has top skills and keeps them serviceable. Technical skills and knowledge of the latest automated equipment are essential.

Confidence of the executive's staff is built slowly and carefully. These are the people who have the responsibility to carry out the objectives of the company or department. The executive secretary's duty is to screen demands on the executives time, not to make the executive as unapproachable as Presidents of the United States have sometimes been made by their staffs.

Decisions must he made promptly; action must be taken swiftly. Anything that slows that action is detrimental to the overall operation of the company. When a member of the staff has to see the boss it may be because that person faces some decision beyond the scope of his or her particular authority. It may seem a simple matter to give notice that the subordinate has to see the executive, but what if the secretary has six or seven calls from different staff members? Who sees the executive first, who next, and who not at all? It is up to the secretary to win the confidence of each member of the staff so that person will be absolutely honest as to the urgency of any particular request. Each has to know that if the employee says, "I must have it five minutes before noon", he or she will have it if it is humanly possible, and that if the employee says, "Tomorrow will be fine", he or she will see the executive tomorrow without any further reminders to the secretary. In such circumstances, maximum use is made of everyone's time. The secretary can work out an orderly plan with the executive to conserve time. The subordinate can attend to other projects without wasting time calling back or attempting to waylay the executive in the hail. In this cooperative atmosphere, everyone realizes that the short-term advantage would not be worth the risk of losing the secretary's confidence.

The secretary must always be aware of being a representative of the executive, and while the staff is subordinate to the executive, the staff is not subordinate to the secretary. As the subordinates' confidence grows, they will ask advice or opinions on how the boss would like something done. The secretary has a responsibility to give accurate advice and to state only opinions that truly represent the executive's feelings. If the secretary's personal opinion is given, the subordinate may be misled as to the executive's actual sentiments on the matter.

The executive secretary cannot play favorites. The executive must view operations as a whole and must be able to depend upon the secretary to reflect this accurately in dealing with subordinates. It is important that each staff member be recognized as an integral part of the team and as making a contribution to the company. Each employee wants the good opinion of the boss, and perhaps even without consciously recognizing it, the secretary's reaction to an employee may be interpreted as a reflection of the boss's opinion. The secretary must remember that a personality trait that is unattractive to the secretary may be exactly the trait that makes the subordinate effective in a particular function. The boss may have a higher opinion of the former than of the latter, and a secretary's favoring of the affable over the precise subordinate might be doing an injustice to both individuals and to the executive. By dampening the enthusiasm of one and giving a false sense of confidence to the other, the executive is misrepresented and the company's objectives may be impeded. The job of executive secretary or administrative assistant is challenging and rewarding and a lot of hard work. Intelligence, interest, dedication, plus experience and training are essential for success.

Legal Secretary

Accuracy and speed are the hallmark of the legal secretary in the one-lawyer office or the large firm with a national reputation. The work of a law office is exacting; an inaccurate record can be extremely expensive to the firm. Terminology is precise. Since many legal procedures have to follow an initial action in exact sequence, timing and organization are essential.

Typing/keyboarding, shorthand, transcription skills, and acknowledge of legal documents and legal terminology are important. Verbal and writing ability are essential because the legal secretary's work is very exacting. The work is also highly varied and involves extensive contact with clients. The legal secretary must, of course, refrain from answering legal questions.

Word-processing systems and microcomputers have been added to most law offices to aid in the preparation of legal documents. The secretary who wishes to remain in the field should take advantage of every opportunity to learn the newest automated equipment.

The legal secretary's job is not easy due to lot of work and pressure, there usually are long hours of work. However, it is one of the most lucrative jobs in the secretarial field. Some advantages in working as legal secretary gets more fringe benefits, and generous vacation. The legal secretary may become a certified professional legal secretary. The Certified Professional Legal Secretary designation is the only certification program for legal secretaries providing a standard measurement of legal secretarial knowledge and skills. Any person who has had five years' experience as a legal secretary and who meets the other application requirements may sit for a rigorous two-day examination. A partial waiver of the five year experience requirement may be granted if the applicant has a bachelor's associate's degree. Seven important areas of legal secretarial practice and procedures are included in the examination: written communication skills and knowledge; ethics; legal secretarial procedures; legal secretarial accounting; exercise of judgment; legal secretarial skills: and legal terminology, techniques, and procedures.

Medical Secretary

Medical secretaries are generally employed in a physician's office, medical clinic, hospital, public health facility, health maintenance organization, nursing home, research center, laboratory, insurance company. Government departments, health services, pharmaceutical company, private agency, publishing company, medical department of a business organization, business that manufactures medical supplies and equipment, or medical transcription service agencies. Earlier each job requires keyboarding skills, machine transcription and acknowledges of word processing but now expect more computers literacy and software programs in addition to familiarity with medical terminology.

The medical secretary may need to know how to perform certain medical tasks, how to complete insurance claim forms, how to take a patient's medical history, how to handle the doctor's billings, and how to perform other clerical duties peculiar to a doctor's office. In addition, the secretary may need to deal with people who are ill, a task requiring patience, sympathy and tact.

Regardless of the setting—a one-doctor office or a large facility— the medical secretary must observe medical ethics. Cases should not be discussed except in the context of office business, and no comments or questions regarding a patient's condition or ailments should be made in the presence of other persons.

The professional medical assistant enjoys an enviable professional status. The medical assistant is eligible to join the American Association of Medical Assistants (AAMA) and can apply for certification. The AAMA offers a certifying examination, the successful completion of which leads to a certificate and recognition as a Certified Medical Assistant-Administrative (CMA-A) or a Certified Medical Assistant- Clinical (CMA-C) or both. The examination is given in January and June of each year at designated centers throughout the United States. As of 1988, revalidation every five years is mandatory, and it can be accomplished through Continuing Education Units (CEUs) or re-examination.

The AAMA provides members the opportunity of attending local, state, and regional meetings and a national convention where one can participate in workshops, learn of educational advances in the field, visit exhibits, hear prominent speakers, and establish a networking system with other medical assistants. The association publishes a bimonthly journal "The Professional Medical Assistant".

The American Association for Medical Transcription (AAMT) member has the opportunity to attend local, state and regional meetings and a national convention where one can participate in workshops, learn of educational advances in the field, visit exhibits, hear prominent speakers, and establish a networking system with other medical transcriptionists. The association publishes a professional journal four times a year, the journal of the AAMT, and publishes a newsletter six times a year, the AAMT Newsletter.

The AAMT offers a certifying examination, with successful completion leading to a certificate and recognition as a Certified Medical Transcriptionists (CMT). The examination is given on the last Saturday in April and a specialty examination on the first Saturday in November at various locations throughout the United States. Certification by examination is valid for three years and may be renewed by paying the annual continuing education assessment fee and earning a minimum of 30 continuing education credits in each three-year period of certification, or achieving a passing score on the certification examination every three years. Of the 30 continuing education units, at least 20 must be in the medical science category. A CMT must continue upgrading skills through attending the Association's lectures and obtaining Continuing Education Units (CEUs).

Technical Secretary

The growth of research, both governmental and private, and the explosion of knowledge have created the need for secretaries with the ability to deal with technical terms and symbols. Typing, editing and proofreading are necessary skills for all secretaries, but technical secretaries must possess the highest level of skills. The ability to accurately type information that can be understood only by the researchers is essential, and the ability to proofread material that makes little or no sense to someone who is not technically trained in the field is indispensable.

The technical secretary must also recognize that the scientists and researchers have been hired for their technical competence, not their writing skill, and frequently the secretary will need to edit material to make it grammatically correct and smooth flowing. This task calls for much tact, patience, and humility in the face of material that is written in English but is often incomprehensible to the layperson. However, for the secretary with the ability to deal with mathematical equations, Greek letters, and so forth, advancement to the level of technical aide and research assistant is possible.

The technical secretary's job is demanding and exacting and requires specialized skills. A strong background in mathematics, science and technical terminology is a definite asset. The remuneration and benefits in these situations are usually quite good.

Educational Secretary

The opportunities for secretaries in educational institutions from the preschool to the graduate level are as varied as the institutions themselves. The secretary in the elementary school may occasionally have to comfort a sick child who is waiting to go home or help a parent deal with the multiple forms that educational systems require. In higher education the secretary may be assigned to a specific academic or administrative area. The educational secretary meets school visitors and has close contact with students, teachers and parents.

The duties of the secretary vary from school to school and often depend on its size. In a small school the secretary may have to handle student records, transcripts of grades, orders for materials and supplies, personnel records, the scheduling of facilities, and many other tasks. In larger institutions the secretary may be assigned just one of these duties or may be responsible for a specific department.

The minimum education requirement for an educational secretary varies. In some institutions a high school education is sufficient, whereas in others, especially colleges and universities, some type of college experience or a degree is required.

Secretary in Advertising, Radio and Television, Journalism, and the Arts

The skills required for these jobs are the same as for a job in any business, but the amount of contact with interesting personalities, public figures, and the public is increased. When dealing with public personalities, the secretary must be able to maintain a professional manner. If the employer does not wish to talk to a local public figure or a network newsperson, the secretary must be firm and diplomatic. Jobs in these fields require the ability to deal with people whose job it is to manipulate responses.

The professional secretary will decide just what kind of job will give the most satisfaction and the kind of atmosphere that will be pleasant. Will the high-pressure atmosphere of an advertising agency or television station make you nervous or will it challenge you? The fact that you are contributing to the success of a museum may be the kind of reward that means the most to you. The excitement of putting any kind of publication "to bed" may be just what you want.

Secretary in US Government

The federal government is the largest employer in the United States and should not be overlooked by the professional secretary. In order to become eligible for most governmental positions, the secretary must take a written civil service examination. Promotions are usually made from within based on availability and the demonstrated skill and industry of the applicant. Government positions offer annual salary increments, job security and retirement systems.

Usually, there are employment opportunities for secretaries in foreign countries. The Department of State has Foreign Service offices in over 300 cities worldwide. Other jobs are also available in the public sector. State, county, and municipal governments, plus the many quasi-governmental agencies, all have need of skilled secretaries.

The secretary who is interested in public service should contact the office of personnel management in the region in which he or she wishes to obtain employment.

Secretary in Travel

Excitement and adventure are the benefits of secretarial work in the travel industry. Airlines, resorts and travel agencies often offer free or reduced rates in transportation, hotel accommodations, and tours to their employees. However, the job requires hard work. One must have a sincere liking for and a desire to help people. You are helping them to spend the money for which they have often worked hard all year. Also, you must deal with concerned offices that may have to get an executive to Europe as quickly as possible.

A secretary in the travel industry must know geography well, he able to read different companies' timetables, plan itineraries, and make reservations through a computer. In short, you must know how to do everything and anything that will contribute to the comfort and enjoyment of your company's customers. Above all, you must he accurate. The pleasure of a vacation or a business opportunity can be lost by a single error. Each year the volume of business and pleasure travel exceeds the previous years. A person with the right combination or interest in people and ability to deal with details will find a bright future as a secretary in the travel field.

SPECIAL EMPLOYMENT SITUATIONS

Most secretaries are employed on a full-time basis in a particular office. However, there are available certain other types of employment situations, among them temporary work and part-time work.

Temporary Secretary

Temporary employment services throughout the country fulfill a need for both employers and employees. The secretary who works on a temporary basis fills in vacancies created by vacations, illness, sudden resignations, or other situations including short-term openings during peak workload periods.

Secretaries take on temporary employment for a number of reasons. Some use temporary employment as an opportunity to explore different industries, organizations, and working conditions so as to determine a preference and a career path. For others, family obligations or other responsibilities make a permanent position inconvenient and a temporary situation ideal. A temporary position also permits a flexible schedule and a choice of job locations, and these considerations may be important to someone pursuing further education or an avocation.

Agencies that engage temporary employees prefer secretaries who have had experience so that they will be able to go into an office and immediately assume the responsibilities of the job. Temporary secretaries must be flexible, confident, and adaptable.

The pay in temporary work is slightly lower in many cases than that of permanent workers who have the same job skills and responsibilities.

Fringe benefits are becoming more available to temporary workers. Some agencies that place temporary secretaries in offices now offer group life and medical insurance, paid holidays, paid vacations, referral bonuses, seniority or longevity bonuses, profit sharing, scholarships and training on word processors, computers and related office equipment.

Part-time Secretary

Physician's offices, Medical Officers, educational institutions, small businesses, and, to a growing extent, large corporations often need part-time secretaries. The individual or firm may require only a few hours of work each day or only a few days per week. In other situations, a few weeks or a few months of the year may be required. Some companies are now willing to divide a full-time job between two part-time secretaries; two secretaries, in other words, share one full-time job. Part-time work enables the secretary to maintain skills while freeing the individual for other responsibilities or interests.

SECRETARY'S DAY

Job descriptions by their nature make the task of organizing the workday a bit easier, but if your job does not have a formal description of duties, organization is the word to keep in mind. Not only must the secretary's desk be organized but also the work that flows across the executive's desk must be ordered. Decisions about what is important must be made constantly, since most secretaries will have more work to do in one day than can be reasonably accomplished. The principle to be used to help one decide what is most important is the principle that keeps the executive and the secretary working together as a team.

The interests of the superior must come first, and the good secretary will be sure to perform tasks that the executive wants completed quickly and thoroughly. Deadlines between the secretary and the executive in the office may be missed because of extraordinary circumstances, but if your boss misses a deadline with higher company executives because your work was not completed on time, do not expect to have an excuse accepted.

The schedule for each day begins the afternoon before when the secretary goes through the tickler or follow-up folder to determine exactly what must be done the next day. The follow-up file should be set up in whatever way the secretary finds most convenient. If the office operates on a yearly schedule with certain meetings, promotions, and correspondence scheduled for the same time each year, the secretary may wish to have monthly tiles with notations about the amount of time it took to plan last year's tall sales meeting and the list of tasks to be performed in connection with that meeting. In an office that does not have this repetitive schedule. The secretary may use a desk calendar to keep track of letters to be answered, telephone calls that must be made, shipments expected and so forth. The secretary should make a list of the items that must be taken care of the next day and a list of appointments for the executive, along with pertinent information and the materials that should be prepared. To conclude the day, the equipment should he turned off and covered and the desk cleared so that the maintenance staff will be able to work.

The morning start with promptness, the office must be ready to function at whatever time it opens and the secretary should be at work in the office, not returning from the washroom or talking in the next office. Certain jobs must be performed each day, and the secretary taking over an office would be wise to make a list of these in the order in which they should be done until the routine becomes second nature.

Scanning the daily mail, and after opening the mail and putting the most important item on top, the trusted secretary may be required to call certain items to the executive's attention. This practice, however, should be begun only when permission has been given. The executive may ask that some of the journals and newspapers the office receives be skimmed and that pertinent articles, notices of new products, promotions, and so forth be marked for special notice.

Mail must be moved quickly from the secretary's desk to the appropriate correspondent; rerouting is done immediately. If some of the letters can be answered by the secretary, the executive may return them with notations about content. This letter-writing and typing task will then be completed as soon as possible.

Priority' of duties the previous afternoon the secretary should have made a list of tasks for the following day by using the techniques of time management. Tasks fall into three categories: those that must be done immediately, those that may be done, and those that may be put off. Just as the executive has a list of appointments, the secretary should have a list of tasks and some notation after each entry to indicate its relative importance. All necessary items can be given an A or 1; the tasks that should be done when there is time, a B or 2; and the tasks that can be left until a slack period, a C or 3. The mental exercise of deciding which items are the most important is the first steps in getting the day's work finished. The trap of putting down jobs which are part of the daily routine or filling the list from the third category must be avoided. Putting down small jobs just for the satisfaction of crossing them out is a dangerous game to play. The executive like to hear what is important and what next to be done, ordered instructions are carried out promptly.

The duties of a secretary are as varied as are jobs and employers. But in any situation it is safe to assume that the secretary is responsible for handling the mail, making calls and answering the telephone, taking and transcribing dictation, following up orders and work in progress, and organizing office work. More often than not, the secretary must keep track of the employer's appointments and maintain a filing system—all in addition to the specifics of the job.

The experienced secretary knows that it is impossible to keep everything in mind. Everything must be written down on the memo pad that is at hand at all times. Every request, every assignment, every message is noted. Nothing is left to memory or chance. The secretary's work procedure depends upon the nature of the job and the size of the company. Some offices have established routines; some employers will specify the methods they prefer; sometimes a departing secretary will train an incoming one. The basic tools of organization are a memo pad, a calendar, an appointment book and a telephone-address book or file.

The memo pad will function as an added memory bank. Notations are made from each phone call, each request for an answer, each new assignment. By writing the information down, the secretary is heed from the need to keep small pieces of information in a mental notebook. Also, by writing all information down, the secretary is able to resume work at the point of interruption.

Keeping an appointment book the appointment book is one of the most important records in the office. There are various methods of recording and following up appointments, but essential to each is the appointment book. In automated offices, there is an electronic calendar.

In some offices the book is kept on the executive's desk. The secretary must maintain an accurate duplicate appointment book so that both members of the office know how each day is to be spent. In other offices the executive assigns the appointment book to the secretary, who makes all of the appointments. To examine the book the executive will have to go to the secretary's desk and read it there or temporarily remove it.

Before making appointments, the secretary must be familiar with office procedure. Such matters as availability of executives, availability of conference rooms for meetings, daily arrival and departure limes and average schedules and length of conferences affect the making of appointments.

The appointment should be entered under the day and the hour agreed upon by the person requesting it and the secretary. The entry includes the names of the persons concerned, some notation of the topic to be discussed, and any other pertinent information. The secretary uses these notes to produce needed documents for the executive to read before the meeting. If the material is complex, the secretary may give it to the executive days ahead of time when the work flow is slow. On the day of the appointment the secretary follows through to be sure that there is no misunderstanding and to be sure that the appropriate materials and notes are on the executive's desk. If the appointment is canceled, arrangements for a new appointment should be made immediately.

Developing familiarity with sources of information the secretary who can find not only the names of those whom the employer must reach most frequently but also the names, addresses, and phone numbers for services, emergencies and sources of information is a valuable asset to the office and is rewarded as such. Many secretaries in education and research organizations will keep a separate file of reference books or sources with notations about the contents and the call letters if they are in the public or the company library. The secretary would do well to become familiar with the area's Yellow Pages and with the various sources of information listed in the section on reference materials in this volume.

Time- and Work-Saving Units

Time is one of a businessperson's most precious commodities. The secretary who learns to organize work and plan time wisely will save minutes out of every hour, hours out of every week. This free time will be used by the professional to expand knowledge and expertise.

Here are a few time- and work-saving suggestions:
- Make efficient use of your desk. Keep the surface clear of everything except your immediate work so you will not have to search through piles of other material when you want page
- Form the habit of using filing folders for anything of a temporary nature—work in progress, incoming or outgoing communications, work being held for additional information—and keep these folders in the file drawer of your desk where they are instantly accessible but not in the way.
- Plan your time; never waste it. When work is slow, one has to plan ahead to complete within the time. Do what can be done to relieve the workload at peak periods? Try to learn more about your company's operations. Consider what you can do to make your part of it run more smoothly. Become familiar with reference materials: learn how to use the reference books your boss consults frequently. The next time you may be able to find that chart or graph that is badly needed. Bring the address book up-to-date. Get to know the filing system.
- Learn to schedule your time realistically. It may take you an hour to type that stack of letters, provided that you are not

interrupted; but you will be. The telephone will ring, your employer will call upon you to take care of something urgent, and people will stop at your desk to ask questions. That one hour may become two or three hours. If you learn to expect interruptions, you will not be flustered by them or lose time trying to pick up where you left off. Interruptions are part of your work and require a place in your schedule.

* Be part of the team. When the workload is heavy, when your employers and other members of the staff are up against a deadline to get a job done, be willing to pitch in and help even if it is a little after closing time. Your ability of function as a professional will be remembered when you have a favor to ask and when you wish a promotion.

FUTURE

The need for skilled secretaries will continue to grow. The secretary of today and the future may be entering the field from high school, vocational school, or college; may be returning to work after many years of gap, or may be making a midlife career change. What all these secretaries have in common is their professionalism and their recognition of the importance of the work they do. The secretary of today and the future recognizes that a life's work deserves to be planned, and the professional secretary chooses a career path carefully. The professional secretary who will assume an important place in business and society will need to be able to respond to the concept and technology of information processing, possess decision-making ability and human relations skills, and be adaptable to learning new skills in a rapidly changing office environment. Secretaries can expect to take more responsibility as the more repetitious aspects of their jobs are automated.

MINUTES OF A MEETING

The executive may ask the secretary to take minutes at a formal or informal meeting. At minutes of meeting (MOM) is a term used to describe an official record of the proceedings of a meeting. Keeping minutes of meetings is always advisable. Although the minutes may not be disseminated, they should be filed in case they are needed at a later date.

Types of Meetings

There are basically two types of meetings: formal and informal. A formal meeting is a preplanned, structured meeting, such as an annual conference or convention and its workshops and symposia. Usually, there is a prepared agenda. An informal meeting may he short and announced only a short time before it is held; it is usually held on company premises. To inform staff members of a quickly scheduled meeting the secretary may use electronic calendaring, if available, or the telephone. Always confirm by sending a follow-up note.

Another type of meeting—a teleconference—has been made possible by modern technology. In a teleconference, two or more persons in different geographic locations communicate electronically (audio, video, and computer). It is effective for informal meetings and serves as an adjunct to more formal, structured meetings. By using audio, video, and/or computer equipment, including the electronic blackboard, meetings can he held simultaneously or on a delayed basis with several groups participating in various locations. Everything in a teleconference is taped.

The minutes of a teleconference can be completed from the recorded media. This allows the secretary time to devote to other duties. The minutes, when completed, can he distributed electronically.

Preliminary Duties

Preliminary duties before a formal meeting may include reserving the meeting room, sending pertinent materials, preparing mailing lists, making calendar notations, preparing an agenda (the order of business), and handling last—minute details, such as supply and equipment needs (e.g. overhead projector or VDT). If you plan to take shorthand notes at the meeting, be sure you have sufficient notebooks, pencils and other supplies. If you plan to record the meeting, check reel-to-reel or cassette recorders to ensure the equipment is operating and that you have sufficient supplies.

Some companies employ technical assistants to be available during electronic transmissions if needed. At a computer conference, the secretary may be asked to keyboard messages and retrieve stored data. These types of conferences should be planned in advance.

Preparing the Minutes

The most important phase of preparing minutes is the accurate recording and reporting of the actions taken. The record should report what was said. At times, it is difficult to report what is done. For informal meetings, the minutes are compact and simple; for formal meetings, the minutes are complex. If you find that grouping the minutes around a central theme is clearer, do so. On the other hand, the executive may prefer chronological order.

Corporate minutes (official minutes of a formal nature) must he prepared in the order of occurrence, showing details and the exact wording of motions, resolutions, and so forth. By law, corporations are required to keep minutes of stockholders' and directors' meetings. These minutes are legal records and should he protect from tampering.

When preparing corporate minutes, use watermarked paper, and place the finalized minutes in key lock binders. Any corrections resulting from a subsequent meeting should be written. Incorrect portions are ruled out in ink and initialed in the margin. The official secretary of the corporation has responsibility for the completeness and accuracy 01 corporate minute, but the secretary may have to type and prepare them.

OFFICE MEMORANDUMS

An office memorandum, almost universally referred to as memo, is basically a letter between company employees and is less formal than a traditional letter. It may be short or long, single or multipage. The secretary may compose memos as well as type them for executives.

Like all other office communications, memorandums transmit information and provide a record that information was transmitted. Office memorandums are used for several purposes: (a) For messages that are complicated; (b) To avoid making unnecessary telephone calls for business that may not be urgent; and (c) When a record is needed. They not only avoid situations that may be misunderstood but also protect people by having a written record. Usually, office memorandums are brief and direct. However, there are exceptions depending upon the nature, purpose, and scope of the subject discussed and the writer's purpose and intent.

The plural form of memorandum may be either memorandums (add "s") or memorandums (add "a"; Latin form). However, when composing or writing, be consistent and use only one form for the plural. Also, when typing from an originator's draft copy, always check for consistency in spelling.

Types of Memos

Interoffice Memorandum

The interoffice memorandum is an in-house communication and is sent to a person in your own firm or department within one location; in other words, it is confined. Forms vary widely from company to company. However, all the principles of writing and business correspondence apply to memorandums as they do to letters.

Intraoffice Memorandum

The intraoffice memorandum is used within the same company between offices in different buildings or locations. For example, Company A may have two offices in New York City and one in Westchester County. Thus, the written communication is external; that is, it is not distributed in one location but must be transmitted elsewhere.

Parts of a Memo

All memorandums, whether printed or not, are composed of similar elements (parts). However, format may differ. These elements include to/from, date, subject, body, and end references (i.e. reference initials, distribution of copies, etc.). There may be slight differences in heading and closing information or in the order of the elements, especially if the forms are printed.

INTRODUCTION

Despite the vast number of devices, methods, and alternatives for communicating information, the telephone remains the most popular means of communication. It allows for communication between two or more persons, and it is the key instrument in initiating tele-communication networks worldwide.

Since the telephone is such an important communication device. It is essential that the secretary use it to its maximum effectiveness and he familiar with its peripheral equipment.

TELEPHONE TECHNIQUES

The secretary is expected to be knowledgeable in the use of the telephone. It is also important to keep up with the constantly expanding and changing services available from the telephone company, as well as the many and varied pieces of equipment that can add to the efficient operation of the business office. The telephone is the most frequently used audio-communication medium in the business world. The dependence upon this instrument has grown so that currently over a billion telephone calls is made daily.

The reputation and good will of the employer and the firm may depend upon the secretary's approach and skill in using the telephone. Although most people in our society begin to use the telephone in early childhood, perhaps the majority of them still need to be trained in proper telephone techniques. An impressive way to point out defects in techniques, and one that results in a rapid and desirable change is to make a recording or tape of a telephone conversation. Such a recording emphasizes the faults in telephone techniques and vividly points out areas needing improvement. Many organizations, even though they are efficiently organized, lose customers, money, and good will simply because employees answering calls are incoherent, curt, or impolite.

Speaking Clearly and Pleasantly

The caller at the other end of the phone cannot see the person who is talking. This should be remembered at all times, for it means that the caller has no visual image on which to base impressions. The telephone caller's attention is focused entirely upon the audio impressions coming over the wires. If these sounds are jarring or unpleasant, a busy executive may quickly lose patience and discontinue association with the firm in question. On the other hand, a pleasant and understanding voice coming over an inanimate instrument can accomplish wonders. The power of the spoken word can and does exert a great impact upon the listener.

The telephone is not a nuisance instrument designed to interrupt the secretary in the midst of some important or complicated task. It is rather, a vital business communication facility that assists the employee in carrying out duties and responsibilities owed to the employer.

In order to enhance one's telephone personality, it is necessary to inject variety and flexibility into the voice, so as to convey mood and attitude in telephone conversations. These qualities can be obtained through pitch, inflection, and emphasis. The development of these qualities is individual. A high-pitched voice may convey an impression of childishness and immaturity or of impatience and irritability. On the other hand, a voice that is well modulated carries the impression of culture and polish. "Pitch" in speaking, like "pitch" in music, refers to the key in which one speaks. Everyone has a range of lone within which a pleasant speaking voice is possible, and it can be consciously controlled. Each person must be conscious of his or her own range and practice utilizing it effectively. An individual is said to speak in a "modulated" voice when the pitch is in the lower half of the possible range. This tonal range carries best and is easiest to hear over the telephone.

In cultivating an interesting individual telephone personality, voice development alone is insufficient; it is essential also that the speaker enunciate clearly and distinctly. A garbled and indistinct speech pattern will annoy the listener who cannot understand what is being said. Do not be afraid to move the lips. One cannot form rounded vowel sounds or distinct consonants unless the lips accomplish their function. It is not necessary to exaggerate or to become stilted; clear enunciation and pronunciation should be made a part of the secretary's natural, daily speech pattern, because it is just as important in face-to-face conversations as in telephone conversations. Above all, be sure that your voice reflects your personality, that it transmits alertness and pleasantness, and that it is natural, distinct, and expressive, and neither too loud nor too soft. Avoid repetitious, mechanical words and phrases, and try to enunciate in a manner that is neither too fast nor too slow.

Answering Promptly

Answering a business telephone call is similar to welcoming a visitor. Therefore, it is essential that each call be greeted by a prompt, effective, and pleasing answer.

The telephone should be placed on the secretary's desk so that it is readily accessible. A pad and pencil or pen should be kept handy in order to jot down necessary information. These should not be used for doodling when speaking on the phone: this habit distracts the secretary from the business at hand and interferes with giving the caller undivided attention.

When the telephone rings, answer it promptly—at the first ring, if possible. Try not to put incoming calls immediately on "hold"; many callers find this practice infuriating. If it becomes increasingly necessary to do this, the employer should be alerted, it may be desirable to install another telephone line and to hire another person, if only for the busiest hours of the day, to help handle incoming calls.

If the secretary finds it necessary to leave the desk, arrangements should be made to have someone else answer the telephone and take the messages during that interval. The instrument should not be left unattended. An unanswered telephone becomes an instrument of failure—failure to the company because of the loss of customers and failure of the individuals responsible. It is well to inform the person who covers the telephone why the secretary will be away from the desk and for how long. Armed with this information, the one who answers the telephone can be more helpful to the caller.

This courtesy, of course, should be extended in both directions. Each secretary should reciprocally cover the calls of colleagues when it becomes necessary for them to be away from their desks so that telephones are never unattended for any period of time.

In many businesses, if the telephone is unattended, an answering unit is used. This machine will record a message after a "beep" usually preceded by a message.

Identifying Who is Answering

For efficiency, the office should be identified immediately when the phone is answered. The secretary's name may also be given, it is correct to say, "Mr Wright's office; Miss Dubrowski speaking", or the firm name may be used, as, "Smith and Grey; this is Mr Lopez". The identification formula depends upon the size and structure of the organization. When the telephone is answered in this fashion, the caller is assured that the proper office has been reached. Avoid answering the business telephone by saying, "Hello". Using this form of greeting is much like saying, "Guess who this is", and is unbusinesslike. Business people have no time to play guessing games, and this form of address can become irritating, particularly if it is necessary to call the office frequently.

In answering calls for others, identify yourself and the office of the person whose calls are being taken. To quote an example: "Miss Laya' office; Mr James speaking." Unless this is done, the caller will not know whether the right person has been reached at all. If the caller expects to hear the voice of Miss Jones' secretary, he or she may be taken aback when an unfamiliar voice comes over the wire. The fact that the correct office has been reached is made clear at once.

Identifying Who is Calling

The wise secretary develops a keen ear and learns to recognize the voices of important or frequent callers. However, a word of caution does not become too sure of an infallible ear, for voices may sound different over the telephone. If the voice is known beyond a doubt, use the caller's name when speaking. If the voice has been identified correctly, the caller will be pleased to be recognized and addressed by name. Then speak to the person at the other end of the wire, not at the telephone. If the secretary was incorrect in identifying the voice before divulging any information, little harm was done. Since the caller will make the correction. Apologize tactfully and take up the business at hand. However, when the name of the caller is not revealed and/or the nature of the business is not identified, the secretary's skill at diplomacy comes into play.

Many executives prefer their secretaries to screen incoming calls. This must be done with tact and discretion. In some cases the executive will speak with anyone who calls but would like to know beforehand who is calling and the nature of the business. It is the secretary's duty to obtain this information before transferring the call to the executive. Curtness and rudeness must be avoided in doing so. It is correct to say, for example, "May I tell Mr Brown who is calling?" or "Mrs Winslow is talking on another line. Would you care to wait, or may I have her call you? I believe her other call may take some time." or "Mr Zobkiw is in conference. May I help you?" Be sincere and courteous in your explanation, but do not divulge information unnecessarily. Your goal is simply to find out tactfully who is calling if you can.

Screening Calls

Although some executives answer the telephone themselves, many depend upon their secretaries to answer all incoming calls. The secretary must, therefore, be familiar with the executive's preferences. It is important to learn which calls the secretary is expected to handle, which are to be referred to the executive, and which should be transferred to someone else. Consequently, the secretary must classify telephone callers accurately and quickly. Every call is important. Enough information must be ascertained to classify the call. A caller cannot be allowed to get to the end of a long inquiry before being referred to the proper person. In order to forestall this, the secretary may make a discreet vocal sound that may cause the caller to pause slightly so that the secretary may say, "Mr Chan in the shipping department should be able to help you with this. Please let me transfer your call to him".

Handling the Call

Generally thc calls that can be handled by the secretary are as follows:

Requests for information: The secretary can handle this type of call if the information is not confidential and if there is no doubt concerning the facts. Sometimes it may be necessary to check with the employer before imparting information. If any complications arise, it is always wiser to turn the call over to the executive, in certain situations; the secretary may ask for a letter of request and, upon its receipt and approval, respond.

Requests for appointments: The secretary is sometimes authorized to make appointments for the employer. However, both the executive's and the secretary's diary should be checked before any appointments are made in order to avoid conflicts. If the employer is out of the office, the appointment should be verified immediately upon return. Commitments could easily have been made about which the executive had either forgotten to inform the secretary or the opportunity had not yet arisen to have had them entered in the desk calendars.

Receiving information: Often the secretary can conserve the employer's time by taking down telephone information. If the message is taken in shorthand, this must be transcribed as soon as possible and placed on the employer's desk.

Transferring calls: If the call cannot be handled by the secretary or the employer, it should be transferred to the office that can give the caller the information sought. This should be done only with the caller's permission, however. If transferal is refused, obtain the information and call hack. If the caller agrees to a transfer, make sure that the right office is reached before hanging up and give the person in that office sufficient information so that the caller will not need to repeat it.

Secretary should know where the executive will be when away from the office, whether urgent messages can be relayed, and the expected time of return to the office.

Also, in taking calls for other persons in the office, as suggested above, it is helpful if one can state when the person called will return or whether the call can be transferred somewhere else. It is best to offer whatever information possible; otherwise the caller may get the impression of being put off with an excuse. Be courteous, and use discretion in explaining an absence from the office. It is less offensive to say, Miss Jones is away from her desk just now. May I have her call you, or would you prefer to leave a message?" than to say bluntly, "She's out", or "This is her coffee break", or "I don't know where she is". The secretary must always use tact in dealing with callers, whether it is for one's own executive or for another secretary whose calls are being taken.

Taking Action

The secretary should promise the caller some definite action and see to it that the promise is kept. If the caller is told that the executive will call back, then this information must be conveyed to the employer so that the call can be made. A broken promise can result in a canceled order or a lost customer, and it may take many months to regain lost good will.

On some calls that the secretary can handle, more information may be needed than is within immediate reach. Therefore, it may become necessary to leave the telephone to look up the necessary information and to inform the caller of this fact and of the length of time it may take to obtain the material. Offer the caller a choice of waiting or of being called back. The customer should never be left waiting for an unreasonable amount of time at the other end of the wire. If a promise is made to call back with the needed information, this promise must be honored.

If the caller is waiting to speak to the executive, the secretary should reassure the caller periodically that the call will be connected as soon as the employer is free. Otherwise the caller will he uncertain as to whether the call is still connected, and a minute's silent delay will seem like a half-hour's wait. When the secretary is ready to transfer the call, thank the customer for waiting.

Completing the Incoming Call

At the completion of the call, indicate readiness to terminate the conversation by summing up the details. Use the caller's name when saying a pleasant "Goodbye". It is courteous to wait for the caller to terminate the call first; the secretary who is too hasty in hanging up the receiver may cost the firm money. The impression may be given that the caller's business is of little importance to the organization because the call is cut short. Permitting the caller to say "Goodbye" first also allows time for last-minute orders or special instructions. The receiver should be replaced gently in its cradle, for the pleasantest "Goodbye" can be spoiled by the jarring sound of a receiver dropped into position. It is like slamming the door after a visitor. The abruptness may not be intentional, but the effect is the same. Do not hang up until your caller has done so first.

Limiting Personal Calls

Because of the secretary's status and the prestige of that position, an example should be set for the office personnel by refraining from making and accepting personal calls during business hours except those that stay strictly within the rules set by the employer. The policy of the company or executive should be determined by the secretary at the very beginning of employment.

Telephone Dictation

Frequently the secretary is called upon to take dictation over the telephone. For this reason a shorthand notebook and pen should be placed near the telephone and ready for use. The caller is always informed of the fact that the conversation will be taken by the secretary. The secretary picks up the receiver and indicates readiness to record the proceedings. In the case of telephone dictation, unlike dictation taken at the employer's desk, the dictator cannot tell whether the secretary is getting all the information. Therefore it is necessary for the secretary to repeat the material phrase by phrase as it is taken down in shorthand.

This informs the dictator as to the rate of dictation, clarity of reception, and errors in grammar or facts. Corrections can then be made immediately instead of waiting until the end of the dictation, which may lead to confusion. If the dictation is too fast, it is best to indicate this immediately. It is a good practice to read back the notes at the termination of the dictation to ensure that the correct information was received and recorded and to correct any misinterpretations. The notes should be transcribed as soon as possible, and a copy should be sent to the telephone dictator. Of course, if the transcription equipment is used is of the type that can be utilized for recording telephoned dictation, the caller will be able to complete the dictation far more rapidly.

Telephone Reference Materials

The efficient secretary must be aware of the available sources of information that will be of help in placing a call expeditiously, skillfully, and economically. Directories and booklets published by the telephone company provide much information. A desk file for frequently used numbers should also be maintained. In the modern automated office, a secretary with a computer terminal at his or her desk may create a database for telephone reference materials and retrieve information from it in a matter of seconds.

Telephone Directories

Telephone directories contain three general sections—the introductory pages, the alphabetical listing of subscribers (which may be divided into subsections), and the classified section, familiarly known as "the Yellow Pages." In many areas of the country, all three sections appear in one volume of the telephone directory. However, in metropolitan areas where the listings are voluminous, the classified section is a separate book.

The introductory section gives instructions on what numbers to call in various types of emergencies, where to place service calls, how to ask for directory assistance, how to make mobile and marine calls, and the different types of calls that can be made. It lists area codes for faster calling and sample rates for long-distance and person-to- person calls. It explains how to make collect calls; how to call overseas; how to call the telephone company's business office and the operators who handle customer information; where to pay bills and transact business in person; and what modern telephone services are available to the customer. A map illustrates area code zones.

The subscriber section lists in alphabetical sequence the names, addresses, and telephone numbers of all the telephone subscribers in a locality, borough, town, village, city, or county. Sometimes the kind of business or the occupation of a subscriber is also shown. In some large directories, business, professional, and organizational listings are given in a separate section from that for residences. Government offices may also be listed in still another section.

At the top outside corner of each page guide, names, or "telltales", indicate the first and last listings on the page for quick location of the page on which a particular name appears. If a name might be spelled in several ways, a cross-reference spelling directs the user to additional listings. The divisions, departments, or branch offices of an organization with separate telephone listings are usually indented under the firm name. Alternate call listings can likewise be found in the telephone directory. These listings indicate telephone numbers to be called when no one answers the regular numbers. Governmental agencies and state, county, and municipal offices are shown with major headings for the principal listing and indented entries for subordinate departments and divisions.

The local alphabetical and classified directories are usually distributed to all subscribers. Out-of-town directories may be purchased by calling the telephone business office.

Street-Address Directories

In some cities, street-address directories are available and may be rented from the telephone company. These directories list telephone numbers according to the alphabetical and numerical arrangements of streets in that city. They are of special value and usefulness to credit and collection agencies and for companies or organizations who desire to make up mailing lists.

Desk Telephone Files

For efficiency and expediency, a desk telephone file of numbers and area codes should be compiled. This list consists of:
1. Business numbers the employer calls frequently and, possibly, taxi, railroad terminal, and airline numbers
2. Emergency numbers for ambulance service, fire department, police department, and so on
3. Personal numbers of the employer's family
4. Extension numbers in other offices
5. Frequently called long-distance numbers, with notations indicating the difference in time zones.

Unlisted numbers should be added to this list, with an identifying mark indicating the nature of such a number. Unlisted numbers arc never revealed without specific instructions from the executive to do so. They were given to the employer for personal use, and this fact should be respected.

It is a good idea when compiling a desk telephone list to make it as informative as possible. The secretary should identify individual names by noting title and company affiliation in addition to the address and telephone number and area code. In entering the name, address and telephone number of an organization, also indicate the name and title or department of the person or persons with whom the secretary or the employer talks most frequently.

The placement of the desk telephone list depends upon its size l quite short, it may be taped neatly to the top or the slide panel of the desk; if long, it may be kept in a book or on a rotary file attached to or near the telephone.

Database Files

Because electronic communication is used in today's automated office, you may have access to or use a terminal at your desk or workstation.

To automate telephonic communications, create databases for telephone reference materials and desk telephone files. Then, you can easily retrieve complete citations for easy reference as well as make changes and additions within seconds. The advantage is that you don't have to handle a book and check via a system to find the data needed. You simply key the data to initiate retrieval. Such databases help speed up directory assistance inquiries. Instead of paging through phone books, operators input a name, and a list of possibilities appears on the screen. Through scrolling, the desired number, if listed, is revealed.

Assembling Data for Outgoing Calls

In order to place outgoing calls quickly for the employer, the secretary should master all the telephone techniques that enable one to do this skillfully. Be absolutely certain of the telephone number before calling. It will save time, trouble, and irritation if the number is checked with the desk list, telephone directory, or correspondence file before calling.

Then assemble all the information that may be necessary to conduct the business transaction when the call is put through. It may be necessary to obtain materials from the files to refresh the executive's memory on previous business or other information that will be of help in making a successful call. All pertinent material should be placed on the executive's desk before the call is made.

It is also a good practice to be sure the executive will be free and available to take the call as soon as it goes through. No one likes to be called and then find that it is necessary to wait because the caller is talking on another line or is otherwise not ready to take the call immediately. Delay may not only lower the prestige of the company and the executive and cause annoyance but also prove costly to the firm making the call.

The question frequently arises as to which executive should answer first. Courtesy prescribes that the caller should be on the line, ready to talk, when the person called is put on the line by his or her own secretary, particularly if the person called outranks the caller. The secretary should put the executive on the line immediately, if possible. This can be done readily if the secretary identifies the employer when the call is answered. The secretary at the other end will then be able to transfer the call to the person called without delay or immediately inform the caller of how to reach that individual.

Telephone Services

In addition to business calls within the local community or surrounding areas, it frequently becomes necessary to place calls to more distant points. The ability to handle long-distance calls capably will enhance the secretary's value to the employer.

Toll Calls

Long-distance calls are those made from one town or city to another town or city outside of a local calling area. A charge is made for such calls in addition to the charge for the regular telephone service. The amount of the charge depends upon the distance, the type of service requested, the time of day or night the call is made, and the time taken for the conversation.

There are two classes of long-distance calls—station-to-station and person-to-person.

Station-to-station calls: Any state in the United States can be reached by direct dialing today. The telephone directory carries a listing of cities and states and their area codes. In order to place a call to any of these localities, dial "I" first, the area code second, and then the local telephone number of the individual. If the city or town is not listed at the front of the telephone directory, refer to the area code directory; then call the directory assistance operator in that area and give the name and address of the party you want to reach. A station-to-station call is made to a particular telephone number, and the caller speaks to anyone who answers the telephone. Therefore, if someone answers the ring, the individual making the call is charged for it, and the charges start as soon as the call is answered. However, this type of call is less costly, is more frequently made, and is usually faster than the person-to-person call.

Person-to-person calls: To place a person-to-person call, the secretary dials zero, the three-digit area code, and then the telephone number; at this point the operator intercepts and the secretary gives the name of the individual being called. When the call is put through the person called may not be present or available to take the call. Then a decision may have to be made as to whether someone else all that number can handle the transaction. A person-to-person call 1 made to a particular person only, and the caller is not charged for the call unless the person called is reached or the caller consents to speak to some other specifically identified individual. Charges start as soon as the caller consents to the call and begins speaking; therefore, the secretary should not start a conversation, but must make sure that the employer is ready to take the call immediately. A "1" is not needed in person-to-person calls because the operator intercepts.

Direct distance dialing: Almost all calls in the United States and abroad may be put through by means of direct distance dialing. A "1" must precede the area code. A list of the area codes one must use for direct dialing is found at the beginning of the telephone directory or in the expanded area code directory available from the telephone company. The direct dialing system works by dialing "1" and a three-digit area code, followed by the local telephone number. There are no two areas that have the same area code, nor are there two identical telephone numbers in an area. The numbers of adjacent geographical area codes are widely different numerically to help avoid confusion and error.

It is a quick and accurate system. If a wrong number is reached, the secretary, before disconnecting, should ascertain the name of the city that was reached. He or she should then dial the operator, or in some cases the credit bureau, and promptly report that an incorrect destination was reached, so that the telephone bill will not reflect a charge for the wrong number. Also, if the transmission was poor or the call was cut off, the operator or the credit bureau should be called in order that the appropriate adjustment may be made. The phone directory also explains how to use direct dialing for credit-card and collect calls and for overseas calls. A "1" must also precede the area code.

Time differences: It is vital to check the differences in time when planning to place a long-distance call. One must be aware not only that this country is divided into time zones, but also that certain regions change to daylight saving time during the summer months and that difference in time exist in all countries. For example, the United States (excluding Alaska and Hawaii) is divided into four standard-time zones: Eastern, Central, Mountain, and Pacific. Each zone is one hour earlier than the zone immediately to the east of it: when it is 12 noon Eastern Standard Time, it is 11 AM in the Central zone, 10 AM in the Mountain zone, and 9 AM Pacific time. Greenwich Mean Time, which is the mean solar time of the meridian at Greenwich, England, is used as the basis for standard time throughout most of the world.

Appointment Calls

The telephone operator is asked to put through a person-to-person call at a specified hour. Contact is established at the time indicated and the caller is then notified that the connection has been made. The charge for such a call is the same as that for an ordinary person-to-person call. This service is not available for international calls.

Sequence Calls

The sequence-calls service is of value when a number of calls are to be made to out-of-town points. Much time is saved by furnishing the operator with a list, oral or written, of the calls to be made at the specified times. The secretary should supply the names of the individuals to be called, the cities and states where they are located, their telephone numbers, if known, and the hour at which the executive wishes to speak to each person on the list. However, it should be noted that this is an expensive procedure, as each call is charged at the "operator-assisted call" rate. If the secretary makes the calls by direct dialing, money is saved.

Conference Calls

Another instance of the various accommodations that the telephone company offers its subscribers is the conference service. It is of particular value to executives of organizations with branches and/or plants located over a wide area who find it necessary to confer speedily with those at the different branches. The telephone company provides two methods for setting up a telephone conference.

1. An arrangement can be made with the conference operator to connect several people in various cities simultaneously for a conference or discussion. No special equipment is required for this hookup.
2. An arrangement can be made with the conference operator whereby a conference call can be placed to a large group of employees. This type of call requires setting up a loudspeaker at the called point in a different city, so that the executive can talk by phone to the entire group at one time.

When placing such a call, the secretary should signal the operator; ask for the conference operator describe the setup desired; and furnish the names of the people to be called, their telephone numbers, if known, the city and slate where each is located, and the time of the conference.

Collect Calls

Calls can be charged to the phone of the person who is being called. The individual called may either accept the call and be charged for it or refuse the call and, of course, not be charged. Collect call rates are higher than direct-dialed station-to-station rates. A subscriber can also charge to his or her own phone long-distance calls placed from other phones. It behooves the efficient secretary to discuss with the employer when collect charges should be accepted. Determine from whom collect charges will be honored. If in doubt, ask the operator to wait while the matter is checked with the executive.

Overseas Calls

You can direct-dial many overseas points. Information on such calls can be obtained from the front pages of the directory, the International Dial brochures, or from the long-distance operator. For person-to-person overseas calls, the secretary must dial the long-distance operator and ask for an overseas operator. The name of the person to be called and the telephone number, if known, must be provided. The charges for this service are higher than those for domestic calls. There are reduced rates for evenings and for nights and weekends. (See section on "Telephoning a Telegram".)

Calls to Ships, Planes, Trains, and Automobiles

Telephone calls to mobile conveyances by way of radio telephone are similarly made by the operator. Such service is not available without the installation of special equipment by the telephone company in the car, plane, or ship, of course. Calls can then be placed directly from the office telephone to the destination desired. (See section on "Satellite Communications Network".)

Returning Long-Distance Calls

Frequently a long-distance call is received when the executive is not in the office to take it. In such a case, the long-distance operator will give the secretary the operator's number, the city calling, and the name and telephone number of the person calling. To return the call, the secretary must dial the operator, ask by number for the operator who placed the call, and identify the city from which the call originated. When the connection is made with the proper operator, the secretary should tell the employer the name and telephone number of the person who placed the call. Collect calls are excluded from this service.

Telephone Record-Keeping

Many organizations require that a record be kept of all long-distance calls made, in order to verify the telephone bill, and have special printed forms for this purpose. The secretary may ask the telephone operator, when placing such calls, to provide the charges when the call is completed. However, the request for charges must be made in advance, not after the call is completed. If you log long-distance calls, record the following: date, time, and caller.

Special Telephone Equipment and Systems

A good secretary should be familiar with the various types of telephone equipment available, in order to meet the needs of the company and those of the executive. Tremendous strides have been made in the field of telephone research. Not only business but also the world in general benefits from the discoveries made by telephone technicians and telephone researchers.

Call director: A push-button telephone that provides the capacity of several ordinary push-button phones in one compact, attractive unit is known as the Call Director. It can handle up to 29 lines and is available in 18- to 30-button models, which can be adjusted as needs change. The Call Director can be combined with the speakerphone feature (see below), which makes it possible to telephone with the hands free when needed. A plug-in headset model is also available; this frees the hands so that the secretary can take notes, consult records, and so forth.

The telephone company has also added the conference feature to the Call Director. This permits an executive to set up an intercom conference by merely dialing a code or pushing a button.

Speakerphone set: The speakerphone consists of a microphone and a loudspeaker and permits the user to convey on a telephone conversation clearly from anywhere in an office without lifting the receiver from its rest. The microphone picks up the user's voice, and the loudspeaker, with an adjustable volume control, broadcasts it to the party at the other end of the line. By sitting around the microphone all members of a group can engage in a telephone conversation at one time. Everybody can talk and offer a viewpoint, and everybody can hear and understand fully what is being discussed.

Direct inward dialing: A setup is available whereby an outside caller can dial the central office designation, followed by the extension needed, and thereby put the call directly to the office desired instead of to the switchboard operator.

Data phone: The data phone is a telephone-computer setup which, after activation by human hands, enables office machines to talk to one another and transmit data at tremendous speeds in various machine-usable forms.

AT & T's Merlin: This system is equipped with a microprocessor and has its own internal software. Programming features are possible. These include automatic dialing, privacy, and "do not disturb" mechanisms. Expansion is possible with other custom features and outside lines.

AT&T's Key 416: The key system links a group of key telephones. Each telephone permits the user to select an intercom or outside line. Paging is possible. The ultimate capacity is 16 stations, 4 central office lines, and 2 intercom paths. It is also possible to set up multilane conferences. Other systems include:

System			Lines	Stations
Com	Key	718	7	18
Com	Key	1434	14	34
Com	Key	2152	21	52

The Com Key system offers many standard and optional features and a choice of telephone sets in various colors.

Custom calling services: These services are available on individual and auxiliary lines for both business and residence telephones. These features can be provided if a customer is served by the central office of ESS (Electronic Switching System). Custom calling services will operate in connection with rotary or touch-tone service. There are four custom calling services.

Call waiting: This service is designed to let the called party know that someone is trying to call while the telephone is in use.

Call forwarding: This service transfers calls to another number when the called party is not at the office or at home.

Three-way calling: A third party may be cut into an existing conversation.

Speed calling: One or two digits can be dialed in order to reach local or long-distance numbers more quickly.

To obtain custom calling services, it is not necessary to install extra equipment or to have an installer visit. These services are available with the regular telephone setup and may be attained by request at the central telephone office.

Dimension PBX: This electronic system uses stored program control, a time division switching network, and switched loop consoles. It is modular in design and has a solid-state system; therefore it saves space, speeds operation, and simplifies installation and maintenance.

There are two types of systems that are available to customers:

1. Dimension 400 has an approximate capacity of 400 lines and 90 trunks.
2. Dimension 2000 has an approximate capacity of 2000 lines and 350 trunks.

However, the capacity of lines and trunks for both dimension 400 and 2000 may change depending upon the line and trunk combinations and how they are used. Information on dimension PBX or any other type PBX telephone system or service may be obtained by calling the local telephone company.

Data speed 40 service: This communication service transmits the written word. It is available for private-line and expanded switched networks. The data speed 40 selective calling system is designed for use with private-line applications in both half duplex and full duplex. ("Full duplex" pertains to a simultaneous two-way and independent transmission in both directions. "Half duplex" service permits communication alternately in either direction or in one direction only.) Data is always prepared on a typewriter prior to transmission. All transmissions are fast, because the data proceeds at a maximum speed rather than the slower keyboard speed. The transmission accuracy is high, since the data is displayed on a monitor in its entirety before it is sent. This permits editing of data before transmission if necessary.

Horizon communications system: This is a microprocessor-controlled system that utilizes stored programs and multi-button electronic telephone (MET) sets. It has a capacity of 32 lines and 79 stations (excluding bridged, not MET, stations). A customer access unit (CAU) provides the ability to make feature changes or telephone-set rearrangements. There are further standard and optional features for both the stations and the system that are too numerous to mention. Local telephone companies can be called for further detailed information.

Picture phone meeting service: With this service a videophone, which is a telephone combined with a television receiver and transmitter, enables users to see, as well as speak to, one another. The service is offered in color in a limited area and in black and white between several large cities. It brings people together for an important meeting so that everyone can participate. It makes it possible to conduct monthly or quarterly administrative reviews, to introduce new products to the sales force, to screen applicants for employment, to resolve production or distribution conflicts, to handle emergencies, etc. Visual aids such as slides, charts, artwork, or graphs may be used to illustrate or clarify facts discussed. Hard copies of information can be transmitted and videotapes can be sent or received. This service has now advanced to video-conferencing, a new technology.

Portable conference telephone set: This permits individuals from an audience to speak directly to the speaker, to ask or answer questions, by means of a standard telephone receiver that may be carried anywhere; it connects to a standard telephone jack.

Computerized Branch Exchange (CBX): This system is used lot large offices. This type of exchange can handle up to 800 stations. It is controlled by a microcomputer that automatically chooses the circuits to use and determines holding times.

Touch-tone telephones: These telephones have buttons. All numbers are used; the symbols and * are for special services. The "tone" permits the transmission of data to computers, similar to voice communications, a new technology. They are much easier to use than rotary-dial telephones.

Touch-automatic: This automatic telephone dialer "remembers" up to 15 (or 31, depending on the type) numbers. It dials them at the touch of a button. Numbers may be added or changed at will.

Wide area telecommunications service (WATS): This service allows subscribers to contract for station-to-station calls within a specified service area at a fixed monthly rate, in lieu of individual call billing. It includes a listing in the National information center records (800-555-1212); by calling this number a subscriber can obtain the number of any other WATS-line subscriber.

Outward WATS provides outgoing direct-distance dialing of long-distance calls by means of a WATS line from the customer's premises to other telephones within a specified service area. Each WATS line has its own WATS number.

Inward WATS allows a subscriber to receive calls over a WATS line without charge to the originating party. The call is automatically charged to the called number without the announcement and acceptance necessary with a collect call.

Service areas number 1 through 7 indicates interstate service. Included within the range of WATS service is all of the United States including Alaska, Hawaii, Puerto Rico, and the US Virgin Islands (St Thomas, St Croix, and St John). The purchase of one service area, 2 through 7, includes the area or areas in the lower numbered service area or areas. Service area "0" is an intrastate service available only in some states. WATS service is available in either of two forms.

Full business day: The initial period allows 240 hours including up to 14,400 completed incoming station-to-station calls a month from any telephone within the specified service area.

Measured: The initial period allows 10 hours including up to 600 completed station-to-station calls a month from any telephone within the specified service area.

Card dialers: A plastic card is inserted in an automatic dialing telephone. The cards are coded with frequently called numbers. The number is dialed rapidly and accurately by the telephone mechanism. In a business that makes a great many calls to the same numbers, the amount of time saved by these cards can be considerable. The telephone that takes the cards may be used in a normal way.

Bellboy: This is a signaling device that may be kept in the pocket, purse, or briefcase. When the user is within a certain range of the office, the Bellboy will beep when the secretary dials its number. The user then goes to the nearest telephone and calls the office to receive the message.

Another name for Bellboy is "Beeper". Due to the advances in electronic communication, beepers may be activated up to 30 miles. Specially manufactured, "high-tech" beepers may range 30 miles plus. These are now common communication devices for top executives.

Telephone Answering Services

Many offices maintain contact with customers or others in the business world through an answering service that takes calls at night and on weekends and holidays. For a small office that closes entirely for vacations, an answering service is valuable.

The answering service may transfer the messages taken by calling at the beginning of the next business day. However, it is more common for the secretary to call in periodically and take the messages that have been received.

Trial and error may be necessary in finding a reliable answering service. If the service does not have enough lines or operators and callers are put on "hold" for unreasonable lengths of time, much good will can be lost. Then again, it is important to have a service that can be trusted to take messages accurately. The secretary planning to engage an answering service will do well to consult other secretaries and take their recommendations. Once the system is in operation, the secretary should check response time regularly.

When it comes time to take the messages from an answering service, the secretary should have pen and paper on hand and be scrupulously accurate in transcribing any messages given and especially so if the answering device does not have playback equipment. A set of priorities may be set up in advance with the employer as to which messages call for immediate action and which may be delayed for a shorter or greater length of time.

A sophisticated service available through the telephone company has an apparatus by which the subscriber can dial a two-digit code and have incoming calls transferred to an answering service. This does not "tie-up" the line, as the subscriber may still make outgoing calls. When the subscriber wishes to disengage the service, a second two digit code will restore the incoming calls to the client's own telephone line. Telephone answering services also provide "wake-up" calls, courtesy calls, and reminder-of-appointment calls at an additional cost.

Telephone Answering Devices

A great variety of telephones answering devices, usually activating a cassette tape recorder, are available. The simplest of these give a recorded message, as for example a statement telling the caller when the person called will be available, telling hours when the business is open, or the like. An equally common type is the recorder in which the person called has prerecorded a message that invites the caller to leave a message. When a tone sounds, the caller can talk for varying lengths of time, depending upon the way in which the recorder is set to operate.

Messages recorded by such a device should be transcribed by the secretary as early as possible at the start of a business day. If it is not possible to understand clearly any portion of a message, a notation should be placed on the transcript to alert the employer that the secretary was not sure of the message given.

A remote-control feature on such devices as the Phonemate allows the user to call the device on any telephone from anyplace in the world and hear whatever messages have been recorded. One phone call plays all messages, and a special feature allows the user to replay any given message without waiting for the entire tape to rewind and replay.

- Assembling data for outgoing calls
- Telephone services
- Telephone record-keeping
- Special telephone equipment and systems
- Telephone answering services
- Telephone answering devices.

Effective and efficient communication is an essential for any business and is required of all employees. Some basic methods of communication have remained largely unchanged; others have changed greatly with technological developments and increasing sophistication. The secretary must be familiar with all communications techniques and how and when to use them. This chapter briefly discusses the major communications techniques: mail, telegrams, cables, radio messages, and the telephone.

OFFICE MAIL

The processing and handling of mail constitutes the most important method of communication between a company and its contacts in the business world. The way in which mail is handled by the secretary affects every phase of a company and its external and internal procedures of information processing. A secretary who can effectively deal with office mail is indeed a valuable asset to an employer.

Electronic Mail Transmission

Electronic mail is the popular term for many of the new forms of communication that use computer and telecommunications technology. Also sometimes called electronic data communication, it is the non-interactive communication of text, data, voice, and image messages between a sender and a recipient using system links.

There are two advantages to electronic mail. One is the high speed with which large amounts of data can be sent from one place to another. The second is that data can be distributed to a specific location and stored in electronic form until it is needed by the recipient.

Electronic mail is rapidly becoming an indispensable tool in communications. Not only do companies use electronic mail for in-house communication but also for many employees who work at home from computer work stations and terminals. With the use of public access networks, such as Tymnet, Telenet, and other digital systems, it is possible to link host computer facilities simply, through a local phone call from almost anywhere in the world.

Electronic mail is implemented with several different technologies, among them facsimile transmission, telex, communicating word processors, microcomputers and other computer-based networks, electronic document distribution systems, and voice technologies. We shall discuss briefly a few of these means.

Telecommunications is the process of transmitting information over a distance, or "at a distance", by electromagnetic or electrical systems. (The prefix tele is derived from a Greek root meaning "at a distance".) Telecommunicated information may be in several forms, including voice, data, image, or message. The transmission systems include telephone lines, cables, microwaves, satellite transmission, and light beams.

Message systems: Message systems send information in data form. Telegrams and teletypewriter messages transmitted through systems as TWX and Telex are examples of message systems. These systems which the secretary may use frequently provide for faster transmission of information than does the postal system.

International electronic postal service: Various networks and services are available for rapid telecommunications. The secretary in an automated office should be familiar with the various network services, know which is best suited for particular purposes, and be able to use them. One such service is the International Electronic Postal Service, usually known as Intelpost.

Intelpost is a computerized network designed for high acceleration of information. The service links the United States, Canada, and Europe. Messages are transmitted by satellites, which use electronic and microwave technology. Documents such as charts, graphs, and photographs, as well as any type of printed text, can be transmitted.

Facsimile Transmission (Table 32.1)

Facsimile transmission is perhaps the oldest form of electronic mail and also a rapidly advancing telecommunications technology. Often known as fax, facsimile transmission is a proven method for sending information in the form of image replication (facsimile). It is flexible, inexpensive, and easy to do. Fax machines are now in many business offices and all secretaries should know how to use them effectively.

Table 32.1: Facsimile standards

Group	Minutes per page	Technology
1	6	Low resolution; analogs*
2	2–3	Low resolution; mostly analog
3	Fraction of a minute	Higher resolution; digital**

*conversion to electric signals
**conversion to binary signals

A fax unit can send a variety of documents—photographs, diagrams, drawings, statistical information, and handwritten or typewritten language messages—to any location that has a telephone line. The telephone line is the connection; without the telephone the system cannot work. The distance between two fax units is irrelevant. Information can be sent to another office in the same building or across the continent.

Fax units can store and forward information. They also have delay features that permit automatic dialing of one or more stations so that unattended transmission to multiple locations is possible on a 24-hour basis.

In 1980 the Consultative Committee on International Telephone & Telegraph (CCITT) set facsimile standards and groupings. The groupings refer to the amount of time it takes to send or receive a standard message over the telephone.

Incoming Mail

A new secretary may find a well-established system of handling mail within an organization. Changes may need to be suggested tactfully. The size of the organization has a great bearing on the system that evolves, in a small office one person may sort and open all mail except that marked "Personal" or "Confidential." (Letters so marked are delivered unopened to the person to whom they are addressed.) A large organization usually has a mailing department, where both incoming and outgoing mail are handled according to a fixed system. In an office where the secretary is assigned the responsibility for opening the mail for the employer, a routine procedure will permit rapid handling of each day's mail.

Necessary Supplies

The secretary will need supplies to open the mail. The following items and others you will need on your desk or work station should be placed there before the mail is processed. You may arrange the items in a circular fashion or another configuration for convenient and easy access. The suggested items are:
- Envelope opener
- Stapler or clips
- Date or time stamp
- Routing slips
- Transparent tape
- Pencils/pens (at least two different colors)
- Memo pad
- Mail register or log, if needed
- Staple remover.

If electric equipment, such as a mail opener or lime stamp, is available, use it. It will save two-thirds of the time as compared to manual equipment.

Opening the Mail

The mail should be opened as soon as it is delivered to the secretary's desk, and an orderly procedure should be followed to ensure that nothing is misplaced or lost, that time is not wasted, and that the executive receives the information needed.

Opening of the envelopes: All the envelopes should be opened before the contents are removed from any of them. To ensure that the contents will not be torn while the letter is being opened, tap the envelope firmly on the edge of the desk so that the contents will slip away from the top. Slit the upper edge of the envelope with a letter opener. If the contents of a letter are cut by the opener, use transparent tape to paste the parts together.

Checking tile contents: After removing the contents of an envelope, check the letter for a return address. If there is none, staple the envelope containing the return address to the contents. (Caution: If the contents include a punched card, use a paper clip for fastening rather than a staple.) The envelope should also be retained if the signature on the letter is not easily distinguishable.

Another check should be made to determine that all enclosures stipulated in the letter are accounted for. If not, a notation should be made immediately on the face of the letter, indicating what is missing.

Even though annotating a letter is one of the procedures encouraged, some companies do not like correspondence marked up, especially legal or business firms that might have to submit a piece of correspondence as evidence in a court of law. Always follow company policy. Some companies prefer that you place a buck slip (adhesive) with the notation on the face of the letter. In theory, it serves the same purpose.

Dating the mail: It is always wise to affix each day's date on incoming mail. The easiest procedure is to use a rubber stamp. Such a procedure is helpful if the letter has arrived too late to meet a deadline requested, has been in transit longer than it should have been, or is undated. In either of the latter two cases, it is well to staple the envelope to the letter in addition to dating the letter. This will give evidence of the date of mailing as well as the date of receipt.

Envelopes: Generally the envelope may be destroyed after it has been ascertained that everything has been removed and that there are no problems concerned with the names, addresses, or dates. However, in certain situations, especially legal matters, envelopes sometimes serve as evidence of date and time received (from the precanceled postage stamp). In such situations, envelopes may be kept and clipped or stapled to the back of the letter.

Preparation of Mail for Employer

In order to save the employer's time, the efficient secretary should take the time to prepare the mail. This involves two basic steps.

1. Read each letter, underlining important points that will aid you and your employer in answering the letter. Underline only those things that are of significance, such as publications, dates, and names of people.
2. Make annotations on each letter. This involves writing notes in the margins. Generally, annotations fall into three categories, namely, a note indicating:
    a. Action required by the letter—date of appointment for correspondent, reservations for a trip the employer may have to make as a result of the correspondence, etc.
    b. Procedures to be followed. These may depend upon former correspondence with the same person or related correspondence, which will have to be sought in the files.
    c. The priority the letter should receive, symbolized by a code. In an agreement with the employer a given place on each letter should be established for this code. For example, a red number may be written in the upper left corner. Such a code might be:
    Code 1: Mail and Reports with high priority and requiring a decision, these should be answered the same day they are received. (It is assumed that personal or confidential mail is delivered unopened to the addressee as soon as it arrives on the secretary's desk.)
    Code 2: Mail for which additional information must be procured, for which answering may have to be deferred for a day or two while data are being collected. All mail should be answered within 48 hours of receipt, except under very unusual circumstances.
    Code 3: Routine mail that the secretary may be able to handle, many employers want to see all mail; it is wise to determine an employer's preference in this regard. After the relationship is well established, many secretaries have their employers' permission to reply to routine letters. In such instances it is usually good procedure to supply the employer with carbons of the letters sent and the original letter.
    Code 4: Letters that require notations but no reply.

As the secretary reads and annotates the mail, it becomes a simple matter to encode and sort the mail as it is prepared for the employer. A fifth or even a sixth category may be added as needed. Usually important reports require a special category, while weekly, monthly, or semimonthly periodicals may require no encoding. Most employers prefer to examine the periodicals before they are made available to others in the office.

Preparing supplementary material. As the letters are being annotated, an efficient secretary will also make a list of files or pieces of correspondence and other information to be looked up before presenting the correspondence to the employer.

Some employers wish to see the mail as soon as it has been opened. In that case the secretary may bring the mail in as soon as it has been annotated. While the mail is being read, the secretary may take the compiled list and seek the necessary files, reports, and other information for acting upon the urgent mail. To keep all papers pertaining to each piece of correspondence together, use file folders or small clips.

Arranging the mail. After the sorting process has been completed, the secretary may arrange the mail either in one pile with the high priority mail on top or in any other arrangement that has been agreed upon. Whenever the mail is placed on the desk of the employer, some provision should be made to prevent others from reading the top letter. Some secretaries simply place the top letter face down.

Absence of the employer. When the employer is away from the office, letters requiring immediate replies may be handled in either of two ways. First, if a decision must be made immediately, it may be necessary to give the mail to the person in charge during the employer's absence. Second, if the employer will be in the office within a day or two and the decision can wait, the secretary should write the sender immediately and explain when a reply may be expected and the reason for the delay.

The efficient secretary to whom the employer has entrusted routine correspondence will maintain a file of materials handled during an absence of the employer. The folder should be readily at hand upon the employer's return.

Outgoing Mail

If the secretary is responsible for the preparation of outgoing mail, as the case may well be in a firm too small to have a separate mailing and shipping department, time and expense can be saved by learning about the various postal and shipping services available and the general regulations and normal charges pertinent to these services. It is important to be alert to frequent changes.

An accurate scale for weighing postal matter is a worthwhile piece of office equipment. It saves time and eliminates guesswork.

Sources of Mail Information

To obtain correct information on postal procedures and rates, which are subject to change, consult the local postal authorities. From them, or from the Superintendent of Document, Government Printing Office, Washington, DC 20402, may be obtained a number of useful pamphlets which are periodically brought up to date. These are some of them:

- Mailers guide
- Packaging pointers
- Domestic postage rates, fees, and information
- How to prepare second- and third-class mailings
- Mailing permits
- International postage rates and fees.

Some of the information in these pamphlets is taken from the Postal Manual, which contains complete data on postal regulations and procedures. Chapters 1 and 2 of this manual, which deal with domestic postal service and international mail, respectively, may be purchased separately.

A monthly publication called memo to mailers is available to business mailers without charge. It tells of rate and classification changes, along with other news of postal matters.

33 | Dictation and Transcription

INTRODUCTION

Physicians offices, clinics, in hospitals and nursing homes, matter of fact wherever medicine is practiced, the busy physicians dictate generally, operation notes, medical reports, discharge summary and some places, history, physical exam, some most of writing by a doctor is dictated for transcribing and producing a typed hard copy. This chapter deals with three types of dictation:

1. In-person dictation
2. Machine dictation
3. Telephone dictation
   - Transcription
   - Rough drafts
   - Envelopes and mailing instructions
   - Signature and follow-up.

For many years secretaries took dictation typed letters, memos, and reports; answered the telephone; and maintained filing systems. Today, secretaries still do many of these same things, but electronic technology has made office work much easier. Offices now use electronic typewriters, word processors, computers, and various types of dictation equipment and telephone hookups. The technology for processing, storing, and communicating information is changing rapidly. Much less time is spent on routine tasks, such as correcting errors and retyping, and greater efficiency has been the result.

The basic secretarial skills of dictation, transcription, keyboarding, and communication are still very much in demand. Shorthand dictation is generally requested at 80 to 100 words a minute, and typing speeds range from 60 to 80 words a minute. However, today's secretary must be able to adapt to the ever-changing technology and to transfer skills to the new office equipment and job requirements. For example, approximately 60 percent of offices now use machine dictation and transcription on word processors.

This chapter discusses the types of dictation, transcription, rough drafts, and final mailing and follow-up procedures for both a conventional and an electronic office.

TYPES OF DICTATION

In some offices an executive dictates to a secretary who takes shorthand. However, in many modern offices, the executive is more likely to dictate into a dictation unit or into a central recorder via a microphone or telephone. Regardless of the equipment used, it is the secretary's responsibility to listen carefully and transcribe the dictated material accurately and in the format desired.

In-Person Dictation

In an office in which in-person dictation is used, the secretary must be prepared at all times to take the executive's dictation and process it. Efficiency is improved if the tools and materials needed for dictation are kept ready, a dictation routine is established, and special signals are used to draw attention to urgent matters or items that need special attention.

Tools

The tools and materials needed for efficient in-person dictation are:
1. A spiral-bound notebook, with a rubber band around the used portion. If dictation is taken from more than one executive, it might be well to have a separate notebook for each, to avoid confusion when transcribing. The first date of dictation should be entered on the front binder and the final date entered when the book has been filled. The dictator's initials can be shown on the cover also. The filled notebooks should be filed in the event there is a question later about a dictated item. The length of time such notebooks are kept will depend upon the policy of the employer.
2. A pen (ballpoint, felt-tip, or whatever is preferred by the secretary); one or two sharpened lead pencils; and a colored pencil usually red. Notes written in ink are easier to read when transcribing than those written in pencil. The lead pencils are used if the pen runs dry; the colored pencil is for special notations.
3. A folder for correspondence and other reference materials.
4. A supply of paper clips, either along the binder of the notebook or clipped to the edge of the folder. These may be used for clipping memos of special instructions or small notes to the pages of the notebook.

5. A pocket-sized calendar, taped to the binder of the notebook or to the front of the correspondence folder. The calendar will be used to check days and dates in the dictated material.

A Dictation Routine

Before dictation begins, enter the date in red pencil at the bottom of the first page to be used that day.

With the permission of the executive, place all dictation materials on a corner of the desk rather than in the lap. (Long periods of dictation can be difficult and very tiring if the secretary has to juggle papers, files, and other materials in the lap or retrieve them from the floor.) The executive's appointment calendar should be close at hand for checking dates so that conflicts in scheduled meetings, travel arrangements, etc. are avoided.

The executive should indicate the number of copies required for each dictated item and, following the dictation, give all related correspondence to the secretary. The secretary may then number the correspondence to agree with the number in the shorthand notebook, place the correspondence in the appropriate folder, and later use to check names, addresses, quoted dates, calculations, and other data prior to transcribing.

Many secretaries use only the left-hand column of the notebook, reserving the right-hand side for corrections, insertions, special instructions, and so on. (Left-handed secretaries reverse this procedure.)

If the dictation becomes too rapid, the secretary should signal the dictator, reading back the last few words taken down. To avoid breaking the dictator's train of thought, the secretary should wait until the end of a sentence or paragraph before interrupting. (The new secretary may be reluctant to interrupt during dictation, but the executive will usually realize a "breaking-in" period is to be expected and will make allowances.)

The secretary should feel free to ask that unusual names or terms be spelled out and then write them in longhand. This can be done at the end of the dictation.

If the dictation is interrupted by a phone call or a visitor, the secretary should use this time to read back over the shorthand notes, inserting punctuation, checking dates on the calendar, or filling in words that may have been missed. If the interruption is extended, the secretary should quietly gather up the materials and return to her or his desk to prepare for transcribing, returning to the executive's office when called.

Special Dictation Signals

The secretary is wise to use special signals to indicate rush or priority items, special instructions, missing items, or other items that need special attention. The following are guidelines used by many experienced secretaries:

- Write the word "RUSH" in red pencil to call attention to urgent letters. It is also a good idea to fold the lower left-hand edge diagonally until the page protrudes one-half inch beyond the edge of the notebook as a signal that this is a priority item.
- Draw a rough box around special instructions and notations of attachments or enclosures to alert you when you are transcribing.
- Leave a blank space in the notes for material to be entered later, such as a date, a name, or other information to be provided by the executive (or secretary), which might not have been available during the dictation period.
- Use a caret or star for small insertions and a circled capital A, B, and so on for longer insertions.
- Use a crosshatch to indicate the end of each dictated item.
- Use standard symbols commonly used by secretaries to indicate special typing or printing instructions—for example, a wavy line under the notes to indicate underscoring; two lines to indicate all capitals; three lines to indicate both underscoring and all capitals. (Note that these are not the standard proofreading symbols used in publishing and many other fields.)
- Draw one or two diagonal lines through the notes after they have been transcribed.

Machine Dictation

Many executives use dictating machines to record some or all of their dictation, since they are able to dictate when no one is available to take notes. This method provides a great deal of flexibility for the dictator, who can dictate while commuting to work, on a business trip, or after working hours.

Types of Dictating Machines

There are several types of dictation/transcription machines available. Desk-top dictation machines are used primarily by executives who dictate frequently. Portable dictation machines, which record on mini-cassettes, are becoming very popular because they are small and lightweight, operate on batteries, and provide a great deal of flexibility for the dictator.

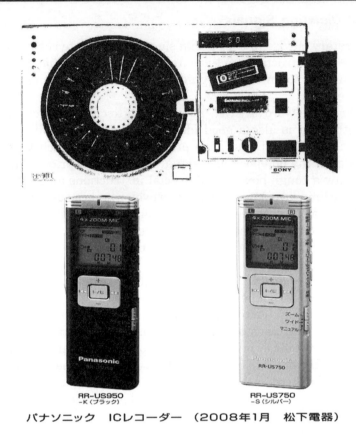

RR-US950
-K (ブラック)

RR-US750
-S (シルバー)

パナソニック　ICレコーダー　（2008年1月　松下電器）

Fig. 33.1: Central dictation system (*Courtesy*: Sony Corporation of America)

With centralized dictation systems, originators call a central recording device to dictate, and a supervisor assigns dictation transcription to an operator (Fig. 33.1).

Dictating to a Machine

With all types of dictation units, the dictator speaks into a microphone (or telephone) and the words are recorded on cassette (or mini-cassette). The dictator must speak distinctly, spell any unusual words, and record the punctuation, capitalization, and paragraphs. For the transcriber's guidance, the number of required copies and other instructions should be dictated at the beginning.

Transcribing from a Machine

The transcriber must learn to adjust the speed, volume, and tone controls of the machine as well as the start, stop, and repeat mechanisms. The machine may be equipped with either a hand or foot control for starting and stopping and a reverse control to replay the dictation when necessary. Some machines are also equipped with an indicator, or index slip, which enables the transcriber to determine easily the length of letters, corrections, or special instructions. Some machines feature electronic scanners that allow the transcriber to scan the dictation for any special instructions the originator/dictator may have included.

The beginning transcriber usually starts the transcribing machine, listens to a few words or a phrase, stops the machine, types the words or phrases, and then repeats the process—start, listen, stop, type. The goal of a good machine transcriber is to keep moving with very few interruptions in the typing process.

The transcriber should be careful not to erase any dictation while transcribing and should be sure that all items are transcribed before returning the cassette (which can be reused) to the dictator's machine. Material transcribed from a dictation unit should be proofread and handled in the same manner as shorthand transcription.

Telephone Dictation

Executives who travel may frequently call and dictate letters, conference notes, instructions, and other messages to the secretary by telephone. The notes, especially names, dates and figures, should be read back to the dictator before the conversation is terminated.

A teleconference is a meeting using electronic technology so that several people in different locations can participate by using telephones and linking computers to communicate and to present and discuss documents. Another advance, video teleconferencing, allows the participants to see one another on a screen as they meet.

The secretary may be asked to monitor an important phone call or teleconference to provide a record of what was discussed. A transcribed summary of what was said is usually sufficient and should be typed immediately while the conversation is still fresh in the secretary's mind.

TRANSCRIPTION

Before transcribing anything, whether it be shorthand or machine dictation, the secretary should establish priorities for the work to be done. Items may be sorted into stacks to be:
1. Handled at once. (This may be a mailgram; a phone call, or a letter to be typed signed, and mailed immediately.)
2. Transcribed before the day is over.
3. Transmitted to others for handling.
4. Handled by the secretary, but under no deadline.

5. Placed in the tickler file for follow-up.
6. Filed.
7. Discarded.

After the sorting has been completed, the secretary should proceed according to the priorities set.

Becoming Familiar with Standard Formats

Many companies have a standard format for correspondence and intra-corporate memos and a different style for letters to customers or clients. The secretary should be familiar with these formats and follow them when transcribing, if there is no company standard, the secretary should use the style preferred by the executive or a style that is generally accepted in an up-to-date style manual.

Checking Notes and Other References

If the secretary has taken in-person dictation, he or she should read through the notes, inserting punctuation where necessary, paragraphing where necessary (if not dictated), checking the calendar for possible conflicts in days and times of meetings or appointments correcting errors in grammar and facts, restructuring poor sentences, and so forth. Many executives rely on their secretaries to make whatever changes are necessary. However, if the secretary notices that a change in fact is necessary, he or she should mention it to the executive. And, if the executive wants the material transcribed exactly as dictated, the secretary should do so.

A dictionary and a current secretarial handbook should be on every secretary's desk so that he or she may check the spelling of unfamiliar words and place names, rules of punctuation, the division of words at the end of a line, and so forth. (One new feature of Webster's New World Dictionary, Third College Edition is a unique system of end-of-line hyphenation.)

Transcribing and Preparing the Final Copies

With experience, the secretary can easily determine the length of a letter to be transcribed and the margins to be set on the typewriter. It is necessary to take into consideration the size of the shorthand notes or the length of the dictation on the machine as well as the type style (pica, elite, and/or proportional spacing) of the typewriter. It may occasionally be necessary to type a rough draft when material not dictated, such as a list of names or a statistical tabulation, is to be inserted.

In a traditional office, the transcriptionist sets the margins, tab stops, and line spacing, and proofreads and edits the documents at the typewriter. Minor mistakes may be corrected with correction tape or correction fluid. More substantial errors may require retyping one or more pages. Today's transcriptionists may occasionally use a carbon packet for copies; however, photocopies and hard-copy originals are more commonly used.

If the transcription process is interrupted, the secretary should put a small check mark in the shorthand notes to indicate the place to resume typing.

In the word processing or electronic office, margins, tabs, and line spacing can be adjusted or changed automatically. Editing tasks such as adding or deleting words, lines, or paragraphs can be accomplished without retyping whole pages. Equipment may have a built-in spell checker or a software program with a dictionary or grammar checking component. The work still should be proofread, however, because the equipment and programs cannot distinguish between homonyms, nor can they determine if the transcript omits a word. The final transcript will be a clean, neat, original document with no trace of revisions.

With modern electronic equipment, the secretary can merge various pieces of information into one document. If you are sending the same letter to several different people, once you have typed the letter, you can merge it with a file that contains a list of names, addresses, and salutations. The computer will then print the same letter with the appropriate inside addresses and salutations.

ROUGH DRAFTS

The executive may request that the secretary type a rough draft of a letter, report, speech, or legal document. This should be done on inexpensive paper. A rough draft of a letter may be single spaced and corrections made in the margins. Speeches and reports should be double or triple spaced, leaving room for editorial changes. Rough drafts are retained until the final draft is approved.

On occasion the secretary may deem it advisable to type a rough draft of a letter without being asked, if experience dictates the probability of a rewrite, it could be diplomatically explained that the rough draft was for the secretary's own guidance in layout or because the shorthand notes were not clear. This will give the executive an opportunity to review the material before the final transcription and to make any changes desired.

Offices equipped with electronic typewriters, word processors, or computers enable secretaries to draft all items, make corrections, or rearrange paragraphs and then push a button to produce a final copy with centered headings, justified margins, and different type styles within the document. These machines are excellent timesavers for secretaries who type manuscripts, technical materials, routine specialized documents, or correspondence for executives who habitually make many changes in their dictation.

ENVELOPES AND MAILING INSTRUCTIONS

Envelopes for letters should be typed as soon as the letter is transcribed. A method preferred by many executives is to place the letter and the enclosures, if any, under the flap of the envelope with the addressed side of the envelope on top. This same procedure may be used with those copies that are to be sent to another party.

Because of the extended use of automated equipment the postal service has made available a leaflet entitled secretarial addressing for automation (Notice 23-B), which may be obtained from customer-service representatives and postmasters. Some suggestions included are:

1. The address area should be in block form with all of the lines forming a uniform left margin. It should be four inches from the left edge of the envelope and on the fourteenth line down from the top edge of the envelope. No print should appear to the right or below it.

2. Mail addressed to occupants of multi-unit buildings should include the number of the apartment, room, suite, or other unit. The unit number should appear immediately after the street address on the same line—never above, below, or in front of the street address.

3. Street addresses or box numbers should be placed on the line immediately above the city, state, and ZIP Code. When indicating a box number at a particular station, the box number should precede the station name. Correct spelling of street names is essential, since some machines match the names in the address to those like it on the machine's memory.

4. City, state, and ZIP Code should appear in that sequence on the bottom line of the address block. Two-letter state abbreviations and nine-digit zip codes should be used. Automatic sorting equipment is instructed to look for this information in that position. Mail presorted by ZIP Codes bypasses many processing steps in the post office and can get to its destination quicker.

5. Type addresses in upper-case letters without punctuation:

GENERAL XYZ CORP
ATTENTION SALES DEPT
1000 MAIN ST
PO BOX 23302 CENTRAL STATION
DALLAS TX 75223-1234

It should be noted that this style of addressing envelopes is not mandatory and the secretary should consult with the executive, before adopting it.

Special mailing instructions should be typed in all capital letters five or six spaces below the area where the postage will be placed or special labels may be used if available.

If a letter states or implies that materials are to be sent separately, the material should be prepared, placed in an envelope or mailing container, and a mailing label typed. If the mailing is to be taken care of by a different person or by another department, the secretary should make a note to check and determine that the mailing was actually done.

SIGNATURE AND FOLLOW-UP

After the dictation has been transcribed and proofread and the envelopes and enclosures have been prepared, the secretary should review his or her notebook to be sure that no items or special instructions have been overlooked.

The secretary should then note any pertinent dates or reminders on the calendar and place follow-up items in the tickler file. The executive's appointment calendar should also be posted, if this was not done during the in-person dictation period.

The completed correspondence should be put in a folder marked: "For Your Signature" and placed on the executive's desk. Rush items should be taken in to the executive immediately. Others may be accumulated and presented to the executive later in the day, but be sure to allow sufficient time for the letters to be signed and mailed on schedule.

Some executives prefer to sign each piece of mail personally. Others authorize their secretaries to sign for them. If authorized to sign, the secretary should place his or her initials after the dictator's/originator's signature, unless otherwise instructed.

SAMPLE DISCHARGE SUMMARIES

General Medicine

ID 1275777
Name: Arnold   Age: 65
DOA: 25.8.2000   DOD: 20.9.2000

Final Diagnosis: Acute pancreatitis-? Alcoholic
            Bronchial asthma-acute exacerbation
            Lower respiratory tract infection
            Type II diabetes mellitus

History
Sixty-five-year-old Mr. Arnold was admitted with complaints of epigastric abdominal pain, radiating to back for 7 days. He did not complain of pain being related to food. He did not give any history of vomiting, hematemesis, malena, diarrhea or constipation. He gives history of developing fever, developing on 2nd hospitalization day, following which he became breathless. He does not give any history of cough or pleuritic chest pain.

Past History
Gives history of pyloroplasty done in 1993. He is a chronic alcoholic on diet and OHA. He is also an asthmatic since 1985 on Tablet Prednisolone 5 mg once daily.

Physical Examination
Pulse 86/min BP 130/80 mm Hg. Peripheral pulses positive.
No pallor, icterus, cyanosis, clubbing or lymphadenopathy
CVS: S1, S2 + No murmurs
RS: Decreased breath sounds on left lower inter-scapular region.
Abdomen: Soft, No organomegaly.
CNS: Normal.

Course in Hospital and Discussion
Sixty-five-year-old Mr. Arnold who has presented with clinical features suggestive of acute pancreatitis. Serum amylase at admission and MRI abdomen was consistent with acute pancreatitis. He was a chronic alcoholic and he is also using steroids for his asthmatic symptoms and both these factors were attributed to the episode. He was stabilized with conservative management by our gastroenterologist. He had an episode of exacerbation of asthma and he was intubated and transferred to our unit. He was stabilized hemodynamically and the possibility of underlying respiratory infection was considered and he was treated with intravenous antibiotics also. He improved and he was extubated. He was treated with beta-2 agonist and steroid inhaler for asthmatic symptom. His blood sugar was under control with OHA. He also a known case of acid peptic disease and had pyloroplasty and he was asymptomatic at present. He was discharged with the following recommendations.

Recommendations
Asthalin inhaler 2 puffs thrice daily
Inhaler Beclamethasione 250 ug puffs twice daily
Capsule Omez 20 mg twice daily
Gastro consult on OPD basis and follow-up in medicine OPD

ID 1515
Name: Richard Age: 50 years
DOA: 11.10.2001 DOD: 17.10.2001

Final Diagnosis:Type II diabetes mellitus with polyneuropathy/nephropathy?
Retinopathy
Essential hypertension

Presenting Complaints
Tingling sensation of both legs and hands for six months. Weakness of both lower limbs for 9 months. Perioral parasthesia for six months.

History
Mr Richard 51-year-old gentleman from Bihar admitted with complaints of weakness of both lower limbs since Jan 2000. He noticed that his shoes slip of his feet without his knowledge and difficulty in getting up from squatting position. Six months back he developed painful burning sensation of both feet and hands, which is more in the night. He has also got sensation of incomplete micturition and constipation. He was on Daonil 2.5 mg twice daily for diabetes and some antihypertensives. Now he was admitted for glycemic control and evaluation.

System Review
Family history: Not significant
Personal history: Working as security personal
Previous treatment history: Was on Daonil 2.5 mg twice daily.

Physical Examination
Weight: 80 Kg
General: Thyroid—bilateral swelling
CVS: S1, S2—normal, No murmurs.
RS: Normal vesicular breath sounds. Bilateral air entry equal.
ABD: Soft, no organomegaly.
Musculoskeletal: DTR decreased bilaterally.

Course in Hospital
Mr Richard was investigated and treated in the ward. He was treated with Gliclazide 40 mg thrice daily, Amitryptyline 50 gm twice daily, Enalapril 5 mg twice daily and Dilantin 100 mg at bedtime. His symptoms were better and blood sugar and blood pressure were controlled. Discharged with advice to continue medications. 24-hour urine protein is planned on follow up.
Referred to neurology for consultation of polyneuropathy.

Recommendations
Activity: Normal
Diet: 1500 Kcal low cholesterol, diabetic diet.

Medications
Tab Gliclazide 40 mg three times daily (½ hours prior to meals)
Tab Enalapril 5 mg twice daily
Tab Amitrypityline 50 mg twice daily
Tab Dilantin 100 mg once daily
Tab Simvastatin 10 mg at bedtime for three months
Continuity of care needs: Nil
Investigation NCV 17.09.2000 IP
Follow-up in medicine clinic after 2 months.

ID 14
Specialty: General Medicine
Consultant: Dr Foster

Episode Summary

History
This 53-year-old man, a known case of alcohol cirrhosis with alcohol dependence, was admitted following a marked deterioration in his condition.
He had previously been admitted on several occasions for alcohol cirrhosis and hypobeta-lipoproteinemia.

On Examination
Unwell, emaciated and jaundiced, with a distended abdomen.

Post-admission
The patient proved to be in an advanced stage of cirrhosis. Ascites were drained. He gradually deteriorated and died one week after admission.

Final Diagnosis
End stage alcoholic cirrhosis.
Complication—ascites.
Alcohol dependence syndrome.
Hypobeta-lipoproteinemia.

ID 13
Specialty: General Medicine
Consultant: Dr Foster

Episode Summary

History
This 50-year-old man was admitted for liver biopsy following abnormal liver function tests. He had drunk 25 pints of beer a week for many years.
He gave a 2-year history of dizziness and abdominal pain.
He had an episode of pain in the first metatarsal joint one week ago due to gout.
Hypertension was diagnosed at a works medical examination 3-year-ago.

On Examination
Hepatomegaly. Blood pressure raised at 180/110.
Slight tenderness over first metatarsal joint.

Post-admission

Final Diagnosis
Chronic alcoholic hepatitis
Gout
Hypertension.

ID 8
Specialty: General Medicine
Consultant: Dr Fletcher

Episode Summary

History
This 50-year-old housewife was admitted as an emergency following collapse and vomiting.
She had experienced a severe occipital headache for 30 minutes prior to collapse, and epistaxes for the past 4 weeks.
Past left sided stroke. Taking anticoagulants and antihypertensive medication.

On Examination
Looked unwell. Slight residual facial weakness, right sided. Blood pressure raised at 180/110.
She was in congestive cardiac failure.

Post-admission
The patient regained consciousness but remained drowsy and confused. She died 2 days after admission.

Final Diagnosis
Cerebrovascular accident.
Congestive heart failure.
Hypertension.

ID 1445
Name: Philip   Age: 20 years
DOA: 30.9.99   DOD: 7.10.99

Final Diagnosis
Rheumatic heart disease with severe mitral stenosis severe aortic regurgitation.
Acute rheumatic fever with carditis.

Presenting Complaints
Breathlessness, right upper abdominal pain, bilateral swelling of leg and decreased urine
output for 10 days.

History
Breathlessness insidious onset, progressively worsening, present at rest associated with
orthopnea.
Abdominal pain-located in right upper quadrant, severe pain, continuous in nature, not
colicky. No vomiting, hematemesis, abdominal distension. Also he had swelling of both
legs for 10 days. There was associated decreased in urine output. No history of facial
puffiness.

Past History
At the age of 13 he had an attack of rheumatic fever but no carditis. He took penidure
prophylexis of 1 year and then stopped. He was well till May 1999 when he developed
fever for 1 month of moderate grade and intermittent along with joint pain but no
swelling. This was followed by proximal muscle weakness of gradual progression, later he
was improving but has worsened over 2 weeks.
System review: Normal.
Family history: Not significant.
Personal history: Not a smoker does not consume alcohol.

Physical Examination
PR: 110/min BP: 160/90 mm Hg. No PICCL. Pedal edema bilateral pitting positive.
He had bilateral flat foot positive, short 4th digit in both legs.

CVS: Elevated JVP, Apex-left 6th ICS 1 cm lateral to mid clavicular line. Hyperdynamic
apex, palpable S3, Sift S, PSM at apex. EDM at aortic area, Soft A2, Lout P2.

RS: Trachea central, bilateral equal air entry bilateral equal air entry. Bilateral crepitating
heard.

Abdomen: Flat abdomen, tender liver 4 cm below right MCL. No free fluids.

CNS: HMF normal. Cranial nerves normal. Motor-proximal and dostal groups in both UL
and LL grade 4/5 power. DTR normal.
Sensory system normal.

Course in Hospital and Discussion
Mr Philip was diagnosed to have rheumatic fever when he was 13-year-old. He did not
have carditis then. He failed to take Penidure prophylaxis subsequently. He came with
breathlessness, palpitations and pedal edema of 10 days duration. On clinical examination
he had mitral and aortic regurgitation and pericardial rub. Because he had involvement of
endocardium and pericardium of short duration he was treated as acute rheumatic carditis and was started on steroids. Because he had pulmonary hypertension it was thought
that it was acute carditis on a pre-existing chronic rheumatic valvular heart disease.
    He also has been having mild proximal muscle weakness of upper limb and lower limb
for 2 months. His CPK was normal. Because he had bilateral short 4th metatarsal bones
hypoparathyroidism was considered but was ruled out by biochemical evaluation. He did
not have... EMG and NCV were normal. Hence the proximal muscle weakness was

thought to be due to severe cardiac failure. In fact with antifailure medications his muscle power improved.

Consultations Obtained

Cardiology unit was consulted for rheumatic carditis and advised antifailure measurements and Penidure prophylaxis.

Neurology unit was consulted for proximal muscle weakness and advised physiotherapy.

Condition on discharge: Improved.

Disposition: Home.

Recommendations

Activity: As tolerated

Diet: Salt restriction diets 4 gm salt and 1 liter of fluid/day.

Tab Envas 5 mg twice daily till review

Tab Prednisolone 50 mg once daily for 3 weeks and then to be tapered over 2 weeks.

Life-long Penidure Prophylaxis

Follow-up in medicine OPD on 20.10.99

ID 833
Name: Haleena   Age: 32 years
DOA: 13.5.98   DOD: 17.5.98

Principal Diagnosis
Pituitary microadenoma.

History
Admitted with an appointment for further investigations for her pituitary problem. No
fresh complaints.

Physical Findings
Obes, facial Cushing, BP 150/75
Systemic examination: NAD

Lab Investigation
Microalbumin	70 mg/L	
Urine creatinine	8.04 mmol/L	
Micralb/creatinine	0.077	
24 hr urine vol	1.187 liter	
Metanephrines	3.5 umol/L	
24 hr metanephrin	4.1 umol/24 h	(Adults less than 4.8)
HDL cholesterol	1.57 mmol/L	
LDL cholesterol	0.6 mmol/L	
Triglycerides	2.8 mmol/L	(Fasting less than 2.3)
Cholesterol	3.5 mmol/L	
Free T4	11.4 pmol/L	(8.4–22.6)
Thyroid stimula	1.484 mIU/L	(.03–4.29)

HbsAg: Positive
X-ray/imaging investigations
CT adrenal: Left adrenal hyperplasia
MRI pituitary: Microadenoma

Treatment and Progress
Put on Nifedipine R, Simvastatin and Humulin N and R.

Condition on Discharge: Stable.

Discharge Medications
Nifedipine, Humulin R and N and Simvastatin.

Follow-up Appointment
On 7.5.98 in medicine OPD.

ID 7
Specialty: General Medicine
Consultant: Dr Foster

Episode Summary

History
This 65-year-old retired civil servant was admitted as an emergency complaining of tight central chest pain of one hour's duration.
10-year history of angina.
On treatment for hypothyroidism.

On Examination
Pyrexial. Otherwise NAD.

Post-admission
ECG and cardiac enzymes were normal. Mrs Dunning was believed to have suffered an anginal attack and was discharged home.

Diagnosis
Angina pectoris.
Pyrexia of unknown origin.
Hypothyroidism.

SAMPLE DISCHARGE SUMMARIES

General Surgery

ID 973
Name: Leo   Age: 39 years
DOA: 25.12.99   DOD: 10.1.2000

Final Diagnosis: Diabetes mellitus
                           Cellulites-right leg
                           Sepsis syndrome

History
Mr Leo presented with pain and swelling of the right leg following a burn injury to the right leg one-week-ago. He also had low-grade intermittent fever for 3 days with no chills or rigors. The swelling and pain in the right leg had progressively worsened and he had difficulty in walking. He also noticed yellowing of the sclera and passed high colored urine for the past 3 days. He is a known diabetic for 5 years. He was diagnosed to have Hansen's disease 10-year-ago and was on multi-drug therapy for one year. He had undergone amputation of the right second and fifth toes 2-year-ago for diabetic cellulites.

On Examination
He was icteric. His pulse rate was 90/min and blood pressure was 110/70 mm Hg. There was edema over the right leg from 2 cm below the tibial tuberosity involving the entire right foot. There was a 3 × 2 cm ulcer over the lateral aspect of the right foot. There was foul smelling purulent discharge from the ulcer.
Cardiovascular and respiratory systems were normal.

Investigations
WBC total counts 12,000/cumm. DC: BF 9 N 86 L5 M2%
Random blood sugar 171 mg% Na 131 mEq/L   K 4.1 mEq/L
LFT: T Bill. 4.6 mg% Dir 3.6 mg% T Prot 6.4 gm% Alb 2.6 gm%
SGOT 38 U/L   SGPT 46 U/L   Alk Phos 219 U/L
Urine sugars present.
Urine bile pigments pos ++
Urine bile salts +
Plasma Glucose: Ac 248 mg% HbsAg and HIV: negative
Random blood sugar 342 mg%
PT 13.4/12.5 sec, INR 1.0
Urine spot Na 108 mEq/L
Urine acetone negative
ECG: Changes consistent with hypokalemia.
Chest X-ray: Normal
ECHO: Mild pericardial effusion seen (laterally 6 mm, posteriorly 6 mm).
Normal LV function. Ejection fraction 57%
26.12.99: Plasma Glucose: AC 235 mg%, PC 321 mg%

Operation Done
Right below knee amputation done under spinal anesthesia on 26.12.99.

Operative Findings
Necrotising fascitis extending up to lower half of right leg.

Postoperative Period
Uneventful.

Recommendations:
Crutch walking
Tab Daonil 5 mg twice daily
Tab Glyciphage 250 mg thrice daily
Inj Actrapid 16–16–20 units
To check sugars after 2 weeks and follow-up in Medicine OPD.

ID 801
Name: Rosaline Age: 40 year
DOA: 10.1.98   DOD: 4.2.98

Final Diagnosis

Chronic calculous cholecystitis with choledocholithiasis noninsulin dependent diabetes mellitus.

History

40-year-old Mrs Rosaline presented with abdominal pain and fever of 3 days duration and pale stools for 1 day. She is not a known diabetic or hypertensive.

On Examination

A moderately built middle-aged lady. There was no pallor, icterus, cyanosis, clubbing, lymphadenopathy or edema detected. Her pulse rate was 92/min and blood pressure was 130/90 mm Hg. Per abdomen: There was tenderness detected in the right hypochondrial region. There was no palpable organomegaly, masses or free fluid detected. Bowel sounds were normal. His cardiovascular system, respiratory system and central nervous systems examinations were normal.

Investigations

Hb   13.0   gm% WBC: TC 15,700/cumm   DC: BF 2 N77 E1 L20%
Na 130mEq/L K 4.8 mEq/L   Creatinine   0.9 mg% Random blood sugar   218 mg%
PT 11/10 sec, PTT   36/30 sec
LFT: T Bill 0.7 mg% Dir 0.4 mg% T Prot   7.9 gm% Alb   3.8 gm%
SGOT   30 U/L   SGPT 36 U/L, Alk Phos   142 U/L   LDH 336 U/L
Serum amylase   25   HbsAg and HIV: Negative
ECG and Chest X-ray: Normal study.
Ultrasound abdomen: Choledocholithiasis casing biliary abstraction and cholangitis.
ERCP: Choledocholithiasis. Proximal common bile duct, common hepatic duct and intra-hepatic biliary radicles were normal.
Sphincterotomy was done. Stone crushed with mechanical lithotripter.

Operation Done

Attempted laparoscopic cholecystectomy and converted to open cholecystectomy under general anesthesia on 29.1.98.

Operation Findings

Hartmann's pouch and proximal cystic duct were adherent to common hepatic duct. Dissection of the calot's triangle could have been dangerous, hence the decision to convert to open cholecystectomy. Subtotal cholecystectomy was performed.

Biopsy Report

Number-1435/98. Chronic cholecystitis.

Discussion

Mrs Rosaline presented with features of cholangitis. Radiologic investigations showed cholelithiasis with choledecholithiasis. ERCP was done and a nasobiliary drain placed *in situ.* She was treated with a course of antibiotics based on bile culture report. After she became afebrile sphincterotomy and stone extraction was done. She underwent open cholecystectomy and had an uneventful postoperative period. She was detected to have diabetes, which was controlled with diet.

Recommendations

1500 calories diabetic diet
Tab Tramadol 100 mg if she has pain
To review in surgery OPD after one month.

ID 184
Name: Muneer   Age: 30 years
DOA: 13.3.95   DOD: 18.4.95

Final Diagnosis
Stricture at the choledochojejunostomy site (postoperation Whipple's operation).
Non-Hodgkin's lymphoma, probably pancreas.

Presenting Symptoms
Mr Muneer presented with jaundice and history of malena for 1 year. Jaundice is intermittent and associated with pale stool. Each episode lasted for about a month. There was
associated abdominal pain mainly in the epigastric region, which was, severs, no radiating
and burning in character. Pain was not associated with food. Dark colored stools started
2-months-ago. He also complains of generalized body aches. He underwent
pancreaticoduodenectomy with choledochojejunostomy and gastrojejunostomy in May
1994 for a mass in the head of the pancreas. Diagnosed previously to have subsequent
non-Hodgkin's lymphoma.

Physical Findings
Young male thinly built. Pulse was 68/min. BP 14/80 mm Hg, No pallor, icterus, pedal
edema or significant lymphadenopathy. Abdomen soft, all quadrants moving well with
respiration. Liver, spleen, gallbladder—not palpable. Systemic examination was normal.

Investigations
PCV   31   RBS   88mg% Creat   0.7 mg% LDH   388
HIV, HbsAg: negative   plat 179,000/cumm   WBC 700/cumm   DC B2 E2 N79 M1

Operation Done
Revision choledochojejunostomy under general anesthesia on 28.2.1995.

Operative Findings
Dense adhesions in the supracolic compartment. Choledochojejunostomy site was
strictured. Adhesions were normal. No evidence of lymphoma in the abdomen. Duodenal
jejunal flexure and C loop of duodenum *in situ*. Other anastomoses no isolated for fear of
causing injury.

Course in Hospital
Uneventful

Recommendations
Tab Atenolol   5 mg   OD
Review in surgery OPD and cancer medicine OPD after 3 months.

ID 514
Name: Francina   Age: 62 years
DOA: 20.12.99   DOD: 17.1.2000

Final Diagnosis
Obstructed incisional hernia

History
Sixty-two-year-old Mrs Francina presented with history of swelling over the lower abdomen for 10 years. She had vomiting and severe pain over the swelling for past 2 weeks. She had not passed motion for 1 week. She had 3 surgeries in the past LSCS done in KSG Hospital, incisional hernia repair in 1985 at Govt Hospital and TAH+BSO at Govt Hospital. She had no history of hypertension or diabetes. She was taking Eltroxin as prescribed elsewhere.

On Examination
She was afebrile. Her pulse was 92/min and BP 170/90 mm Hg.
Examination of CVS was normal.
RS-there was bilateral basal crepitations heard.
Abdomen: There was a subumbilical lines scar 7 cm long. There were 2 swellings. One swelling 4 × 4 cm in size on the right side just below the umbilicus which was not reducible, another swelling above the putis on the left side of midline which had a cough impulse. Bowel sounds were heard normal.

Investigations
Hb 11.4   TC: 8000/cumm   DC: N69   E1 L23 M7
RBS: 155 mg% AU and HIV: Negative creatinine   1.0
Na   138   K+ 3.2
ECG: Sinus tachycardia. Probable old inferior wall myocardiac infarct.
ECHO: normal LV function
TFT: T4 8.7   FTC 1.39   PFT Normal

Treatment
Incisional hernia repair with mesh under general anesthesia on 6.1.2000.

Operation Findings
Infraumbilical midline defects 2 × 1 cm in upper end and another 7 × 4 cm in lower part of scar. Upper sac contained omentum. Lower sac contained small bowel loops, which were adhered to the neck of the sac and were viable.

Post of Period
Uneventful.

Recommendations
Tab Combiflam whenever necessary for pain thrice daily.
Review in surgery OPD next week.

ID 065
Name: Nancy   Age: 31 years
DOA: 2.9.2000   DOD: 14.9.2000

Final Diagnosis
Nodular hyperplasia.

History
Mrs Nancy noticed a swelling in front of the neck for the past six years. There were episodes of increase and decrease in the size of the swelling. There were no features or hypothyroidism of hyperthyroidism. For the past one year she developed pain over the swelling. She was diagnosed to have rheumatoid arthritis ten-year-back for which she took medicines for six years. She is not a know diabetic but was diagnosed to be a hypertensive for which she was not on regular medication. No history of loss of weight or appetite.

On Examination
Her pulse rate was 80/min and blood pressure was 120/70 mm Hg. There was no pallor or icterus. She had a swelling in front of the neck in the region of thyroid, which moved with deglutition. On the right side, the lobe measures 4 × 4 cm and was soft. On the left side, the lobe was 5 × 5 cm and firm. On the right side a 0.5 × 0.5 cm hard nodule was felt. The swelling had a retrosternal extension. The carotids were normally placed. There were no cervical lymph nodes palpable.
Respiratory system: Bilateral equal air entry. No crepts or wheeze present.
Cardiovascular system: S1 and S2 normal.
Abdomen: There were no masses palpable.

Investigations
Hb 10.5 gm% Random blood sugar   163 mg% S Creatinine   0.9 mg%
LFT: T Bill   0.5 mg% Dir   0.2 mg% T Prot   7.2 gm% Alb 3.2 gm%
SGOT 47 U/L SGPT   32 U/L   Alk Phos   187 U/L
HIV and HbsAg: Negative
PCV   27% Platelet counts   1,27,000/cumm
PT   15.1/10.8 sec, INR 1.3   PTT 30.8/28.6
Calcium   5.5 mg%
Barium swallow: Tertiary contractions of esophagus—nonspecific esophageal motility disorder. Soft tissue density mass 6 × 4 cm in lower neck goiter.
ECG and chest X-ray: Normal.

Operation Done
Near total thyroidectomy done under general anesthesia on 4.9.2000.

Operative Findings
Bilateral nodular thyroid swelling in the left lobe larger than the right. Most of the thyroid was nodular.

Biopsy Report
Number 15917/00. Nodular hyperplasia, both lobes of thyroid.

Post of Period
Following near total thyroidectomy, Mrs Nancy developed hypocalcemia. Postoperative calcium was 5.5 mg%. She was treated with parenteral and oral calcium supplements.

Recommendations
Normal diet.
Tab Sandocal 2 thrice daily for 1 month
Cap Proxyvon 1 thrice daily for 7 days.
Tab Eltroxin 0.15 mg once daily
Yearly follow-up.

ID 16
Specialty: General Surgery
Consultant: Miss Shackleton

Episode Summary

History
Mary Staples is a 78-year-old widow, living with her 54-year-old daughter. She has been referred as an urgent case by her GP with bleeding per rectum.
She has a history of myocardial infarction with congestive cardiac failure. 2-year-previously, she suffered a cardiac arrest and has recurrent chest pains. She also suffers from folate deficiency anemia.

On Examination
Sigmoidoscopy in outpatients indicted malignant tumors of the rectum. The biopsy was reported as adenocarcinoma. No signs of congestive cardiac failure. No ECG changes.

Diagnosis on Admission
Admitted for resection of rectal carcinoma.

Procedure
Abdominal resection with colostomy.

Postoperative
Uneventful postoperative course.
Discharged after 12 days.

Final Diagnosis
Primary: Adenocarcinoma of rectum
Secondary: Folate deficiency anemia
    Angina
    History of healed myocardial infarction.

ID 15
Specialty: General Surgery
Consultant: Mr Bridge

Episode Summary

History
This 65-year-old lady was admitted with increasing tiredness and shortness of breath.
She had been feeling unwell for the past 10 days.

Previous Medical History
Gastrectomy for carcinoma stomach 2-year-ago.

On Examination
Large Irregular mass in the upper abdomen.
Large right pleural effusion.

Procedure
Pleural aspiration.

Post-admission
Generalized carcinomatosis
Right pleural effusion indicative of a secondary malignant neoplasm of the pleura.
2 liters of fluid were removed via a pleural tap with some benefit.

Final Diagnosis
Secondary malignant neoplasm of pleura
Carcinomatosis
Previously resected carcinoma stomach.

ID 718
Name: Fathima Age: 40 years
DOA: 6.10.2000   DOD: 10.10.2000

Principal Diagnosis
Presented with 5-month history of diarrhea, heat intolerance, palpitation with chest discomfort and shortness of breath, occasional difficulty in swallowing, generalized body ache and weight loss (around 10 kg). She did not notice any neck swelling. She menopausal since more than 12 years. No eye changes and no mood changes.

Physical Findings
Not in pain or distress. PR: 100/min regular BP: 130/90. No myxedema, JVP not raised. Tremor ++, peripheral pulses: felt. No exophthalmos, no carotid bruit. Thyroid: diffuse smooth swelling, no tenderness, and no bruit. Systemic examination: unremarkable.

Investigations
HB 13.2   WBC 7.0   Plt   301
UE1+LFT+Bone: WNL
OGTT: Impaired glucose tolerance
Antithyroglobulin: Negative
Antithyroid microsomal antibodies: Positive
TFT: Free T4 62.9 TSH 0.003
X-ray/imaging investigations: 7.10.2000: Ultrasound thyroid: Echotexture of both thyroid lobes are mixed heterogeneous of non-specific. Size of the thyroids are within normal however. 9.10.2000: X-ray right hand: No evidence of bone of joint abnormality. Soft tissue swelling around the proximal IPJ of the index finger.
ECG: sinus tachycardia.

Consultation Findings
She was seen by surgeon for a small abscess in her right index finger. For that she was started on Augmentin.

Treatment and Progress
She was started on Carbimazole 15 mg tid and Propranolol 40 mg tid. After that she felt well and improved.

Follow-up Care and Advice
To be followed up at Chennai Hospital. TFT to be repeated after two month, and the dose of Carbimazole to be readjusted.

Discharge Medications
Carbimazole 15 mg tid × 1/12
Propranolol   40 mg tid × 1/12
Augmentin   375 mg tid × 5 days

Follow-up Appointment
The patient has appointment on next weak in surgical OPD.

SAMPLE DISCHARGE SUMMARY

Psychiatry

ID 9
Specialty: Mental Illness (Psychiatry)
Consultant: Dr Houghton

Episode Summary

History
This patient was admitted for assessment under section 2 of the Mental Health Act. John was unsure why he was in hospital but he had been suffering severe paranoid delusions and believed his neighbors were trying to kill him.
He is alcohol dependent and his paranoid ideas coincide with periods of heavy drinking. He had been admitted on three previous occasions.
His father suffered from schizophrenia before his death.

Post-admission
He remained deluded and was irritable and abusive on the ward. He accepted drug therapy and two weeks later was feeling better and was demonstrating no psychotic features. Following two event free periods of weekend leave he was discharged home.

Final Diagnosis
Paranoid schizophrenia
Alcohol dependence
Family psychiatric history.

SAMPLE DISCHARGE SUMMARIES

Orthopedics

ID 607
Name: Nicholas   Age: 26 years
DOA: 4.4.99   DOD: 7.4.99

Final Diagnosis
Disk prolapse L3-4 with Left L4 radiculopathy.

History
26-year-old man presenting with low back pain since 4 months. Radiating pain over left lower limb for past 1 month. Pain in sharp, shooting type over left thigh, by relieved by sitting for 10 minutes. No history of chronic cough. Treated in Muscat with NSAID and bed-rest. No history of bladder or bowel disturbance. No history of weakness of lower limbs. Occasional paresthesia of left foot. Past history—not a known hypertensive or diabetic.

On Examination
Young adult thinly built. CVS and RS: normal. BP: 126/84 mm Hg, spine-no deformity (Paraspinal spasm positive). Tenderness present. Range of movement: flexion possible upto midthigh level extension painful limitation. SlRT – right negative/45° left side.

Investigations
PCV—45 AU and HIV—Negative.

Treatment and Discussion
Surgery done discectomy L3-4 on 5.4.98 and left L4 root canal decompression under general anesthesia. Postoperative neurology same as preoperation.

Recommendations
Cap Cephalexin 500 mg every 6th hourly for 7 days.
Bed-rest for 2 weeks.
To review in orthopedic OPD after 3 weeks.

ID 605
Name: George   Age: 25 years
DOA: 10.5.99   DOD: 13.5.99

Final Diagnosis
Maluniting fracture shaft of left femur.

History
Alleged history of road traffic accident 3-months-ago when he sustained closed injury to left thigh and left leg with inability to stand or walk on left leg. He was treated with a pop cast till toes. Not a known diabetic or hypertensive.

On Examination
Not pale, pulse 86/min. Other systems: normal.

Local Examination
Apparent shortening, left lower limb present with muscle wasting left thigh varus deformity at mid femur present, skin hyperkeratosis present, stress tenderness present, left knee flexion 0-10 degree. Actual shortening 4 cm infratrochanteric (+), left leg normal. There is no distal neurovascular deficit.

Investigations
PCV 50 %, RBS 108 mg%, Creatinine   0.9 mg%, AU, HIV – negative. X-ray maluniting fracture left shaft of femur.

Treatment and Discussion
On 11.5.99 under spinal anesthesia osteoclasis and open "K" nailing with 13 × 42 cm and distal interlocking with local bone grafting done.

Recommendations
Cap Cloxacillin 500 mg four times daily × 1 week
Tab Voveran 50 mg one prn.
Non-weight bearing crutch walking × 6 weeks.
Review in orthopedic OPD on 21.5.99.

ID 231
Name: Catharine   **Age: 35 years**
DOA: 1.1.2001   **DOD: 5.1.2001**

Final Diagnosis
L5-S1 Disc prolapse.

History
35-year-old Mrs Catharine presented to the OPD with pain in the low back for the past one year aggravated for the past one-month and radiation down the left thigh and leg and is grossly interfering with her activities of daily living.

On Examination
She is an obese lady. BP 130/80 mm Hg. Gait-cautious with a list to the left. Straight leg rising test positive at 60. Spine: Decrease in lateral flexion to the left. Lasigues positive at 50. Motor: Grade 4 power left EHL, EDL. Sensory: No deficits. DTR: left ankle jerk: Absent.

Investigations
PCV 48%, Creatinine 0.9 mg%, RBC 127 mg%, AU and HIV negative, Chest/ECG within normal limits.

Surgery Done
Discectomy L5-S1 under general anesthesia on 16.2.2000.

Postoperative Period
Uneventful.

Recommendations
Tab Combiflam one twice daily.
Tab Rantac 150 mg twice daily.
Back care.
Lumbar spine strengthening exercises.

ID 12
Specialty: Orthopedics
Consultant: Mr Morris

Episode Summary

History
This 15-year-old boy sustained a knife laceration to the left thumb one month previously. Exploration was carried out at that time, but it was subsequently felt that deeper structures were involved and the patient was readmitted.

Procedure
Exploration of the muscles of the left thumb was carried out and the damaged flexor pollicis muscle was repaired.

Post-admission

Final Diagnosis
Open wound of finger with tendon of thumb involvement.
Accident caused by knife.

ID 11
Specialty: Orthopedics
Consultant: Mr David

Episode Summary

History
This 24-year-old motorcyclist was involved in a collision with a car.

On Examination
Closed fracture mid shaft right femur
Compound fracture mid shaft right tibia.

Post-admission

Final Diagnosis
Closed fracture mid shaft right femur
Compound fracture mid shaft right tibia
(Fracture involving multiple body regions)
Road traffic accident.

ID 10
Specialty: Orthopedic
Consultant: Mr David

Episode Summary

History
This 19-year-old golfer sustained a twisting injury to his left knee on the golf course.

On Examination
Knee swollen with effusion
Patient unable to extend knee
Marked tenderness medical aspect of joint

Procedure
Arthroscopy of left knee revealed tear of medical cartilage, which was repaired.

Postoperative

Final Diagnosis
Medical cartilage tear.
Overextension and strenuous movements.

SAMPLE DISCHARGE SUMMARIES

Neurosurgery

ID 100
Name: Paul   Age: 3 years
DOA: 11.11.90   DOD: 13.11.90

Final Diagnosis
Post-traumatic left partial motor seizures with secondary generalization.

History
Three-year-old Paul was brought to casualty with an alleged history of fall while playing
on 11.11.90 at 8 pm. He had 2 episodes of partial motor seizures involving left upper and
lower limbs with secondary generalization. He also developed decreased movement of the
left side since then. There was no history of vomiting, ENT bleed or any other external
injuries.

On Examination
His pulse rate was 130/min and BP was 120/70 mm Hg. Saturation was 99% on O_2. Pupils
were equal and reacting to light. There was left sided gaze paresis. He was in postictal
state. GCS was E4 M5 V3 12/15. There was mild left sided hemiparesis. There was
bilateral equal air entry and abdomen was soft. There were no other external injuries.

Investigations
PCV   32   sodium 134 mEq/L   potassium 3.6 mEq/L S creatinine 0.5 mg%
HIV and HbsAg were negative.
Chest X-ray: Cervical spine X-rays and skull X-rays were normal.
CT scan brain was normal. There were no focal lesions. The subarachnoid spaces and
basal cisterns were seen well. There were no fractures seen.

Discussion
Three-year-old Paul was brought to casualty around on hour following fall while playing
at 8 pm on 11.11.90. He had 2 episodes of posttraumatic left partial motor seizures with
secondary generalization. He had developed mild left hemiparesis following the seizures
CT scan did not show any focal lesions. He was admitted for observation. During the next
day there was improvement in his weakness. He was advised to continue syrup phenytoin 20 mg twice daily till further advice.

Condition at Discharge
He was afebrile, alert and active. GCS was 15/15. There were no further seizures. The
power was grade 5 in all 4 limbs. Gait was normal.

Advice
Syrup Phenytoin 20 mg twice daily till further advice.
Syrup Salbutamol 0.9 mg thrice daily till further advice.
Normal saline nasal drops 6th hourly for 1 week.
To follow-up in neurosurgery OPD after 1 month.
To follow-up in child health OPD.

ID 96
Name: Dr Barbara   Age: 55 years
DOA: 8.11.95   DOD: 16.11.95

Final Diagnosis
Left anterior tentorial meningioma
Diabetes mellitus
Disseminated choroiditis.

History
This fifty-five-year-old lady presented with a history of episodic lancination pain in the left side of the face, for the past two years. The pain was severe and worsened with slight touch or with facial movements. There was no history suggestive of diplopia, or other cranial nerve dysfunction. No history of difficulty in chewing. No other neurological system. She had very gradually progressive hearing loss in the left ear for the last three years. No history of associated vertigo or tinnitus. She is a known diabetic on Daonil. She also to disseminated choroiditis. No history of recent worsening in visual symptoms. She had undergone vaginal hysterectomy for uterine prolapsed in May 95, when she had a hypertensive reaction during anesthesia.

On Examination
General and systemic examination: Unremarkable. Pulse rate 94/min. BP 120/80 mm Hg. No significant lymphadenopathy.

Neurological examination: Mental functions normal. Visual acuity: Right finger counting at three feet with large central scotoma, left is normal. Fundus revealed degenerative changes around maculae bilaterally. No papilledema. Pupils right 3 mm, left 3.5 mm, reacting to light. Eye movements were normal. Left corneal reflex was diminished. There was anesthesia in left V2, V3 territory. Mild masseter wasting on left side. No jaw deviation. No facial weakness. Mild hearing impairment in left ear, bone conduction better than air conduction. Weber lateralized to left. Lower cranial nerves normal. Sensory-motor examination revealed no deficits. Deep tendon jerks were normal. Planters were flexor. No cerebellar or meningeal signs.

Investigations
PCV 32   WBC Total   7700/cmm   Diff N 72% L 18% E 3 % ESR (1 hr) 45   Creatinine 0.9 mg% Pl Glucose   AC 140 mgm%
X-ray chest: Normal
ECG: Normal
Echocardiogram: Normal
CT scan brain (June 95): Shows a partly calcified, irregular, hypo dense mass (3 × 2 cm) along the anterior edge of the tentorium on the left side. There was minimal effacement of the left crural cistern. No hydrocephalus.
MRI scan brain (August 95): Shows a 3 × 2 × 2, ill-defined, irregularly outlined lesion in left anterior tentorial edge, adjacent to Meckel's cave, bulging in to the left ambient cistern without significant compression of the brainstem. No other parenchymal lesions. No hydrocephalus.

Discussion
This patient presented with trigeminal neuralgia in left V2, V3 distribution. Peripheral nerve avulsion had been done elsewhere for temporary pain relief. Imaging studies revealed a small calcified, enhancing mass in the region of the anterior tentorial edge. A possibility of a tentorial meningioma or inflammatory lesion was considered. The surgical approach to the lesion involved retraction of the dominant temporal lobe and as most of the lesion appeared calcified there was a possibility of inconclusive biopsy. Considering the small size of the lesion and the totally a symptomatic present status she was advised follow-up after six months, to assess radiological or clinical progression of the disease.

Condition at Discharge
Neurological status quo.

Advice
1500 calories Diabetic diet.
Tab Danonil 5 mg with breakfast.
              2.5 mg with dinner.
To come for follow-up after six months.

ID 579
Name: Patrick   Age: 45 years
DOA: 4.8.98   DOD: 6.8.98

Final Diagnosis
Left glomus jugular tumor.

History
This 45-year-old gentleman presented with pulsatile tinnitus in the left ear since 1-½ years. This was followed by gradual diminution of hearing in his left ear. There was no history of headache, vomiting, loss of consciousness, seizure or vertigo. There was no history of fever, trauma or weight loss. He had no weakness or sensory impairment. There was no difficulty in maintaining balance while walking. There were no known medical risk factors.

On Examinations
Average built. PR was 70/min. BP was 110/80 mm Hg. General examination was normal. Both carotid pulsation was felt normally with no palpable thrill and no bruit was heard. CVS, chest and abdomen were normal. Higher mental functions were normal. Pupil was bilaterally equal in size and normally reacting to the light. Fundus was normal. Rinne's test was positive on the right side and negative in the left ear. Weber test was lateralized to the left ear. Rest of the cranial nerves was normal. Motor examination was normal. All the sensory modalities were well-preserved. There was no cerebellar sign. No meningeal sign was present. Skull and spin were normal.

Investigations
Platelets   3153000/ccumm   BT 2.0   MIN mts PT pt/cont   14/12 sec
MRI brain-showed a contrast-enhancing lesion in the left jugular fossa and was seen eroding the petrous bone adjacent to it.
Angiography brain—the lesion was seen to be supplied by the left ascending pharyngeal and left carotico-tympanic artery.
Procedure: CT guided stereotactic radiosurgery done on 5.8.98.
A 15 gray radiation, 80% of isodose, was given to the lesion.
The size of the collimeter was 2.5 cm.

Discussion
This 45-year-old gentleman presented with pulsatile tinnitus and gradual loss of hearing in the left ear since 1-½ years. Clinically patient had severe conductive hearing loss in his left ear. MRI brain showed lesion in the left jugular fossa and was seen eroding the surrounding petrous bone, which was suggestive of glomus-jugular tumor. He underwent CT guided stereotactic radiosurgery of the lesion on 5.8.98. Post-radio surgery there was no fresh complaint and patient was discharged with the advice for follow-up after 1 year.

Condition on Discharge
Afebrile. No fresh complaint. Neurologically as before.

Recommendation
Tab Paracetamol 1 tablet for pain as and when required.
Review in neurology surgery OPD after 1 year.

ID 37
Name: Leona   Age: 50 years
DOA: 5.7.99   DOD: 26.7.99

Final Diagnosis
Closed head injury, left temporal contusion, left humerus fracture.

History
50-year-old lady was brought to casualty at 3 pm on 5.7.99, 3 hours following an alleged fall from 10 feet height. She had loss of consciousness for 10 minutes followed by altered sensorium. She had vomited 4 times. No seizures or ENT bleed. No significant systemic history or past medical risk factors.

On Examination
Afebrile. Pulse 90 /min   BP   110/70 mm Hg SaO$_2$ 99% on room air. She had no scalp lacerations. She had closed fracture of left humerus. GCS   12/15: E4/M5/V3. Pupils were bilaterally equal and reacting to light. She had no motor deficits. Systemic examination was normal.

Investigations
PCV 31   sodium   135 mEq/L   potassium 4.9 mEq/L   creatinine   1 mg% random glucose sugar 99% HIV and HbsAg were negative.
Chest X-ray: Normal.
X-ray cervical spine lateral showed no fracture or dislocation.
X-ray of left arm showed a fracture of proximal one-third of humerus.
CT scan (5.7.99) showed a left posterior temporal contusion with effaced temporal horn. The brainstem cisterns were normal.

Discussion
50-year-old Mrs Leona was brought to casualty 3 hours following trauma with a GCS of 12/15. CT scan showed a left posterior temporal contusion. She also had a closed fracture of the left humerus. She was treated with anticonvulsants, antiedema measures, analgesics and intravenous fluids. The orthopedics doctors who had applied a plaster cast for the fracture saw her. Her GCS improved to 13/15, she was found to be aphasic. She was started on nasogastric tube feeds. She was discharged and was advised to continue anticonvulsants, and also nasogastric tube feeds till she was able to take oral feeds.

Condition at Discharge
Afebrile. GCS 13/15: E4/M5/V4. Pupils bilaterally 2 mm and reaction to light. No cranial nerve, motor or sensory deficits. On plaster for the left humerus fracture. On nasogastric tube feeds. On urinary catheter.

Advice
Cap Dilantin   100 mg thrice daily till further advice.
Paracetamol 2 tablets for pain or fever.
Nasogastric tube feeds as demonstrated: 3000 ml, 2000 cal, 40 gm protein, 16 gm salt, in sitting position.
Change urinary catheter after 3 weeks.
Review in orthopedics OPD and neurology surgery OPD.

ID 478
Name: Catharine   Age: 40 years
DOA: 5.7.2000   DOD: 26.7.2000

Final Diagnosis
D8-9 intradural extramedullary meningioma.

History
This 40-year-old lady presented with difficulty in walking and weakness of both lower limbs for the past 3 months. She had stiffness of both lower limbs for the past 3 months. She had impaired sensation in both lower limbs for the past 2 months. She had low back pain, no radicular pain. There were no bowel or bladder abnormalities. There were no medical risk factors.

On Examination
She was a moderately built, middle-aged lady. Her pulse rate was 86/min and blood pressure was 130/80 mm Hg. The general and systemic examination was normal. The higher functions were normal. The visual acuity and fields were normal. There was no papilledema. The pupils were equal and reacting to light. There were no other cranial nerve abnormalities. The motor power and tone was normal in the upper limbs. Both the lower limbs were spastic. The touch, pain and temperature sensation were impaired by 30 % below D9 level bilaterally, no sacral sparing. The joint position sense was impaired in digits of both the lower limbs. The upper limb reflexes were normal. The lower limb reflexes were exaggerated bilaterally. The plantars was up going. The superficial abdominal and cremasteric reflexes were absent. There were no signs of meningeal irritation or of cerebellar dysfunction. Gait was spastic. There was no spinal deformity or local tenderness.

Investigations
PCV 38   Creatinine   0.8 mg% Random Glucose sugar   170 mg%. The chest X-ray was normal.
The ECG showed occasional ventricular premature complexes.
X-ray of the thoracic spine showed scoliosis with convexity to the left.
HIV and HbsAg were negative.
The MRI dorsolumbar spine revealed the presence or a nodular, intradural mass at D8 and D9 levels, enhancing with contrast and compressing the spinal cord.

Operation Done
D8-9 right hemilaminectomy, right D8-9 facectomy and total excision of the tumor under general anesthesia on 17.7.2000.

Operative Findings
Right D8-9 facers were drilled out followed by right.
D8-9 hemilaminectomy. Dura was opened laterally. There was grayish red, moderately vascular, soft to firm extramedullary tumor. The right D9 root was sacrificed. Dura was not closed and was covered with gelfoma.

Biopsy Impression
Number 12742/00: Meningioma, D8-9 level, and vertebral canal.

Discussion
Forty-year-old Catharine presented clinically with progressive spastic paraparesis. MRI thoraco-lumbar spine showed contrast enhancing mass lesion at D8-9 level. She underwent D8-9 right hemilaminectomy, right D8-9 facectomy and total excision of tumor under general anesthesia on 17.7.2000. Postoperatively, there was subjective improvement of power in both lower limbs and spasticity also improved. She had low back pain. She was walking with support. She was given physiotherapy.

Condition on Discharge

Afebrile. She was taking normal diet and voiding normally. Neurological status remained same in both lower limbs. She was walking with support. Wound was healthy.

Advice on Discharge

Normal diet.

Tab Paracetamol 2 tab for pain.

To continued physiotherapy.

To come for review in neurosurgery OPD after 3 months.

ID 6
Specialty: Neruosurgery
Consultant: Mr Foley

Episode Summary

History
Mr Jackson is a 35-year-old man who has suffered with hypertension for some years. He is a driving instructor who works long and irregular hours. He presented with paralysis of the left side of the face, left arm and left leg. He was very drowsy and confused.

On Examination
Cerebrovascular accident was diagnosed caused by the rupture of a congenital cerebral aneurysm.

Post-admission
Mr Jackson was discharged after 5 weeks.

Procedure
Clipping of aneurysm

Diagnosis
Main condition: Cerebrovascular accident.
Other conditions: Hypertension.
                  Ruptured congenital aneurysm.

SAMPLE DISCHARGE SUMMARIES

Pediatric Surgery

ID 732
Name: Teena   Age: 8 years
DOA: 20.5.99   DOD: 24.5.99

Principal diagnosis
Right hydronephrosis with proximal hydroureter.

Operation/Procedures
Cystourethroscopy, right retrograde pyelography 24.5.99.

History
This 8-year-female child was referred from Government hospital because of right flank pain since 3 months ago. There was dysuria but no hematuria. For the last 1 month she was pain free. IVP done in Govt hospital right hydronephrosis with proximal hydroureter because of? Stone at level of L4. She was booked for ESWL.

Physical Findings
Look well, vital signs stable, chest clear, normal heart sounds, abdomen soft, no tenderness, and normal female external genitalia.

Lab Investigations
FBC, UE1, coagulation screen all normal. Urine showed no growth.
X-ray/imaging Investigations
Ultrasound showed dilatation of the right pelvicalyceal system but no calculus seen.

Consultation Findings
The adult urologist saw her. Taken for ESWL but procedure was abandoned because no calculus was visualized.

Treatment and Progress
Underwent Cystourethroscopy, right retrograde pyelography. Tolerated procedure well. Findings as noted. Probably there was a small stone before that was passed out.

Operation Findings
Urethra, bladder, both ureteric openings all-normal. Dye study-showed dilated calyceas as in IVP, but normal looking pelvis and ureter right side.

Condition on Discharge: Stable.

Follow-up Care and Advice
Review after 6 month with DTPA at the same clinic visit.

Discharge Medications: Paracetamol.

Follow-up Appointment
The patient has appointment on 12.6.99 at 11.00 am pedartic surgery OPD.

ID 680
Name: Prince   Age: 6 years
DOA: 21.6.2001   DOD: 25.6.2001

Principal Diagnosis
Rectal mucosal proplapse, post PSARP for high anorectal anomaly.

Operation/Procedures
Excision of mucosal prolapse + circumcision 22.6.2001.

History
This 6-year-male child with rectal Mucosal prolapse post PSARP for high anorectal anomaly was admitted this time for excision of the mucosal prolapse. Known case of high anorectal anomaly. Underwent colostomy here at day 2 of life and much later definitive surgery followed by closure of the colostomy. Developed rectal mucosal prolapse right after the surgery, which persisted. Otherwise passing stools normally.

Physical Findings
Looks well, chest, normal heart sounds, abdomen flat, no fecal loading, uncircumcised, penis rotated 90 degrees to the right, testes descended, slight rectal mucosal prolapse.

Lab Investigation
Within normal limits.

Treatment and Progress
Underwent excision of the Mucosal prolapse + circumcision. Tolerated procedure well. Postoperative course unremarkable.

Operation Findings
Preoperative titanic stimulation revealed lesser contractions on the (L). Prolapsed anal mucosa on the left half of the anal orifice. Easily admits little finger. Perianal skin mobilized to see the muscles all around. Mucosectomy done. Anteriorly interrupted stitches (mattress) taken to approximate the muscles over the mucosa. One stitch taken similarly at the 6 o'clock position. Skin edges freshened and mucocutaneous interrupted sutures taken. Hemostasis achieved. Postoperative titanic stimulation revealed much better contractions on the (L). But still lesser than the (R). Penis found to be rotated 90 degrees to the (R), normal meatus. Excess foreskin excised to complete the circumcision.

Condition on Discharge: Stable.

Follow-up Care and Advice
Site bath 4–5 times daily. Review after 3 months.

Discharge Medications
Paracetamol. Lactulose 10 ml bid for 1 month.

Follow-up Appointments
Review on 30.9.2001 in paedartic surgery OPD.

ID 541
Name: Idaline's Baby   Age: 0 month
DOA: 14.5.95   DOD: 21.5.95

Principal Diagnosis
Lumbosacral myelomeningocele.

Operation/Procedures
Repair of lumbosacral myelomeningocele 14.5.95.

History
This male neonate with lumbosacral myelomeningocele was transferred from MEDIC Hospital at day 1 of life. Full term, normal home delivery. Birth weight 2.050 kg, head circumference 32 cm, height 45 cm. No abnormal features noted. He was admitted in MEDIC Hospital at 4 hours of age. Small tear developed at the sac before reaching the hospital. He was started on penicillin and gentamicin and was transferred here. Mother is G10 P9 L8.

Physical Findings
Active, pink, fontanelle soft, head circumference 32 cm, chest clear, CVS NAD, abdomen soft, normal foreskin, testes descended, anus patulous, 3 × 3 cm lesion at the Lumbosacral area, bilateral CTEV, good movements at the hips, knee and ankle.

Lab Investigations
Hb 17.7   urea, creatinine, electrolytes normal.
X-ray/imaging investigations
Both kidneys are normal. Mild dilatation of both lateral ventricles. Cortical mantle thickness of 2.2 cm. Third and fourth ventricles not dilated. No midline shift.

Treatment and Progress
Underwent back closure. Tolerated procedure well. Antibiotics continued. Postoperative course unremarkable. Head circumference of discharge 34.5 cm.

Operation Findings
Neural plaque at the dome of the sac.

Condition on Discharge: Stable

Follow-up Care and Advice
Twice weekly head circumference measurement at KMC hospital. Review after 1 month at the OPD.

Follow-up Appointments
The patient has appointment on 21.6.95 in pedartic surgery OPD.

ID 434
Name: Pauline's Baby   Age: 3 months
DOA: 10.5.99   DOD: 22.5.99

Principal Diagnosis
Meconium peritonitis.

Operation/Procedures
Laparotomy, adhesiolysis, resection of small bowel, end-to-end anastomosis 10.5.99.

History
This female neonate was transferred from KGN hospital at day 2 of life because of meconium peritonitis. Pre term, 35-36 weeks normal delivery to a G2P1 28 year's mother. Antenatal ultrasound showed polyhydramnios with features suggestive of hydrops. At birth, baby was cyanosed and needed head box oxygen. Abdomen was distended with signs of free fluid. Paracentesis was done because of respiratory distress and obtained 45 ml of ascitic fluid. Abdominal X-ray showed areas of calcification. Cefotaxime and gentamicin were started.

Physical Findings
Sick looking, afebrile, tachypneic, no dysmorphism, chest clear, abdomen markedly distended, no redness, tense all over, reducible swelling at the right inguinal area, normal female genitalia, anus patent.

Lab Investigations
Routine blood investigations with in normal limits. Blood and peritoneal fluid cultures no growth.

Treatment and Progress
Posted for surgery. Antibiotics continued. Underwent
Laparotomy, adhesiolysis, resection of small bowel, end-to-end anastomosis. Tolerated procedure well. TPN started. Later feeds was gradually introduced which was tolerated well till full feeds reached. Passing stools.

Operation Findings
On opening the peritoneum, a segment of ileum (about 20 cm from the IC junction) was adherent to the anterior abdominal wall and to transverse colon and omentum. This was inadvertently opened during the incision of the peritoneum. This segment ills the site of volvulus with perforation. Lots of greenish fluid with meconium was sucked out from the peritoneal cavity particularly in the right and left gutter. The small bowel was matted with plenty of yellowish green fleks adherent to the wall. The terminal ileum was full of grayish pellets. The site of anastomosis was good color and bleeding well (good blood supply).

Condition on Discharge: Stable.

Follow-up Appointment
Review on 29.6.99 in pedartic surgery OPD.

SAMPLE DISCHARGE SUMMARIES

Neurology

ID 79
Name: Kevin   Age: 50 years
DOA: 5.1.98   DOD: 16.1.98

Final Diagnosis
Myeloradiculopthy due to involvement of vertebrae with poorly differentiated metastasis adenocarcinoma.

Presenting complaint
Sudden onset paraplegia
Acute retention of urine   2 months.
Bowel incontinence

History
Mr Kevin not a known hypertensive or diabetic presented with sudden onset paraplegia from 2-months-ago. Along with this he had retention of urine and incontinence of bowel. His compliance of no sensory loss though there were paresthesias present. His condition has remained the same since then with no improvement or deterioration. There was a history of fall from 12 feet height 4-year-back and since then he has been having lower back pain, which radiated down the lateral aspected of both thighs. Pain used to increase while walking for a long distance.
System review: Sleep, appetite, weight, vision: Normal.
Bowel, micturition: Incontinence.
Past history: No history of hypertension/diabetes/previous history in the past.
Family history: Nothing significant.
Personal history: Smokes/not a consumer of alcohol.

Physical Examination
PR: 72/min BP 140/80 mm Hg.
No pallor, icterus cyanosis, clubbing or generalized lymphadenopathy.
No neurocutaneous markers positivie.
CVS: S1, S2 normal. No murmurs.
RS: Trachea shifted to the right. Apex at right 6th intercostals space, left sided mild and lower zones dull to percussion.
Decreased air entry in the left med and lower zone.
Abdomen: Soft, liver, spleen-normal.
CNS: Higher functions: Normal. Cranial nerves: Normal.
Motor: UL: Right and left—Normal.
LL: Right and left—Increased in breath.
Power: UL: Normal bilaterally. Bewers test: Positive.
Reflexes: UL reflexes normal. Right knee jerk not elicit able. Both plantar were up going. Abdominal reflexes are absent in all four quadraints.
Sensory: Touch sensation. Decreased upto T12 no meningeal or cerebellar signs are present. Funduscopy was normal.

Discussion
This 50-year-old gentleman was admitted with history of sudden onset paraparesis. On clinical examination he had a myeloradiculopthy with the highest level at T7 vertebral spine. Thoracic and lumbar spine X-ray showed diffuse osteosclerosis bony metastasis. Poorly differentiated metastasis adenocarcinoma of the bone. As carcinoma prostate is the most common cause for osteosclerotic bone metastastis a per rectal examination was done which revealed a normal size prostate with normal consistency. Prostatic specific

antigen level was 3.9, which was just above the upper limit of normal range. At the urologist were consulted and they felt that the PSA should have been very high if there is such an extensive disease. Hence a search was conducted of other sites of primary tumors. The second site, which was considered, was the lung as this patient had a left sided pleural effusion. Pleural tap showed hemorrhagic exudate fluid but the cytology for malignant cell were negative. Pleural biopsy revealed non-specific chronic inflammation of pleura. A further search for the primary site could not be done as patient wanted to go home due to social and financial reasons. Antituberculous treatment was continued, as there had been some documented radiological improvement in the pleural effusion. He was advised to come back for further evaluation.

Recommendations
The prognosis of recovery of function to the lower limbs is poor.
Activity: Restricted due to the
Diet: Normal.

Medications
Tab Tegretol 200 mg twice daily.
Tab Isoniazid 300 mg once daily.
Tab Rifampicin 450 mg once daily.
Continuity of care needs: Catheter drainage.

ID 1091760
Name: Nixon   Age: 50
DOA: 9.5.2001   DOD: 23.6.2001

Final Diagnosis
Cerebrovascular accident—Left gemiplegia
Diabetes mellitus type II with nephropathy and background retinopathy.

History
Mr Nixon presented with a history of bifrontal headache with vomiting and right ear discharge for 15 days. He had drowsiness and slowness of movements for 5 days before admission. There was no history of fever. Ex-smoker (stopped 10-year-ago). He was a known diabetic on treatment with oral drugs and a case of ischemic heart disease.

Physical Examination
General examination: Good BP: 100/70 mm Hg. Pulse: 92/min
CNS: Drowsy, slow response, well oriented.
Minimal right VII nerve UMN palsy.
Right ptosis.
Right otitis media positive
Absent deep tendon reflex both knee and ankle joint.
Plantars: Down going.
Fundus: Background retinopathy.
Palmomental reflex and Gabellar tap absent
Systemic exam: Normal.

Discussion
Mr Nixon a known diabetic presented with a history of drowsiness and altered sensorium for 15 days. Possibilities considered were metabolic encephalopathy (in view of high sugars more than 500 mg% and very low sodium of 114 mg%). A brain abscess was also considered (as he had right otitis media). He developed fever one week after admission. CT scan was done to rule out brain abscess and CVA and showed cortical atrophy but no other lesions. CSF examination was normal, thereby eliminating the possibility of meningitis. While in hospital he was noticed to have decreased movement of left upper and lower limbs with up going plantar. Hence, the possibility of small brainstem infarct, which was not picked up by CT scan, was considered. A repeat MRI showed multiple lacunar infarcts. Due to rapid correction of sodium, sodium levels increased to 150 mg% and hence possibility of central pontine myelinolysis was thought of. His sugars were initially difficult to control and he was started on thrice daily Actrapid injections and at discharge his sugars were under control. He also developed a urinary tract infection, which was treated with Ceftazidime with which fever subsided. His sensorium did not improve much. He was discharged at request.

Recommendations
1500 Cal. Diabetic diet + 4 L fluids through Ryle's tube
T Sorbitrate 5 mg thrice daily
T Diltiazem 30 mg thrice daily
T Becosules one daily
Moisolseye drops every 3 hours tape down eyelids at night
Position change daily every 2 hours
To change urinary catheter every month.

SAMPLE DISCHARGE SUMMARIES

Dermatology

ID 2
Specialty: Dermatology
Consultant: Dr Jones

Episode Summary

History
Miss Stephens is 59-year-old and works as a cleaner at the Technical College. She has been referred by her GP who has been treating her without success. She was admitted as a day case.

On Examination
Red scaly patches on elbows neck and back of hands.

Post-admission
Biopsy of lesion, not yet reported.

Provisional Diagnosis
• Systemic lupus erythematosus.
• Discoid lupus erythematosus.

ID 5
Specialty: Dermatology
Consultant: Dr McKenzie

Episode Summary

History
Gary Bennell is a 45-year-old man who presented with pain over the right eye.

On Examination
Unilateral pustular eruption over right eye with reddening. Some corneal ulceration.

Procedure
Antibiotics prescribed.

Diagnosis
Herpes zoster of ophthalmic nerve with some keratitis.

SAMPLE DISCHARGE SUMMARIES

Pediatrics

ID 923
Name: Jenny   Age: 10 years
DOA: 10.9.99   DOD: 13.9.99

Presenting Complaints
10-year-old Jenny was admitted with a history of high-grade intermittent fever for 6 months progressive pallor and palpitation for 3 months. He had two blood transfusions prior to admission.

Salient Clinical Findings
He was afebrile and drowsy. He had severe pallor, had generalized lymphadenopathy and in respiratory distress. The lymph node size was 1-2 cm, discrete and smooth nodes. Heart rate was 100/mt, respiratory rate was 24/mt and blood pressure was 100/70 mm Hg.
CVS: Soft cystolic murmur at the apex
Abd: Soft and liver was just palpable
Other systemic examination was within normal limit.

Clinical Diagnosis at Admission
Lymphoproliferative disorder.

Investigations

Hb (gm%)	: 2.9
TC (cumm)	: 6,000
DC (%)	: Blast 45, P2, M1, M1, N3, BF2, L47
Platelets (cu.mm)	: 4,000
Retics	: 0.2
S sodium (mEq/L)	: 136
S potassium (mEq/L)	: 4.8
Liver function test	: Total bilirubin 0.6 mg%
	Direct bilirubin 0.2 mg%
	Total protein 7.8 g%
	Albumin 3.8 g%
	SGOT 29 U/L
	SGPT 22 U/L
	Alk Phos 200 U/L
LDH	: 223
Uric Acid	: 7.1
Smear	: Acute lymphoblastic leukemia.

Treatment Given
Packed cell transfusion
Platelet rich concentrate × 3

Course in Hospital
10-year-old Jenny was admitted with a history of high-grade intermittent fever for 6 months, progressive pallor for 3 months. He had generalized lymphadenopathy and severe anemia. The diagnosis considered was lymphoproliferative disorder. Investigation revealed severe anemia, thrombocytopenia and peripheral smear study was suggestive of lymphoblastic leukemia. He was given an emergency packed cell transfusion and platelet rich concentrate. After which bone marrow examination was done which confirmed the diagnosis of acute lymphoblastic leukemia. The prognosis and the need for chemotherapy were explained to the parents in detail and he was discharged at request.

Condition at Discharge
He was pale. He had no active bleeding manifestation.

Recommendations
Chemotherapy elsewhere.

Final Diagnosis
Acute lymphoblastic leukemia.

ID 974
Name: Kenneth Age: 2 months
DOA: 23.2.89   DOD: 26.2.89

Presenting Complaints
Two-month-old infant was admitted with history of fever, breathing difficulty, cough and poor feeding for 2 days. History of oil installation into the eyes ears, nose and mouth 5 days back.

Salient Clinical Findings
Infant was moribund, dyspneic with marked chest retractions. His heart rate was 184/min, respiratory rate was 70/min, sat 96% on 5 liters of head box oxygen, temperature was normal. No cyanosis peripheral pulses well felt. Weight was 4 kg.
Cardiovascular system: S1 S2 heard normal
Respiratory system: Bilateral vesicular breath sounds. Bilateral crepitations and rhonchi heard.
Central nervous system: Anterior fontanelle was flat. No neurological deficit.
Abdomen: Soft Liver was 2 cm below the right costal margin.

Clinical Diagnosis at Admission
Lipoid pneumonia.

Investigations
HB (gm%)	: 8.5
Total WBC count (cumm)	: 5,800
Differential WBC count (%)	: BF1, N66, L33%
Platelets (/cumm)	: 7,62,000
S calcium (/cumm)	: 9.2
S sodium (mEq/L)	: 144
S potassium (mEq/L)	: 3.4
S creatinine (mg%) .	: 0.6

ABG		
	pH	: 7.2
	PCO_2	: 39.6
	PO_0	: 33.2
	HCO_3	: 14.9
	ABE	: −12.5
	SPO_2	: 99.8

Chest X-ray: Hyperinflated chest bilateral pneumonitis.

Treatment Given
Inj Calcium gluconate 6 ml with equal amounts of 10% dextrose stat IV
Inj Lasix 8 mg IV stat
Inj Hydrocortisone 40 mg IV stat.
Inj Cloxacillin 100 mg IV Q6H.
Inj Gentamicin 15 mg IV once daily
Syp Paracetamol 40 mg whenever necessary.
Bricanyl nebulization.

Course in Hospital
Kenneth was admitted with diagnosis of lipoid pneumonia. X-ray showed hyperinflation with bilateral pneumonitis. A blood gas revealed metabolic acidosis, for which sodium bicarbonate correction was given. Child was kept NPO treaded with O_2, IV fluids, cricanyl nebulization and antibiotics after blood culture. Child showed improvement clinically and was started on nasogastric feeds followed by oral feeds. Blood cultures were sterile and discharged on oral antibiotics.

Condition at Discharge
Child was alert and afebrile.

Recommendations
Syp Cloxacillin 100 mg Q6H for 5 days
Hovite drops 0.3 ml once daily.
Syp Salbutamol 0.4 mg QBH for 3 days.

Final Diagnosis
　　Lipoid pneumonia
　　Metabolic acidosis.

ID 4
Specialty: Pediatrics
Consultant: Dr Patterson

Episode Summary

History
Male 10-year-old admitted with high temperature, complained of chest pains and had a persistent cough. He had lost weight over the past few weeks. He had recently returned to England after living abroad with his grandparents for a few months.

On Examination
Swelling and tenderness of neck gland was detected and there were some painful red lumps on his shins.

Post-admission
Suspicion of tuberculosis
Sputum and urine specimens taken and sent for analysis, tuberculosis confirmed.
Sent for X-ray.

Procedure
Drug treatment given. Discharged to a convalescent home after 2 months.

Diagnosis
Main condition: Cervical lymphadenopathy.
Other condition: Miliary tuberculosis.
                   Bilateral corneal ulcer.

ID 3
Specialty: Pediatrics
Consultant: Dr Johnson

Episode Summary

History
Maureen Snow, a 9-year-old girl with recent impetiginous rash, presented with a high temperature, severe headache, stiff neck and vomiting.

On Examination
Pyogenic meningitis was diagnosed.

Procedure
Treated with antibiotics. Apart from some chest infection she made a complete recovery and was discharged after 22 days.

Diagnosis
Main condition: Pyogenic meningitis
Other condition: Impetigo
                   Pneumonitis.

SAMPLE DISCHARGE SUMMARIES

Cardiothoracic Surgery

ID 948
Name: Jones   Age: 63 years
DOA: 2.5.2001   DOD: 21.5.2001

Principal Diagnosis
CAD and aortic regurgitation.

Operation/Procedures
CABG × 3 and Aortic valve replacement done on 16.5.2001.

History
Chest pain on exertion. No history of dyspnea, syncopal attacks. Echo and cardiac cath showed severe calcific aortic stenosis and triple vessel disease. He was admitted for elective surgery.

Physical Findings
Patient comfortable, vitals stable, no pallor, cyanosis, edema, JVP not raised, CVS: S1 S2 normal, Ejection systolic murmur present, RS: clear, B/L air entry normal and equal, P/A: soft, no organomegaly.

Lab Investigations
Blood group: A positive, sickling Negative, INR at the time of discharge 2.3
ECHO: showed severe calcific aortic stenosis and mild AR
Angiogram/cardiac cath: Cath done on 23.4.2001 showed triple vessel disease and aortic regurgitation.

Operation Findings
ABG × 3 and aortic valve replacement done on 10.5.2001. Hypertrophic LV. Good LIMA flow. Vein of reasonable quality. Aorta calcified throughout. Aortic valve severely calcified and stenotic.

Treatment and Progress
Patient had uneventful postoperative recovery and his INR levels were titrated with Warfarin dosages. At the time of discharge his sternal and leg wound were healing well.

Condition on discharge: Satisfactory.

Discharge Medications
Tab Warfarin 2 mg OD
Tab Tenormin 50 mg OD

Follow-up Appointment
Review in cardiothoracic on 13.6.2001.

ID 067
Name: Tony   Age: 35 years
DOA: 30.4.99   DOD: 12.5.99

Principal Diagnosis
Severe MR, endocarditis.

Secondary Diagnosis
Post-thecoperitoneal shunt.

Operation/ Procedures
Mitral valve replacement done on 5.5.99.

History
This patient had mitral valve disease since birth and developed infective endocarditis. As a complication of this he developed mycotic aneurysm of middle cerebral artery, which bled. He was operated and aneurysm was clipped. Subsequently he developed meningitis, which was treated, and further he developed hydrocephalus for which a thecoperitoneal shunt was made. It was explained to the patient that the primary pathology is the mitral valve regurgitation and infective endocarditis. He was admitted for mitral valve replacement.

Physical Findings
Patient comfortable, vitals stable, no pallor, cyanosis, edema, JVP not raised, CVS: S1 S2 normal, systolic murmur present, RS: Clear, B/L air entry normal and equal, P/A: Soft, no organomegaly.

Lab Investigations
Blood group: A positive, sickling negative, INR at the time of discharge 1.98.
ECHO: Showed severe MR, AML prolapses.

Operation Findings
Mitral valve replacement done on 5.5.99. Large heart. Dilated LA. The mitral valve was incompetent. The anterior leaflet thickened at it is edge. Prolapsing ruptured charade of the post-papillary muscle. The posterior leaflet looked normal. There was small area of vegetation at the edge of the anterior leaflet. The valve thought to be amenable to repair.

Treatment and Progress
Patient had uneventful postoperative recovery and Warfarin dosage was titrated with INR.

Condition on Discharge
Satisfactory.

Discharge Medications
Tab Warfarin 4 mg OD
Tab Digoxin 0.124 mg OD
Tab Lasix 40 mg OD.

Follow-up Appointment
Review in cardiothoracic after 3 weeks.

ID 125
Name: Regina   **Age: 30 years**
DOA: 14.3.98   **DOD: 25.3.98**

Principal Diagnosis
Aortic dissection.

Secondary Diagnosis
Postdelivery.

Operation/Procedures
Dissecting aortic aneurysm repair done on 14.3.98.

History
This lady delivered 5 days back and subsequently had severe back pain. She was discharged from OG side but her back pain never stopped. She was investigated at KMC hospital, CT scan was done and it revealed aortic dissection. Patient was shifted to cardiology and aortogram was done which showed aortic dissection form just below subclavian extending to right iliac. Right renal artery was not seen and right lower limb vessels were not pacifying.

Physical Findings
Patient comfortable, vitals stable, no pallor, cyanosis, edema, CVS-S1 S2 normal, no murmur, RS-clear, BL air entry normal and equal, P/A-soft, right femoral pulses were weak.

Lab Investigations
Blood group AB positive, sickling negative
X-ray/imaging investigation
CT scan done on 14.3.98 at KMC hospital showed dissection of thoracic aorta DTPA reno gram: 25.3.98.
Reduced and delayed right renal uptake of 29% – probable consequence of aortic dissection. Mild left hydronephrosis – washes out well? Cause.
Angiogram/cardiac Cath
Aortogram showed aortic dissection starting just below left subclavian and extending to right iliac artery.

Operation Findings
Dissecting aortic aneurysm repair done on 15.3.98. There was a dissection of the thoracic aorta starting just below the left subclavian. The intima upto the middle of the thoracic aorta was completely destroyed. The false lumen was extending downward into the abdominal aorta. The aortic wall very frible.

Treatment and Progress
Patient was initially put on antihypertensive drugs and than taken for surgery. Postoperative recovery was uneventful and her wound is healing well. Her BP in postoperative period was on higher side and it was thought that it is renal hypertension DTPA scan was done which showed reduced and delayed right renal uptake of 29%—probable consequence of aortic dissection and mild left hydronephrosis.

Condition on Discharge
Satisfactory.

Discharge Medications
Tab Dilzem   60 mg tid
Tab Tenormin 100 mg OD
Tab Olfen 100 mg prn

Follow-up Appointment
Review after 2 weeks in cardiothoracic OPD.

ID 396
Name: Titus   Age: 29 years
DOA: 1.2.2000   DOD: 6.2.2000

Principal Diagnosis
Fracture of ribs left side 1st to 5th, minimal hemothorax, fracture neck of scapula left side. Road traffic accident.

Operation/Procedures
Aspiration of hemothorax/LA.

History
Alleged RTA, was hit by a "showel" when he was driving his pick-up van according to the patient. No history of loss of consciousness, no breathing difficulty.

Physical findings
Patient conscious, oriented, no focal neurological deficits, PEARL, PR   80/min, BP 130/80 mm Hg moving all limbs. Difficulty in moving the left upper limb, apparently due to pain. Chest–B/L good air entry, normal breath sounds. CVS-S1 S2 normal, no murmur. Abdomen: Soft, no area of tenderness or guarding, no free fluid, BS positive. No fracture long bones clinically. Skull and spine normal. Abrasion on the left lateral chest wall.

Lab investigations
Hb 14.5   gm/dl, Blood group A positive, other all investigations are with in normal limit.
X-ray/imaging investigations
X-ray chest (On admission) showed fracture ribs 1st to 5th on the left side. X-ray left shoulder showed a # of the neck of the scapula. X-ray chest after 2 days showed minimal fluid on the left side with obliteration of the left costophrenic angle.

Consultation Findings
He was seen by Orthopedics specialist on 1.2.2001. He advised conservative management of the fracture scapula with collar and cuff. Also advised to review in fracture clinic in MMC hospital on a Sunday after 2 weeks.

Discharge Medications
Tab Olfen SR 100 OD × 5 days
Tab Ranitidine 150 mg bd × 5 days.

Follow-up Appointments
Review in thoracic surgery OPD after 1 week.

SAMPLE DISCHARGE SUMMARIES

Cardiology

ID 608
Name: Mathew   Age: 38 years
DOA: 13.3.98   DOD: 23.3.98

Final Diagnosis: Chronic obstructive pulmonary tuberculosis disease
Drug induced hepatitis
Ischemic heart disease

History
Thirty-eight-year-old man diagnosed to have TB (based on chest X-ray) and was treated with ATT for 1 year. He was irregular and discontinued treatment for 2 months. He presented with high-grade fever dyspnea—progressively increasing and swelling of the limbs.

On Examination
In respiratory distress, respiratory rate 40/min. BP 120/86 mm Hg supine, pulse 100/min regular, bilateral pitting pedal edema present, mucous membranes
Clubbing present, JVP elevated.
RS: Trachea shifted to right bilateral expiratory wheeze heard. Bronchial breath sounds in right apical area vacal resonance increased on right apical area. Few crepitations over right
Lower lobe. Apex normal
CVS: S1 S2 heard normally, no murmur heard
CNS: Gross deficits
Abdomen: Distended soft, liver palpable 0.3 cm below right costal margin. Free fluid present in abdomen. Bowel sounds heard normally.

Investigations
Hb   16.9 gm%   WBC   6000/cumm   N 76   L22   M2
PT   22/14   MP/MF: Negative
Sodium 135 mEq/L   Potassium 4.3   mEq/L   Bicarb   29 mEq/L   Creatinine 1.3   mg%
Random 109   mg% HbsAg: Negative   T Bilirubin 14.3   5.1 mg% Direct   11.1   3.1 mg%
T Protein 7.2 6.9 g% Albumin   3.6 3.4 g% SGOT   499   43U/L   SGPT   85   36 U/L Alk Phos   95 99 U/L
CXR: Bilateral apical infiltrates and right lower zone bronchiectasis consistent with TB cardiomegaly present, few apical calcification seen.
U/S Abdomen: Normal study
ECG: 'P' pulmonzale seen T wave inversion in lead II. No definite ischemic changes.

Discussion
This patient presented with features of COPD with cor pulmonale. Chest X-ray showed active tuberculosis. He was started on ATT. While in ward he developed jaundice and was investigated for viral etiology. It was considered to be due to drug allergy and if subsided after stopping hepatotoxic drugs. The COPD was well controlled with bronchodilator.

Recommendations
Salt free diet + 4 g salt 1.51 fluids/day
Inj Streptomycin 0.75 mg   IM once daily
Tab Ethambutol 800 mg 1-0-0
Tab Lasix   40 mg 1-0-0
Tab Ciprofloxacin   500 mg 1-0-1   for 5 days
Tab Deriphylline R 300 mg 1-0-1

Tab Sorbitrate 5 mg 1-1-1
Tab Disprin ½-0-0
Ipratropium inhaler 2 puffs twice daily.
Asthalin inhaler 2 puffs whenever necessary
Becoride forte 2 puffs twice daily
To have ENT consult in ENT OPD on 27.3.98
To recheck LFT after 2 weeks add on Bifampicin and INH gradually.

ID 037
Name: Aaron   Age: 14 years
DOA: 11.8.2001   DOD: 15.8.2001

Final Diagnosis
Type III aortoarteritis
Secondary hypertension
Bilateral renal artery stenosis
PTA with stinting to bilateral renal artery done on 14.8.2001.

History
Mr Aaron, presented with accelerated hypertension since 3 months. USG (abdomen) with renal Doppler showed bilateral renal artery stenosis. No history of fever/body ache.

Examination
PR 80/min   BP   190/100 mm Hg
JVP: Normal
CVS: S1 S2 normal: LV S4   +: Soft abdominal bruit +
R/S: Clear.

Investigations
Blood: Report enclosed
ECG: Left ventricular hypertrophy
X-ray: Cardiomegaly. CTR   13.5/23.5
ECHO: RV 9   FS 22   LVID (D) 49   (S) 38   PW 8 AR Mild (3.4/19) Mod MR (3.8/99) Mod.
TR TRG   39 mm Hg   EDV 78   ESV   39   EF 59 Aortic gdt 17 mm Hg
CO_2 Angio
Proximal 99% eccentric stenosis right RA
Occluded Left RA filling from collaterals
Occluded SMA. SMA territory supplied by large Drummond's artery
Aorta appears normal.
Procedures
Left RA PTA and Stenting : RFA – 7F
                          : GC – 7F RCA
                          : AW – 018" RR
                          : Balloon UTD 4 × 20 mm
                          : Stent – Intrastent 16 mm
Deployed at 12 atm distal vessel seen filling well: probably a posterior branch pinched
Right RA PTA and stenting RFA 7F – 7.5-flong sheath (40 cm).
GW-018" RR-ASS   1 cm ST
Balloon UTD   6 × 40 mm
Stent – Intrastent 16 mm
Deployed at 14 atm good results.

Discussion
He underwent bilateral renal PTA with stenting on 19.8.2001. Postprocedure stay was uneventful and his BP was well controlled with reduced dose of antihypertensive.

Advice on Discharge
Tab Atenolol   50 mg   once daily   till review
Tab Nicardia R   10 mg   twice daily   till review
Tab Prednisolone   30 mg   once daily   till review
Tab Colpidogrel   75 mg   once daily   1 month
Tab Ecosprin   75 mg   once daily   till review
Salt free diet + 4 gm salt/day
To check ESR and mail the report to us for adjustment of prednisolone dosage
Review after 6 months in cardiology OPD.

ID 889
Name: Thomas   Age: 50 years
DOA: 1.3.2000   DOD: 14.3.2000

Final Diagnosis
　　Coronary artery disease
　　Triple vessel disease
　　Old inferior wall myocardial infarction
　　Diabetes mellitus type II
　　Dyslipidemia
　　Coronary artery bypass graft surgery done on 7.3.2000.

Investigations
Blood: Reports enclosed
ECG: Old inferior wall myocardial infarction
X-ray: CTR-PA-within normal limits
ECHO: EF 55   No RWMA   Normal LV Systolic and diastolic function.

Discussion
50-year-old gentleman with coronary risk factors of diabetes mellitus type 2, smoking and dyslipidema who had an inferior wall in 96 presented with effort angina. Coronary angiogram revealed triple vessel disease with an occluded left anterior descending artery and he was admitted for coronary artery bypass graft surgery.

Surgery Done
Coronary artery bypass graft surgery done on 7.3.2000. Postoperative period was uneventful.

Advice on Discharge

Tab Biduret	1 tab	once daily	1 month
Tab Colsprin	100 mg	once daily	till review
Tab Atorvastatin	10 mg	once daily	at bedtime till review
Tab Dilzem	30 mg	thrice daily	till review
Tab Metoprolal	12.5 mg	twice daily	till review
Inj Mixtard	20 units	subcutaneously	with breakfast
	12 units	subcutaneously	with dinner

Low fat, low cholesterol, 1500-calorie diabetic diet.
Restricted physical activities for 6 weeks
To collect detailed surgical notes from cardiothoracic office.
To check sugars periodically and adjust the dosage of insulin in consultation with physician.
Review after 6 months in cardiology department.

ID 815
Name: Vincent   Age: 45 years
DOA: 6.10.98   DOD: 10.10.98

Final Diagnosis
Noninsulin dependent diabetes mellitus
Dyslipidemia
Severe mitral regurgitation
Pulmonary artery hypertension
Normal coronaries.

History and Examinations
45-year-old male presented with history of PND/pain one-month back. Since then effort dysp. Class I symptomatic. Not known case of hypertension. Diabetes mellitus/ischemic heart disease/rheumatic fever. P 96/min. BP 130/80 mm Hg, CVS-Mitral regurgitation. Pulmonary artery hypertension? Chest-clear.

Investigations
Blood: Hb   12.5 gm%, ESR: 20 mm 1st hr, S Creatinine   1.4 mg% WBC: TC 7300/cumm, DC: N-63% E-5% M-6% L-26%, Na   136 mEq/L, K   4.5 mEq/L, Glucose PL: AC   138   mg% PC   284 mg%, Lipid Profile Fasting: Cholesterol   277 mg% Triglycerides   155 mg% HDL Cholesterol   39 mg% LDL Cholesterol   207 mg% HbsAg and HIV: Negative
ECG: Sinus rhythm. No evidence of ischemia.
X-ray: Cardiomegaly. Lung fields clear.
ECHO: AO 22   LA 30   RA 11   IVS   11 EDV 83   ESV 38   E 133   A 76 PW 9
EF 56   FS 33   EPSS 4   Dect 130   AO gdt 11
Cath and Angiogram
Left main: Normal
Left anterior decending: Normal
Left circumflex: Normal
Right coronary artery: Normal
Aortic root angio: Tricuspid competent valve
LV angio: 3 + MR. Normal LV function
Impression: Severe mitral regurgitation, normal coronaries
Recommendation! Mitral valve replacement at the earliest.

Discussion
Patient had undergone coronary angiogram on 8.11.99. That showed severe mitral regurgitation with normal coronaries. Patient was discharged with following advice.

Advice on Discharge
Tab Digoxin   0.125   mg once daily   5 days a week
Tab Envas   1.25   mg once daily   till review
Tab Daonil   2.5   mg once daily   till review
All infection, dental and surgical procedures to be covered by appropriate antibiotics under medical supervision.
Elective mitral valve replacement/mitral valve repair within 3 month.

ID 129
Name: Bruce   Age: 53 years
DOA: 6.11.97   DOD: 7.11.97

Principal Diagnosis
Unstable angina, DV disease.

History
53-year-old male admitted with left sided chest pain radiating to the left arm at around 4.00 pm. Pain was relieved promptly after receiving Tab Angised in A and E after 2 hours. No other associated symptoms.

Past History
No history of DM or HTN. Coronary angiography 1997: 70% RCA lesion in the LAD. Normal LCx. Normal LV AS and mild AR gradient 55 mm Hg.

Physical Findings
Stable vital signs, JVP not raised, no edema.
Chest few fine basal crepts B/L
CVS: S1 S2 and AS AR Abdomen NAD.

Lab Investigations
Normal CBC, U/EL and card. Troponin negative.
ECG: SR, HR 100/min, LAD, St depression in C4 and C5, small Qs in C2-C4

Treatment and Progress
Remained pain free thought admission.

Condition on Discharge
Stable, pain free.

Physical Activity Advice
Light physical activity.

Discharge Medications
T Tenormin 50 mg OD, T Aspirin 150 mg OD, T Angised 0.5 mg S/L Prn, T Isordil 10 mg tid.

Follow-up Appointment
To admitted on 10.11.97 for angio on 11.11.97
For surgical review thereafter for CABG and AVR.

ID 950
Name: David   Age: 55 years
DOA: 11.4.99   DOD: 17.4.99

Principal Diagnosis
    Triple vessel disease
    Hypertension.

Operation/Procedures
55-year-old male patient known case of hypertension but not known diabetic and no family history IHD. Admitted c/o of recent onset exertional angina followed by rest angina. No history of claudication or tia and no history of palpitatin or syncopal attacks.
Family History: No significant family history of IHD

Physical Findings
Clinically and hemodynamically stable, BP 150/90 unremarkable systemic examination

Lab Investigations

Triglycerides	1.1 mmol/L	Fasting < 2.3
Cholesterol	5.0 mmol/L	
HDL cholest	0.7 mmol/L	
LDL cholest	3.8 mmol/L	
AST (SGOT)	68 IU/L	(10-42)
CK	438 IU/L	(22-269)
Ckmb	28.5 IU/L	(<10)
%CKMB of total	6.5%	(< 3.5%)
PT	13.7 secs	(11.5–14.5)
APTT	49.6 secs	(28.0–43.0)
FIBL	4.54 g/L	(1.5–4.0)
Urea	6.2 mmol/L	(2.5–7.5)
Sodium	133 mmol/L	(137–148)
Potassium	4.0 mmol/L	(3.6–5.0)
Creatinine	91 umol/L	(60–120)

ECG: SR, ST depression in the lateral lead
Angiogram/cardiac cath: Angiography on 16.4.99 showed RCA 40-50% distal plaque, lmca N, Cx 75%, LAD   100%. Discussed with cardiothoracic, the patient is a candidate of CABG to LAD, LCx, RCA.

Treatment and Progress
This patient admitted initially as a case of unstable angina and treated with Clexane, Aspirin, Lipostat, Carvidalol added later, angisid, Inhibace 1.25 mg OD, his condition improved, angiography done, at present this gentleman is free of pain at rest.

Condition on Discharge
Patient condition improved. He is free of pain at present time. The possibility of CABG and angio result discussed with the patient and his relative. Cardiothoracic accepted the patient for CABG and advice appointment in the concern clinic for discussion arrangement and evaluation.

Follow-up Care and Advice
Cardiothoracic clinic after 4 month.

Physical Activity Advice
To avoid any strenuous exercise, diet education given.

Discharge Medications
Aspirin   150 mg od
Carvidalol 25 mg   bd
Isordil   20 mg   tid
Lipostat   20 mg   hs.

Follow-up Appointments
The patient has appointment on 20.5.99 in cardiology OPD.

SAMPLE DISCHARGE SUMMARIES

Hematology

ID 976901B
Name: Nancy   Age: 30 years
DOA: 2.12.99   DOD: 20.01.2000

Final Diagnosis
Acute promyelocytic leukemia relapse on arsenic
Impacted left wisdom tooth with secondary infection.

History
Thirty-year-old Ms Nancy was diagnosed (out side) to have APML in November 1999 when she developed fever and ecchymotic spots. She had received Dauno and ATRA in December 1999 – I cycle. The second, third and fourth cycle was given with Inj Daunorubicine and Cytosine. The fourth cycle of chemo was received in June 2000. She was put on maintenance with ATRA on 8.8.99. In the month of December 99, she had drop in her platelet counts with and ecchymotic spot on the left arm and bone marrow outside revealed relapse APML. She was admitted for treatment with arsenic. At the time of admission patient was asymptomatic.

Physical Examination
Patient a febrile, no pallor, no icterus, no lymphadenopathy. No pedal edema, no ecchymotic spot, no active bleeding from any site. Pulse: 96/min. BP: 100/70. Chest, CVS: clear, normal, abdomen: No organomegaly. CNS: normal.

Discussion
Patient was started on Inj arsenic 10 mg daily from 30.12.99 and did not develop any arsenic toxicity except rise in her total WBC count to 37600 for which hydroxyurea was added on 8.1.2000 for 10 days till count dropped to 9000. During hospital stay patient developed jaw pain left side and was found to have impacted left wisdom tooth for which analgesics and antibiotics were given. She was asymptomatic at the time of discharge. She received support with platelets (30 units), 8 FFP, 3 packed cells last one on 26.1.99. She was advised to continue treatment with arsenic on an OPD basis.

Recommendations
Inj   Arsenic 10 mg I/V once daily in 500 ml DNS (to follow OPD)
Tab   Primolut 5 mg once daily to complete 21 days.
Tab   Paracetamol 2 tab when necessary.
Tab   Tydigesic 0.2 mg s/l when necessary.

ID 007742B
Name: Lilly   Age: 40 years
DOA: 24.7.2000   DOD: 24.8.2000

Final Diagnosis
Hypoplastic anemia.
Disseminated tuberculosis.

History
40-year-old lady presented with history of fatigue and generalized weakness of 1-month duration with history of fever of 10 days duration and breathlessness of 2 days duration. No history of pedal edema. History of dry cough present. No history of bleeding symptoms. History of blood transfusion 2 days ago. No history of hypertension/tuberculosis/diabetes mellitus.

Physical Examination
Pallor present, no icterus, lymph nodes, edema. BP: 120/70 mm Hg. Pulse: 92/min. Temperature: 101F. CVS: S1, S2 normal. PA: Liver, Spleen. RS: Creps present. Right side: No rhonchi

Discussion
Patient was admitted for evaluation of pancytopenia. Bone marrow was consistent with hypoplastic anemia. However patient bad elevated LDH and alkaline phosphates, which was unlikely to be related to the aplastic anemia. Since she had persistent high fever with chest infiltrates the possibilities considered were granulomatous infiltrates of the marrow and collagen vascular disease. Connective tissue work-up was negative. A Bronchio alveolar lavage was done which was negative and liver biopsy showed only iron overload. A CT guided FNAC of mediastinal nodes was planned but deferred to later date. Patients fever gradually subsided and patient's platelet counts improved with Danazol. Emperical ATT was not started since the fever settled with antibiotics. Patient was discharged with the advice to be followed up in OPD after 1 month.

Recommendations
Tab Folic acid 2.5 mg once daily.
Tab Danazol 200 mg thrice daily.
Cap Omez 20 mg once daily.

ID 040000B
Name: Mathew   Age: 50 years
DOA: 23.7.99   DOD: 23.8.99

Final Diagnosis
Multiple myeloma.

History
History of low backache for 1-½ months, increased in intensity for 3 weeks. Difficulty in sitting, lying down for 2 weeks. No history of preceding trauma, fever, weakness, fatigability. No history of oliguria, bowel/bladder disturbances. No history of weakness in lower limbs. Known case of diabetes mellitus for 13 years, on oral hypoglycemic agents. History of surgery for 17 varicocele 13-year-back.

Physical Examination
Afebrile. Pulse: 92/min. BP: 130/80 mm Hg. CNS, RS, P/A, and CNS: Normal. Lower thoracic tenderness present. X-ray outside: collapse.

Discussion
Mr Mathew was diagnosed to have multiple myeloma based on his investigations and was given the 1st cycle of CVAD regime. (VCR 0.4 mg, Cyclophos 500 mg. Adriamycin 17.5, Dexamethasone 40 mg × 4 days then tapered over next 2 days) from 6.8.89 to 11.8.89 and he tolerated the chemotherapy well. He developed foot drop right side during hospital stay for which he was investigated. The foot drop was attributed to diabetic neuropathy / compression neuropathy.

Recommendations
Tab Folic acid 2.5 mg once daily.
Tab Tidigesic 0.2 mg s/c when necessary.
Physiotherapy as advised.
Alkathine brace to be worn.
Revisit to hematology OPD on 9.9.89 for his second cycle of chemotherapy.

ID 477
Name: Stephen   Age: 26 years
DOA: 20.5.2000   DOD: 25.7.2000

Final Diagnosis
Hemophilia A.
High titer inhibitor.
Pseudotumor excision over right lower end of thigh.
HCV positive.

History
26-year-old male known case of hemophilia A with high titer inhibitor was admitted for excision of pseudotumor of right thigh.

Physical Examination
Afebrile, no pallor, no icterus, no lymph node. CVS, RS: Normal. Abdomen: Soft. CNS: Normal.

Investigations
Hemogram at admission: Hemogram at discharge
Hb   11.5 g/dL   Hb   11.0 g/dL
Inhibitor Assay: 96 BU.
Pus; Enterococci + NFGNB, sensitive to Amoxycillin, Ciprofloxain.

Discussion
Patient was a known case of severe hemophilia A with high titer inhibitor presented with pseudotumor of right thigh. Excision of the pseudotumor was performed on 20.5.2000 under FEIBA cover and fibrin glue. Postoperatively, he was supported with FEIBA. On 30.5.2000, he developed core from local site dropped his hematocrit. FEIBA support was increased and packed cell transfusions as necessary was given. He developed a large hematoma at the local site for which he was started on short wave diathermy. Suture removal was done on 10.6.2000. The hematoma evaded through the skin resulting in the formation of a large ulcer. On 20.6.2000, he complained of foul smelling discharge – pus cultures grew GNB and enterococci sensitive to 1st line antibiotics. He received ciproflox and Amoxycillin for 10 days for the same and daily dressings were done by the orthopedic surgeons.

He received a total of about 56,000 units of FEIBA. He was started on physiotherapy post-operation. He was well at discharge. He needs to continue physiotherapy on operative basis and go to orthopedic OPD on alternate days for dressing.

ID 039
Name: Saron   Age: 35 years
DOA: 8.7.2001   DOD: 10.7.2001

Final Diagnosis
Mediastinal large B cell lymphoma for chemotherapy.

History
This 35-year-old lady diagnosed to have mediastinal large B cell lymphoma was admitted for 5th dose of chemotherapy MACOP – B protocol. There was no history of fever, cough or bleeding from any sites.

Physical Examination
She was afebrile. PR was 88/min. BP was 120/80 mm Hg. There was no pallor. There was no lymph node enlargement. Systemic examination revealed no abnormalities.

Investigations
Hemogram at admission
Hb   11.2 g/dL
Platelet   340000/mm^3
WBC   9900/mm^3
Differential Count: N: 41 L: 43 BF: 7 Myelo: 9

Biochemistry at Admission
Creatinine 0.9 mg/dL
Sodium   135 mEq/L
Potassium 4.4 mEq/L
Liver function test: T.Bill. 0.3 mg/dL Dir. 0.1 mg/dL, T.Pro. 6.9 g/dL, Albumin 3.9 g/dL, SGOT   24 U/L   SGPT 32 U/L   Alk. Phos.   53 U/L

Discussion
This lady diagnosed to have mediastinal large B cell lymphoma was admitted for her 5th week chemotherapy according to the MACOP B protocol. She was given Inj. Adriamycin and Cyclophosphamide. She tolerated the chemotherapy well.

Recommendations
Cap Fluconazole 200 mg.
Cap Omez 20 mg twice daily.
Tab Prednisolone 75 mg once daily.
Tab Sortaline 25 mg once daily.
Tab Folic acid 5 mg once daily.

SAMPLE DISCHARGE SUMMARIES

Gastroenterology

ID 822
Name: Sam   Age: 40 years
DOA: 4.7.99   DOD: 5.7.99

Principal Diagnosis
NSAIDs-induced duodenal ulcer with positive *H. pylori*.

Operation/Procedures
OGD on 4.7.99.

History
He was having headache during the last 10 days for which he was taking different types of analgesics mainly NSAIDs. Presented with 3 days history of passing dark black color stool and feeling generally weak with mild epigastric discomfort. No hematemesis/fever/jaundice.

Physical Findings
Clinically stable, however, looks pale but no jaundice/lymphadenopathy.
Afebrile. BP: 150/100 mm Hg later was normal PR 110/min regular
P/A: Soft with mild epigastric tenderness, No mass, BS +
Chest/CVS/CNS: unremarkable

Lab Investigations
CBC: Hb   6.4   Plt. 363   WBC   10.1   Coag: PT   12.8", APTT   33.3"
UE1: Urea 4 Na 140 K 4   Cl 108 Co_2 27 Creatinine   87   Blood sugar 6.2
Blood group: O positive

Treatment and Progress
Patient started on IV fluid along with Ranitidine 50 mg IV tid and PRBCs transfusion was arranged and kept nil by mouth till OGD done for him. Underwent OGD on 4.7.99: there is an ulcer on the inferior wall of the bulb, with slough covering it. There were no stigmata of high-risk of rebelled on the base hence no therapeutic procedure required. There were 2 to 3 broad flat erosions in the bulb on the opposite wall too. No stigmate of bleed noted. CLO test: positive, he had no further bleeding. With the above results he is started on triple therapy and advised to stop NSAIDs.

Discharge Medications
Omeprazole 20 mg bd for 10 days
Clarithromycine 500 mg bd for 10 days
Amoxylline 1 g bd for 10 days
Followed by ranitidine 300 mg HS for 2 months.

ID 684
Name: Elizabeth   Age: 58 years
DOA: 1.5.2001   DOD: 10.5.2001

Principal Diagnosis
Obstructive jaundice secondary to periampullary carcinoma
(By USG/CT diagnosis).

History
Referred from Government hospital for ERCP and further management as patient was admitted in Government hospital for 10 days with one history of upper abdominal pain and yellowish discoloration of the eyes with history of watery loose stool.

Physical Findings
Elderly sick looking but hemodynamically stable
Afebrile. BP: 100/60 mm Hg   PR 80/min regular
Jaundice ++ No pallor/lymphadenopathy
Chest: Clear
CVS: Regular HS
P/A: Right hypochondrial tenderness with hepatomegaly
CNS: Blind lady but no focal deficits/meningeal signs.

Lab Investigations
CBC: Hb 12.6 Plt. 233 WBC 7.5   Coagulation: PT 13" APTT   54.8"
UE1/Bone: normal
LFT: TB 270   TP 57 Alb. 11   ALP   292
X-ray / imaging investigations
3.5.2001: Ultrasound abdomen
Dilated intrahepatic biliary radicles, CHD and CBD (15 to 17 mm) till lower end with delated pancreatic duct, highly suggestive of a lower CBD
Tumor /periampullary tumor. A large oval structure with echogenic areas within noted below the liver? Distended gallbladder filled with sludge.
Moderate as cites noted. Spleen, both kidneys are normal.

Treatment and Progress
Patient started on conservative management with IV fluid and nutritional support. Planned for ERCP, however cannot be done due to her condition as assessed by the anesthetist. And with this view of her age and her disease planned for supportive care with transfer to her local hospital. And she is for transfer to Government hospital on 11.5.2001 as per discussion with Dr Ninan.

Condition on Discharge
Hemodynamically stable, however, GC is same.

ID 058
Name: Annie   Age: 72 years.
DOA: 10.8.2000   DOD: 17.8.2000

History
Mrs Annie, a 72-year-old housewife presented with pain abdomen for 1 year, vomiting for 5 months and anorexia, significant physical examination revealed mild pallor. Pulse: 84/min, Resp: 16/min, BP: 150/80 mm Hg. Per abdomen examination revealed a hard, non-tender mass palpable in the epigastrium. There were no other organomegaly or free fluid. Chest and CVS examination was within normal limits.

Investigations
Hb 9.4 g%, Blood picture: Aniso +, Total WBC: 6900 cumm, Platelets; 173000 cumm, MCV 88.5, PTT P10.3 / C10.3 INR 1.0. Chest X-ray: NAD. ECG; Normal.
Ultrasound abdomen: 11.9 cm, moderate echogenic mass in right and left lobe of liver. PV is displaced but no thrombus. GB contracted, mild IHBD int he left lobe peripheral to mass. Stomach wall thickened at antrum and duodenal wall thickening with ill-defined mass in the region.
Gastroscopy: Esophagus – normal, stomach-GJ at 49 cm, both loops entered normal, duodenum normal.
Impression: Post GJ, deformed pyloroduodenal complex.

Discussion
Mrs Annie was admitted for evaluation of palpable mass. USG abdomen revealed a space-occupying lesion involving both the lobes of liver. An ultrasound-guided biopsy was done. Postprocedure hospital stay was uneventful. She is being discharged with an advice to follow-up in gastroenterology OPD with the report.

Diagnosis
Hepatocellular carcinoma.
Postgastro-jejunostomy state.

Recommendations
Normal diet.
Tab Ranitidine 150 mg twice daily.
Follow-up in gastroenterology OPD.

SAMPLE DISCHARGE SUMMARY

Plastic Surgery

ID 17
Specialty: Plastic Surgery
Consultant: Mr Eadie

History
Marie Johnston is a 15-year-old girl who has planned admission for plastic surgery to her face. She has scarring of her face following accidental burning. She has had previous skin grafts.

On Examination
Scarring of face.

Diagnosis on Admission
Scarring of face, for plastic surgery.

Procedure
Excision of scar tissue and skin graft.

Postoperative
She was discharged after 5 days.

Final Diagnosis
Primary: After-care involving plastic surgery to scar.
Secondary: Late effects of burn on face.
              Late effects of accident caused by fire.

SAMPLE DISCHARGE SUMMARY

Renal Transplantation

ID 877
Name: John   **Age: 22 years**
DOA: 30.9.90   **DOD: 1.10.90**

A case of chronic renal failure on maintenance hemodialysis transferred from nephrology department for renal transplantation.

Preoperative Investigations
Hb   11.1 gm% S. Creatinine   3.6 mg% Total count 7,600/cumm Blood urea 36 mg%   HIV
and HbsAg, HCV: Negative

LFT:	T. Bilirubin	0.4 mg%	T. Protein	3.6 mg%
	Direct	0.2 mg%	Albumin	3.2 gm%
	SGOT	19 U/L	SGPT	19 U/L
	Alk Phos	59 U/L		

Cultures: Blood, Urine: No growth
Doppler study of iliac and femoral vessels: Bilateral patient iliac and femoral veins arterialized flow in both iliac and common femoral veins.
Femoral angiogram: No AVF noted bilaterally. Normal study

Operation
Renal transplantation, right iliac fossa done on 30-9-90. Donor's Name: Raman. Hospital No. 234445A. Relationship with Recipient: Father. DST: No X.Match: Negative. HLA: Haplo
Donor's Kidney: Left No. of arteries: One. Veins: One   Ureter: One
Renal artery anastomosed end to end to internal iliac artery. Renal vein anastomosed end to side to exernal iliac vein. Ureter reimplanted into the bladder by Roy-Calne's interrupted suture technique and DJ stent kept.

Postoperative Investigations
PCV   31% Total Count   12,400/cumm   Creatinine   1.1 mg%

LFT:	T Bilirubin	0.6 mg%	T Protein	6.1 gm%
	Direct	0.2 mg%	Albumin	3.2 gm%
	SGOT	26 U/L	SGPT	19 U/L
	Alk.Phos	52 U/L		

Cultures: Urine: No growth. SC contaminants

Postoperative Period
Rejection episodes if any   : No
Treatment of rejection   : No
Urinary complication if any   : No

Final Diagnosis
Renal transplant recipient

Advice
To continue triple drug immunosuppression
To attend transplant clinic
To get DJ stent removed on 2.11.90 and attend urology OPD on 10.11.90 for admission and investigation.

SAMPLE DISCHARGE SUMMARIES

Endocrinology

ID 426
Name: Angelin   Age: 38 years
DOA: 6.9.2000   DOD: 13.9.2000

Principal Diagnosis
Primary aldosteronism.

History
Not known DM, HTN since 1994, admitted for further evaluation of high BP. No complaints. Not smoker. Married with 5 children.

Physical Findings
Not in acute distress, BP 185/105, PR 80/min, regular, temp 37C,no jaccold. CVS: S1 S2 RS clear P/A soft no organomegaly. CNS intact.

Lab Investigations
HB 13.9 WBC 4 Plat 194 Urea 3.1 Na 138 K2.6 Creat. 49 Glucose 4.9, TB 26, TP 77, Plasma Renin 0.3 ng/ml, $K^+2.8$, Na^+ 137
X-ray/Imaging investigations
CT upper abdomen: a small well-defined low density rounded mass, less than 2 cm in diameter arising from the medial limb of right adrenal gland, suggesting an adenoma. Left adrenal appears normal.
ECG: Left axis deviation, LVH.

Treatment and Progress
Prazocin	0.5 mg tds
Nifidipine R	20 mg bd
Slow K	600 mg tds

Condition on Discharge
BP   150/90, mobile.

Follow-up Care and Advice
Readmission after one month
To check K^+ level after one week at nearest health center, if it's normal, discontinue slow K tablets.

Discharge Medications
Spironolactone 200 mg bd for one month
Nifedipine 20 mg bd for one month
Prazocin 0.5 mg tds for one month
Slow K 600 mg tds for one month.

Follow-up Appointments
The patient has appointment on 5.10.2000 in endocrinology OPD.

ID 918
Name: Nafiza   Age: 45 years
DOA: 9.9.99   DOD: 17.9.99

Principal Diagnosis
HTN and Addison's disease for investigation and further assessment.

Secondary Diagnosis
Hypertension, Addison's disease, recurrent pancreatitis, hyperlipidemia and osteoarthritis.

History
A known case of above conditions c/o epigastric burning pain not associated with nausea and vomiting. Admitted for investigation.

Physical Findings
Comfortable, BP: 196/80 PR: 80/min, afebrile, left carotid bruit+
P/A: Mild epigastric tenderness, no mass.
Chest/CVS/CNS: Unremarkable.
X-ray/imaging investigations
CT pituitary fossa with contrast (2.7.00): Normal.

Treatment and Progress
Continued on her old treatment.

Follow-up Care and Advice
Follow-up in Endocrinology OPD on third week of next month.

Discharge Medications
Inhibase 2.5 mg OD
Hydrocortisone 10 mg bd
Motilium 10 tds
Fefol 1 cap OD.

SAMPLE DISCHARGE SUMMARY

ENT

ID 895
Name: Jacob   Age: 25 years
DOA: 9.4.2000   DOD: 12.4.2000

Final Diagnosis
Bilateral CSOM–TUBO tympanic disease.

Presenting Symptoms
Bilateral mucopurulent, intermittent ear discharge since 10 years. No discharge for 4 years. Previous surgery done in 95 in the left ear at Government hospital. Chennai.

Physical Examination
Healthy female.
Right ear: No mastoid tenderness. Subtotal perforation
Left ear: Large central perforation
Nose: Deviated nasal septum to right
Oral cavity/oropharynx/IDL: normal

Investigations
Hb   12.5 gm% RBS   93 mg% TC   9300/cumm   HIV and HbsAg: Negative audiogram: Bilateral mild conductive hearing loss
X-ray mastoids: Bilateral sclerosing mastoiditis.

Operation Done
Right cortical mastoidectomy and tympanoplasty under GA on 10.4.2000.

Operative Findings
Subtotal perforation. Antrum filled with granulations and thickened mucosa. Aditus blocked with granulations. Incus enclosed with granulations and fibrous tissue. Middle ear squamous epithelium present. Ossicular chain intact. Graft placed by underlay technique.

Biopsy
Number 14469/00. Non-specific inflammation, connective tissue from right middle ear and right mastoid antrum.

Course in Hospital
Uneventful.

Recommendations
Tab Ciprofloxacin 500 mg twice daily × 1 week
Tab Paracetamol 2   whenever necessary
Tab MVT   1 once daily × 1 week
No head bath for 2 weeks (can wash the hair with wet towel)
After 6 weeks can take a bath with cotton in the ear for 3 months
Check-up in ENT outpatients after 3 months.

HUMAN BODY

Exercise 1

Complete the following:

1. The basic unit of the life is _____.
2. Groups of similar cells working together to do a specific job is _____.
3. Several _____ combine to form a system.
4. There are _____ chromosomes in a mature sex cell.
5. The three types of muscle tissues are _____, _____, and _____.
6. The four planes of the body are _____, _____, _____, and _____ planes.
7. The vertical plane which divides the body or structure into anterior and posterior portions is _____.
8. The directional term "efferent" refers to _____ the structure.
9. The directional term " afferent" refers to _____ the structure.
10. The medical term for one thousand is _____.

Exercise 2

Match the following:

—	1.	Prone	A. Standing up
—	2.	Ventral	B. Front
—	3.	Caudal	C. Flavus
—	4.	Pneumo	D. Lower end of body
—	5.	Lateral abdominal	E. Sex
—	6.	Distal	F. Albus

—	7.	Cranial	G.	Right and left epigastric area
—	8.	Erect	H.	Lungs
—	9.	White	I.	Face up
—	10.	Six	J.	Aurus
—	11.	Hypochondriac	K.	Face down
—	12.	Supine	L.	Either side of umbilical region
—	13.	Mammary	M.	Breast area of chest
—	14.	Golden	N.	End of fingers
—	15.	Yellow	O.	Head

Exercise 3

Explain the meaning for the following terms related to roots, prefix, and suffix with an example:

S. No	Term	Meaning	Example
1.	belphar		
2.	cerebro		
3.	chir		
4.	cost		
5.	gastr		
6.	hemat		
7.	hyster		
8.	pyo		
9.	pyel		
10.	neph		
11.	an		
12.	bi		
13.	dys		
14.	epi		
15.	hemi		
16.	tri		
17.	–cele		
18.	–malacia		
19.	–oma		
20.	–rhexis		

MUSCULOSKELETAL SYSTEM

Exercise 1

Complete the following:

1. The skeleton is made up of _____ bones.
2. Bones are classified according to shapes, which are _____
   _____.

3. The humerus is an example of a _____ bone.
4. A sharp projection in the bone is called _____.
5. The spinal column is made up of vertebrae, _____, and
   _____.
6. There are _____ pairs of ribs.
7. All skull bones are immobile except for the _____.
8. The three groups of vertebrae in the spinal column are the
   _____, _____, _____.
9. The long bones of the arm are _____, _____,
   _____.
10. The patella is the _____.
11. The seven ankle bones are called _____.
12. The eight carpal bones are located in the _____.
13. Fibrous joint allow _____ movement, cartilaginous joints
    allow _____ movement, and synovial joints allow
    _____ movement.
14. The bending of joint is called _____.
15. The most movable type of joint in the body is the _____
    joint.

Exercise 2

Give the meanings of the components of the following:

1. Anencephalia:
   An _____
   encephal/ia _____
2. Osteoarthritis:
   Osteo _____
   arthr _____
   itis _____
3. Osteodystrophy:
   Osteo _____
   dys _____
   trophy _____
4. Osteolysis
   Osteo _____
   lysis _____
5. Sacroiliac
   Sacro _____
   iliac _____

Exercise 3

Match the following:

1. Sacrum		A.	Extreme tip of vertebral column
2. Clavicle		B.	Jawbone
3. Femur		C.	Smaller bone of lower leg
4. Humerus		D.	Large weight-bearing bone of lower leg
5. Sternum		E.	Collar bone
6. Zygomatic (or malar)		F.	A nasal bone
7. Patella		G.	Shoulder blade
8. Coccyx		H.	Next to last vertebral bone
9. Scapula		I.	Thigh bone
10. Vomer		J.	Kneecap
11. Tibia		K.	Medial long bone of the forearm
12. Mandible		L.	Breastbone
13. Fibula		M.	Lateral long bone of forearm
14. Pubis		N.	Small, lower, strongest portion of pelvic bone
15. Ischium		O.	Broad upper portion of pelvic gridle
16. Carpals		P.	Ankle bones
17. Ilium		Q.	Most anterior part of pelvic gridle
18. Tarsals		R.	Wrist bones
19. Radius		S.	Upper arm bone
20. Ulna		T.	A cheek bone

Exercise 4

Complete the following:

1. The study of muscles is called _____.
2. Movement is produced by the ability of muscle to _____ and _____.
3. Three types of muscle tissue are _____, _____ and _____.
4. The buccinator muscle is also called the _____.
5. The diaphragm is a muscle of respiration located in the _____.
6. Muscles for chewing are the _____.
7. The auricular group of muscles moves the _____.
8. The muscle around the eye is called _____.
9. A broad, flat, superficial muscle of the back of the neck and trunk is the _____.
10. _____ muscles contract when we cough or sneeze.

Exercise 5

Give the meanings of the components of the following:

1. Myalgia:
   My _____
   algia _____
2. Myoma:
   My _____
   oma _____
3. Myorrhaphy:
   Myo _____
   rrhaphy _____
4. Tenosynovectomy:
   Teno _____
   synov _____
   ectomy _____
5. Myosclerosis:
   Myo _____
   sclero/osis _____

CARDIOVASCULAR SYSTEM

Exercise 1

Complete the following:

1. The cardiovascular system includes the _____,
   _____, _____ and _____.
2. The external layer of the saclike membrane covering the heart is
   called the _____.
3. The heart is divided into _____ chambers.
4. The valves of the heart prevent a _____ of blood into
   the atria.
5. Arteries carry _____ blood from the heart throughout the
   body, and _____ transport it back to the heart.
6. The four blood types are _____, _____, _____ and
   _____.
7. _____ veins are the only veins carrying oxygenated
   blood.
8. The _____ is the largest artery in the body.
9. The three branches of the aorta are the _____, _____
   and _____.
10. The _____ drains into the right atrium.

Exercise 2

Match the following:

— 1. Cardiosclerosis   a. Pacemaker
— 2. Atrium   b. Contraction of the heart
— 3. Systole   c. A lower heart chamber
— 4. Sinoatrial node   d. Hardening of heart tissues and vessels
— 5. Diastole   e. Inflammation of the heart muscle
— 6. Ventricle   f. Bluish skin color caused by reduced
      amounts of hemoglobin in the blood
— 7. Pulmonary value   g. Relaxation of heart
— 8. Myocarditis   h. Inflammation of the veins
— 9. Phlebitis   i. Valve between the heart and the lungs
—10. Cyanosis   j. An upper chamber of the heart

Exercise 3

Give the meaning of the components of the following medical terms:

1. Aortitis:
   Aort _____
   itis _____
2. Pericarditis:
   Pericard _____
   itis _____
3. Arteriosclerosis:
   Arterio _____
   sclerosis _____
4. Cardiomegaly:
   Cardio _____
   megaly _____
5. Myocarditis:
   Myo _____
   card _____
   itis _____
6. Hemothorax:
   Hem _____
   thorax _____
7. Dextrocardia:
   Dextro _____
   cardia _____
8. Cyanosis:
   Cyano _____
   sis _____

9. Bradycardia:
   Brady _____
   cardia _____
10. Tachycardia:
    Tachy _____
    cardia _____

BLOOD AND LYMPHATIC SYSTEM

Exercise 1

Complete the following:

1. The three major types of blood vessels are _____,
   _____ and _____.
2. Arteries carry _____ blood from the heart
   throughout the body and _____ transport it back to
   the heart.
3. Erythrocytes contain an iron-containing pigment called _____.
4. Lack of iron in erythrocytes results in _____.
5. Leukocytes are divided into two groups, _____ and
   _____.
6. The lymphatic system plays roles in the _____
   and _____ systems.
7. Five areas where lymph glands are located are _____,
   _____, _____, _____, and
   _____.
8. The largest structure of lymphoid system is the _____.
9. There are _____ pairs of tonsils.
10. The important functions played by the tonsils in the immune system
    is _____.

Exercise 2

Match the following:

—	1.	Spleen	A. Hardening of walls of a vessel
—	2.	Complement	B. Decrease of leukocytes
—	3.	Thymus	C. T-cells
—	4.	Lymphatic vessels	D. Decrease of granulocytes
—	5.	Lymph nodes	E. Palantine
—	6.	Leukocytopenia	F. Decrease of erythrocytes
—	7.	Pyrogens	G. Hypersensitivity
—	8.	Tonsils	H. Production of granulocytes

—	9.	Cisterna chyli	I. Storage sac
—	10.	Granulocytopenia	J. Gland like
—	11.	Null cells	K. Fire like chemicals
—	12.	Erythropenia	L. Filters
—	13.	Allergy	M. Protein group
—	14.	Angiosclerosis	N. Natural killer
—	15.	Granulocytopoiesis	O. Beaded appearance

Exercise 3

Give the meaning of the components of the following medical terms:

1. Lymphadenitis:
   Lymph _____
   aden _____
   itis _____
2. Splenectomy:
   Spleen _____
   ectomy _____
3. Lymphocytopenia:
   Lympho _____
   cyto _____
   penia _____
4. Lymphadenectasis:
   Lymph _____
   aden _____
   ectasis _____
5. Lymphostasis:
   Lymph _____
   ostasis _____
6. Leukemia:
   Leuk(o) _____
   emia _____
7. Phlebitis :
   Phleb _____
   itis _____
8. Septicemia:
   Septic _____
   emia _____
9. Thromboangitis:
   Thrombo _____
   ang _____
   itis _____

10. Hematorrhea:
    Hemat _____
    orrhea _____

NERVOUS SYSTEM

Exercise 1

Complete the following:

1. The nervous system is divided into the _____ and
   _____.
2. Threadlike dendrites and axons are also called _____.
3. The three meningeal membranes are the _____,
   _____ and _____.
4. The brainstem consists of the _____, _____ and
   _____.
5. The four lobes of the cerebrum are the _____,
   _____, _____, and _____.
6. _____ is found inside the spinal cord.
7. There are _____ pairs of spinal nerves along the
   spinal cord.
8. The peripheral nervous system includes the _____
   system, the _____ nerves and the _____
   nerves.
9. There are _____ pairs of cranial nerves.
10. The first cranial nerve, for the sense of smell, is the _____
    nerve
11. The second cranial nerve, the _____ is the nerve
    of vision.
12. _____ is the eight cranial nerve which maintains the
    balance and equilibrium.
13. The nerve which controls the muscles of the tongue, and functions
    in speech and swallowing is _____.
14. _____ nerve is the longest of the cranial nerves, which
    has extensive distribution over the pharynx, larynx, trachea,
    esophagus etc. and stimulates the secretion of hydrochloric acid
    for the process of digestion.
15. The autonomic nervous system has two division: _____
    and _____.

Exercise 2

Give the meaning of the components of the following medical terms:

1. Arachnoiditis:
   Arachnoid _____
   itis _____

2. Polioencephalomeningomyelitis :
   Polio _____
   encephalo _____
   meningo _____
   myel _____
   itis _____

3. Anencephalia:
   An _____
   encephal _____
   ia _____

4. Heterotopia spinalis:
   Heterotopia _____
   spinalis _____

5. Encephalocele:
   Encephal _____
   cele _____

6. Craniomeningocele:
   Cranio _____
   meningo _____
   cele _____

7. Macrocephaly :
   Macro _____
   cephaly _____

8. Encephalomalacia:
   Encephalo _____
   malacia _____

9. Cephalgia:
   cephal _____
   algia _____

10. Dysphasia:
    Dys _____
    phasia _____

Exercise 3

Match the following:

____ 1. Long nerve cell processes that carry impulses from the cell body

____ 2. Numerous short nerve cell processes that conduct nerve impulses toward the cell body

____ 3. Neurons concerned with muscle or gland action

____ 4. Peripheral neurons that conduct afferent impulses from the sense organs to the spinal cord

____ 5. Region of connection between process of two adjacent neurons for transmission of impulses

____ 6. Peripheral nerve endings

____ 7. Space between the pia mater and the arachnoid

____ 8. Space between the dura mater and arachnoid

____ 9. Centrally body of the cerebellum, shaped like a worm

____ 10. A furrow, or groove, separating folds of the brain

____ 11. Second cranial nerve, which innervates the retina of the eye

____ 12. Third cranial nerve, which innervates the eye muscles and the sphincter of the pupil and ciliary processes

____ 13. Interlacing network of spinal nerves

____ 14. Nerve that originates in the spinal cord and innervates the diaphragm

____ 15. A so called wandering nerve, both motor and sensory, with an extensive distribution, with some gastric, pyloric, hepatic and celiac branches

A. Subarachnoid

B. Vagus

C. Sulcus

D. Synapse

E. Oculomotor

F. Dendrites

G. Terminal twigs

H. Axon

I. Subdural

J. Plexus

K. Sensory neurons

L. Optic

M. Vermis

N. Motor neurons

O. Phrenic

DIGESTIVE SYSTEM

Exercise 1

Complete the following:

1. The wavelike movement of the intestines is called _____.
2. The _____ serves a dual purpose in the respiratory and gastrointestinal systems.

3. The stomach is divided into _____, _____ and _____.
4. The three divisions of the small intestine are the _____, _____ and _____.
5. The colon is divided into _____ sections.
6. The accessory organs of the digestive system are _____, _____ and _____.
7. The _____ both an exocrine and endocrine gland.
8. The largest gland in the body is _____.
9. _____ stores the bile.
10. The four types of the teeth are _____, _____, _____ and _____.
11. The thin lubricating, serous fluid secreted by the salivary glands is called _____.
12. Two hormones secreted by the islets of Langerhans are _____ and _____.
13. The two main functions of the tongue in digestive system are _____ and _____.
14. Most of the water absorption of the body take place in the _____.
15. The last segment of the large intestine is _____.

Exercise 2

Match the following:

_____ 1. Rigid body structure in the roof of the mouth   A. Chyme

_____ 2. Musculo membranous tube from pharynx to stomach   B. Lesser curvature

_____ 3. Lower left margin of the surface of the stomach   C. Uvula

_____ 4. Upper right margin of the surface of stomach   D. Greater curvature

_____ 5. Very hard substance that covers the exposed part of the tooth   E. Sphincter

_____ 6. Semi fluid material produced by gastric digestion of food   F. Hard palate

_____ 7. Any one of the four front teeth of either jaw   G. Molars

_____ 8. Broad teeth used in grinding food   H. Enamel

_____ 9. Pendulum of the soft palate   I. Esophagus

_____ 10. Ringlike muscles that contract to close an opening   J. Incisor

Exercise 3

Give the meaning of the components of the following medical terms:

1. Enterogastritis:
   Entero _____
   gastr _____
   itis _____
2. Gastroenterocolitis:
   Gastro _____
   entero _____
   col _____
   itis _____
3. Hepatitis:
   Hepat _____
   itis _____
4. Ileocolitis:
   Ileo _____
   col _____
   itis _____
5. Procitis:
   Proc _____
   itis _____
6. Gingivitis:
   Gingiv _____
   itis _____
7. Hepatomegaly:
   Hepato _____
   megaly _____
8. Gastrolith:
   Gastro _____
   lith _____
9. Hypersplenism:
   Hyper _____
   spleen _____
   ism _____
10. Proctoptosis:
    Procto _____
    ptosis _____
11. Hepatoma:
    Hepat _____
    oma _____
12. Herniorrhaphy:
    Hernio _____
    rrhaphy _____

13. Colotomy:
 Col _____
 otomy _____
14. Sailolithotomy:
 Sailo _____
 lith _____
 otomy _____
15. Cholecystotomy:
 Chole _____
 cyst _____
 otomy _____

ENDOCRINE SYSTEM

Exercise 1

Complete the following:

1. Endocrine gland secretions are called _____.
2. The endocrine system is made up of _____ glands of internal secretion.
3. The two parts of the pituitary gland are the _____ and _____ lobes.
4. The islands (islets) of Langerhans in the pancreas secrete _____ and _____.
5. Two little cap like glands on top of the kidneys are the _____ gland.
6. The two distinct parts of the adrenals whose functions differ are the _____ and the _____.
7. The _____ of the adrenal gland secretes epinephrine and norepinephrine.
8. The _____ lobe of the pituitary gland secretes an antidiuretic hormone that stimulates water re-absorption by tubules of the kidneys.
9. The pineal gland secretion is _____.
10. The essential element of the thyroid hormone is _____.

Exercise 2

Match the following:

____ 1. Melatonin   A. Male hormone producing secondary sex characteristics

____ 2. Oxytocin   B. Hormone secreted by the islands of Langerhans, which increases blood glucose

____ 3. Prolactin

____ 4. Glucagons

____ 5. Calcitonin

____ 6. Testosterone

____ 7. Glucocorticoids

____ 8. Parathyroid hormone

____ 9. Epinephrine

____ 10. Insulin

C. Adrenal cortex hormones concerned with fat, protein, and carbohydrate metabolism

D. Thyroid hormone that helps to regulate calcium levels in the blood

E. Hormone secreted by the posterior lobe of the pituitary gland that stimulates uterine contractions

F. Hormone that reduces glucose in the blood

G. A skin lightening hormone of the pineal gland

H. Hormone secreted by the adrenal medulla that helps the body to meet stresses by stimulating the sympathetic nervous system

I. Hormone regulating calcium and phosphorus in blood and bone

J. Hormone responsible for development of breast in pregnancy

Exercise 3

Give the meaning of the components of the following medical terms:

1. Hypothyroidism:
   Hypo _____
   thyroid/ism _____
2. Thyrotoxicosis:
   Thyro _____
   toxic/osis _____
3. Hemithyroidectomy:
   Hemi _____
   thyroid _____
   ectomy _____
4. Hyperthyroidism:
   hyper _____
   thyroid/ism _____
5. Acromegaly:
   Acro _____
   megaly _____

RESPIRATORY SYSTEM

Exercise 1

Complete the following:

1. The organs of the respiratory system are _____, _____, _____, _____ and _____.
2. The process of respiration generally involves _____ and _____.
3. The pharynx is divided into _____ parts.
4. The trachea is also known as the _____.
5. The diaphragm separates the _____ and _____ cavities.
6. The diaphragm descends during the _____ phase of respiration.
7. The _____ side of the lung is composed of three lobes.
8. The main function of trachea is to _____.
9. The volume of inhaled air during ordinary respiration is called _____.
10. The respiratory center is in the _____.

Exercise 2

Match the following:

___ 1. Air sac of the lung   A. Diaphragm
___ 2. Branch of trachea going to each lobe   B. Oxygen
    of the lung
___ 3. Warms and moistens entering air   C. Carbon dioxide
___ 4. Odorless, colorless gas formed in   D. Mucous membrane
    tissues and excreted by the lungs
___ 5. Has a role in respiration, digestion,   E. Bronchiole
    and speech
___ 6. Potential space between the parietal   F. Pleural cavity
    and visceral pleural membranes
___ 7. Muscular and membranous partition   G. Bronchus
    that separates the thoracic cavity
    from the abdominal cavity
___ 8. Epithelial lining of the nose   H. Alveoli
___ 9. Small branch of bronchial tree   I. Nose
    extending from secondary bronchi
___ 10. Gas present in air, necessary for   J. Pharynx
    survival

Exercise 3

Give the meaning of the components of the following medical terms:

1. Rhinitis:
   Rhin _____
   itis _____
2. Bronchorrhagia:
   Broncho _____
   rrhagia _____
3. Laryngoptosis:
   Laryngo _____
   ptosis _____
4. Nasopharyngitis:
   Naso _____
   pharyng _____
   itis _____
5. Mediastinitis:
   Mediastin _____
   itis _____

SENSE ORGANS

Exercise 1

Complete the following:

1. The transparent portion of the fibrous coat of the eyeball is _____.
2. The innermost of the three coats of the eyeball is _____.
3. Tears are secreted by _____.
4. The receptors of light stimuli are the _____ and _____.
5. The "white of the eye" is called the _____.
6. The divisions of the ear are the _____, _____ and _____.
7. The ear has two functions _____ and _____.
8. The three ossicles are the _____, _____ and _____.
9. The tympanic membrane is also known as the _____.
10. Hair cells transmit sound stimulation to the brain by way of the _____ nerve.
11. The _____ is the organ for smell.
12. The organs of taste are located mainly on the _____.

13. Skin is composed of two principal layers _____ and _____.

14. The skin is the receptor for _____, _____, _____ and _____.

15. Sebaceous glands secrete _____.

Exercise 2

Match the following:

____ 1. Special cylindrical neuroepithelial cells in the retina, highly sensitive to low light

____ 2. The partition separating the external nares

____ 3. The projecting posterior part of the ear that lies outside the head

____ 4. Structure leading from the ear to the throat

____ 5. Structure that separates the middle ear from the external ear

____ 6. Sebaceous glands

____ 7. Dermis

____ 8. Areola

____ 9. Melanin pigment

____ 10. Sebum

A. Dense, gibbous connective tissue

B. Secretions of sebaceous glands

C. Rods

D. Pinna

E. Septum

F. Tympanic membrane

G. Area around the nipple

H. Glands with ducts opening around hair follicles

I. Eustachian tube

J. Pigment of skin or hair

Exercise 3

Give the meaning of the components of the following medical terms:

1. Retinoblastoma:
   Retinoblast _____
   oma _____
2. Blepharitis:
   Blephar _____
   itis _____

3. Conjunctivitis:
   Conjunctiv _____
   itis _____

4. Diplopia:
   di _____
   opia _____

5. Dacryoadenectomy:
   Dacryo _____
   aden _____
   ectomy _____

6. Dacryocystitis:
   Dacryo _____
   cyst _____
   itis _____

7. Retinitis:
   Retin _____
   itis _____

8. Keratitis:
   Kerat _____
   itis _____

9. Aphakia:
   A _____
   phakia _____

10. Microophthalmos:
    Micro _____
    ophthalmos _____

11. Myringitis:
    Myring _____
    itis _____

12. Tympanomastoiditis:
    Tympano _____
    mastoid _____
    itis _____

13. Otalgia:
    Oto _____
    algia _____

14. Otorrhea:
    Oto _____
    rrhea _____

15. Microtia:
    Micro _____
    otia _____

16. Labyrinthectomy:
    Labyrinth _____
    ectomy _____
17. Stapedectomy:
    Staped _____
    ectomy _____
18. Anosmia:
    An _____
    osmia _____
19. Dermatosclerosis:
    Dermato _____
    sclerosis _____
20. Albinism:
    Albin _____
    ism _____

EXCRETORY SYSTEM

Exercise 1

Complete the following:

1. The organs of the urinary system are the _____,
   _____, _____ and _____.
2. The concave depression on the medial margin of the kidney is
   called the _____.
3. The _____ is the functional unit of the kidney.
4. The main function of the kidney is to _____ the blood.
5. The wrinkles on the mucous membrane lining the bladder are
   called _____.
6. The twisted cluster of capillary channels called the _____
   is contained in the _____ capsule.
7. Sectioning of kidney shows it to have an internal _____.
8. Sectioning of kidney shows it to have an external _____.
9. The process of muscular contractions so as to pass urine is called
   _____.
10. _____ endocrine glands are located above each kidney.

Exercise 2

Give the meaning of the components of the following medical terms:

1. Anuria:
   An _____
   uria _____

2. Dysuria:
Dys _____
uria _____
3. Glomerulonephritis:
Glomerulo _____
nephr _____
itis _____
4. Hematuria:
Hema _____
turia _____
5. Pyelitis:
pyel _____
itis _____
6. Urethroplasty:
Urethro _____
plasty _____
7. Nephrectomy:
Nephr _____
ectomy _____
8. Nephropexy:
Nephro _____
pexy _____
9. Nephrotomy:
Nephro _____
otomy _____
10. Ureteropyelostomy
Uretero _____
pyelo _____
ostomy _____

REPRODUCTIVE SYSTEM

Exercise 1

Complete the following:
1. The male reproductive cell is called _____.
2. The chief male sex hormone is _____.
3. The vase deferens are encased by the _____.
4. The female reproductive cells are called _____.
5. The functions of the ovaries are _____.
6. The onset of menstruation is called _____.
7. The cessation of the menstrual cycle is called _____.

8. The smooth muscle, elastic tube extending from the uterine is called the _____.
9. The _____ stage last from the second through the eight week of pregnancy.
10. The only connection between the mother and the fetus is the

_____.

Exercise 2

Match the following:

— 1. Pair of tubes encased by spermatic cords	A. Testis
— 2. Secretion discharged by male reproductive organ	B. Endocervix
— 3. Foreskin of penis	C. Vagina
— 4. Male gland producing spermatozoa	D. Mons pubis
— 5. Reproductive cells of the female	E. Vas deferens
— 6. External female genitalia	F. Prepuce
— 7. Mucous membrane lining of the uterus	G. Areola
— 8. Interior of cervix	H. Vulva
— 9. Saclike male structure	I. Ova
— 10. Neck of uterus	J. Spermatozoa
— 11. Elastic muscular tube below cervix, extending to body exterior	K. Fetus
— 12. Developing human beginning with ninth week	L. Cervix
— 13. Pad of fat in front of symphysis pubis	M. Endometrium
— 14. Pigmented portion of nipple	N. Semen
— 15. Reproductive cells of the male	O. Scrotum

Exercise 3

1. Anarchism:
   An _____
   archism _____
2. Hydrocele:
   Hydro _____
   cele _____
3. Prostatomy:
   Prosta _____
   otomy _____
4. Orchotomy:
   Orch _____
   otomy _____

5. Hydrosalpinx:
   Hydro _____
   salpinx _____
6. Mastitis:
   Mast _____
   itis _____
7. Menorrhagia:
   Meno _____
   rrhagia _____
8. Oopheritis:
   Oopher _____
   itis _____
9. Salpingooophorectomy:
   Salpingo _____
   oophor _____
   ectomy _____
10. Vulvectomy:
    Vulv _____
    ectomy _____

ANSWERS

HUMAN BODY

Exercise 1

1. Cell
2. Tissue
3. Organs
4. 23
5. Skeletal, voluntary, or striated; visceral, involuntary, nonstriated, or smooth; cardiac, involuntary, or striated
6. Frontal or coronal; median, midsagittal, or midline; sagittal; transverse
7. Frontal
8. Away from
9. Towards the
10. Milli

Exercise 2

1. K	6. N	11. G
2. B	7. O	12. I
3. D	8. A	13. M
4. H	9. F	14. J
5. L	10. E	15. C

Exercise 3

1. Belphar:eyelid; belpharitis
2. Cerebro: brain; cerebrospinal
3. Chir:hand; chiromegaly
4. Cost:rib;costosternal
5. Gastr:stomach;gastritis
6. Hemat:blood;hematuria
7. Hyster:uterus; hysteropexy
8. Pyo:pus; pyometritis
9. Pyel: pelvis; pyelitis
10. Neph: kidney; nephritis
11. An: without/no; anesthesia
12. Bi:two/both/double; bilateral
13. Dys: bad/difficult/painful;dysuria
14. Epi:around/upon/at;epidermis
15. Hemi:half; hemiplegia
16. Tri: three; tricuspid
17. –cele: hernia/protrusion; hyrdocele
18. –malacia:softening;encephalomalacia
19. –oma:tumor;cardinoma
20. –rhexis:rupture; cardiorhexis

MUSCULOSKELETAL SYSTEM

Exercise 1

1. 206
2. Long, flat, short, irregular
3. Long
4. Spine
5. Sacrum, coccyx
6. 12
7. Mandible (lower jaw bone)
8. Cervical, thoracic, lumbar
9. Humerus, ulna, radius

10. Kneecap
11. Tarsals
12. Wrist
13. No, slight, free
14. Flexion
15. Ball-and-socket

Exercise 2

1. *Anencephalia:* No or not; brain—developmental anomaly with absence of cranial vault and cerebral hemispheres
2. *Osteoarthritis*: Bone; joint; inflammation—degenerative joint disease; inflammation of bone joint
3. *Osteodystrophy:* Bone; bad; difficult, disordered; nutrition or nourishment—defective bone formation
4. *Osteolysis :* Bone; dissolution—dissolution of bone
5. *Sacroiliac:* Sacrum; ilium—joint between sacrum and ilium

Exercise 3

1. H	6. T	11. D	16. R
2. E	7. J	12. B	17. O
3. I	8. A	13. C	18. P
4. S	9. G	14. Q	19. M
5. L	10. F	15. N	20. K

Exercise 4

1. Mycology
2. Extend, contract
3. Skeletal, visceral and cardiac
4. Trumpeter (muscle)
5. Thorax
6. Masseters
7. Ear
8. Orbicularis oculi
9. Trapezius
10. Abdominal

Exercise 5

1. Myalgia:muscle; pain—painful muscle
2. Myoma: muscle; tumor—tumor of muscle
3. Myorrhaphy: muscle; suturing—suturing of muscle

4. Tenosynovectomy:tendon; synovial sheath; excision—surgical excision of tendon sheath
5. Myosclerosis:muscle; hardening—hardening of muscle

CARDIOVASCULAR SYSTEM

Exercise 1

1. Heart, blood, arteries, veins
2. Pericardium
3. Four
4. Backflow
5. Oxygenated, veins
6. A, B, O, AB
7. Pulmonary
8. Aorta
9. Ascending aorta, aortic arch, descending aorta
10. Inferior vena cava.

Exercise 2

1. D		6. C	
2. J		7. I	
3. B		8. E	
4. A		9. H	
5. G		10. F	

Exercise 3

1. Aortitis:aorta; inflammation—inflammation of aorta
2. Pericarditis:pericardium; inflammation—inflammation of pericardium
3. Arteriosclerosis: artery; hardening —hardening of the arteries or an artery
4. Cardiomegaly: cardio; enlargement; enlargement of the heart
5. Myocarditis:muscle; heart /cardio; inflammation—inflammation of the heart muscle
6. Hemothorax:blood; thoracic cavity—accumulation of blood in the pleural cavity
7. Dextrocardia:right side; heart—heart is displaced to the right side of the thoracic cavity
8. Cyanosis: blue color; condition—bluish skin color caused by reduced amounts of hemoglobin in the blood
9. Bradycardia:slow; heart—slow heart beat
10. Tachycardia:fast/rapid; heart—rapid heart beat

BLOOD AND LYMPHATIC SYSTEM

Exercise 1

1. Arteries, capillaries, veins
2. Oxygenated, veins
3. Hemoglobin
4. Anemia
5. Granulocytes and agranulocytes
6. Cardiovascular, immune
7. Lower jaw, neck, axilla, groin, knee (or any other known areas)
8. Spleen
9. Three
10. Filters our bacteria and foreign matter

Exercise 2

1. J	6. B	11. N
2. M	7. K	12. F
3. C	8. E	13. G
4. O	9. I	14. A
5. L	10. D	15. H

Exercise 3

1. Lymphadenitis:lymph; gland; inflammation—inflammation of lymph glands
2. Splenectomy:spleen; surgical removal—surgical removal of spleen
3. Lymphocytopenia:lymph; cell; deficiency—deficiency of lymphocytes
4. Lymphadenectasis: lymph; gland; enlargement—enlargement of a lymph gland
5. Lymphostasis:lymph; stand till—obstruction of the lymph flow
6. Leukemia:white cells; blood—malignant diseases of the blood
7. phlebitis:vein; inflammation—inflammation of vein
8. septicemia:septic; blood—general systemic blood infection caused by pathogenic
9. thromboangitis: clots; vessel; inflammation–blood clots accompanying inflammation of the interior blood vessel
10. hematorrhea: blood; flow—profuse hemorrhage

NERVOUS SYSTEM

Exercise 1

1. Central, peripheral
2. Nerve (fibers)
3. Dura mater, arachnoid, pia mater
4. Medulla oblongata, pons, midbrain
5. Frontal, temporal, parietal, occipital
6. Cerebrospinal fluid
7. 31
8. Autonomic, cranial, spinal
9. 12
10. Olfactory
11. Optic
12. Auditory
13. Hypoglossal
14. Vagus
15. Sympathetic, Parasympathetic.

Exercise 2

1. Arachnoidits: arachnoid membrane; inflammation—inflammation of the arachnoid membrane
2. Polioencephalomeningomyelitis: gray matter of the brain; brain; meninges; spinal cord; inflammation;inflammation of the gray matter of the brain, spinal cord, and meninges
3. Anencephalia: no; brain; absence of cerebral hemispheres and cranial vault
4. Heterotopia spinalis: other; place; spinal—displaced spinal cord or spinal cord displaced to other than normal position
5. Encephalocele: brain; protrusion—protrusion of a part of the cranial contents through a defect in the skull
6. Craniomeningocele: skull; meninges; protrusion—herniation of the cerebral membranes through a defect in the skull
7. Macrocephaly: large; skull—excessively large size of head
8. Encephalomalacia: brain; softening—softening of brain tissue caused by reduced blood supply
9. Cephalgia: head; pain—headache
10. Dysphasia: difficulty; speech—speech impairment caused by central nervous system lesion

Exercise 3

1. H	6. G	11. L
2. F	7. A	12. E
3. N	8. I	13. J
4. K	9. M	14. O
5. D	10. C	15. B

DIGESTIVE SYSTEM

Exercise 1

1. Peristalsis
2. Pharynx
3. Fundus, body, pylorus
4. Duodenum, jejunum, ileum
5. Four
6. Liver, pancreas and gallbladder
7. Pancreas
8. Liver
9. Gallbladder
10. Incisors, canines, premolars, molars
11. Saliva
12. Insulin, glucagons
13. Keeps food between teeth during chewing, aids in swallowing
14. Large intestine
15. Rectum.

Exercise 2

1. F	6. A
2. I	7. J
3. B	8. G
4. D	9. C
5. H	10. E

Exercise 3

1. Enterogastritis: intestine;stomach; inflammation—inflammation of intestines and stomach
2. Gastroenterocolitis: stomach; small intestine; colon; inflammation —inflammation of stomach, small intestine and colon
3. Hepatitis: liver; inflammation—inflammation of liver
4. Ileocolitis: ileum; colon; inflammation—inflammatioin of ileum and colon

5. Procitis: rectum; inflammation—inflammation of rectum
6. Gingivitis: gums; inflammation—inflammation of gums
7. Hepatomegaly: liver; enlargement—enlarged liver
8. Gastrolith: stomach; stone—stone in the stomach
9. Hypersplenism: excessive, abnormal; spleen; condition—abnormally increased hemolytic function of spleen
10. Proctoptosis: rectum; downward displacement—rectal prolapse
11. Hepatoma: liver; tumor—malignant tumor of the liver
12. Herniorrhaphy: hernia; suture or repair—suture or repair of a hernia
13. Colotomy: colon; incision—incision into the colon
14. Sailolithotomy: salivary gland; stone; incision—removal of stone from salivary gland
15. Cholecystotomy: gallbladder; cyst or stone; incision—incision into the gallbladder for exploration of cyst/stone

ENDOCRINE SYSTEM

Exercise 1

1. Hormones
2. Ductless
3. Anterior, posterior
4. Insulin, glucagons, and pancreatic polypeptide
5. Adrenal
6. Cortex, medulla
7. Medulla
8. Posterior
9. Melatonin
10. Iodine

Exercise 2

1. G	6. A
2. E	7. C
3. J	8. I
4. B	9. H
5. D	10. F

Exercise 3

1. Hypothyroidism: under, decreased; thyroid—decreased function of the thyroid gland
2. Thyrotoxicosis: thyroid; toxic; condition—toxic thyroid condition; thyroid crisis

3. Hemithyroidectomy: partial or half; thyroid—surgical excision of part of the thyroid gland
4. Hyperthyroidism: over, increased; thyroid—overproductioin of thyroid hormone
5. Acromegaly: extreme or extremities; enlarged or huge—enlarged bones of hands, feet, and facial bone

RESPIRATORY SYSTEM

Exercise 1

1. Nose, pharynx, larynx, trachea, bronchi, lungs
2. Inspiration, expiration
3. Three
4. Wind pipe
5. Thoracic, abdominal
6. Inspiration
7. Right
8. Maintain its part of airway
9. Tidal
10. Brain

Exercise 2

1. H
2. G
3. I
4. C
5. J
6. F
7. A
8. D
9. E
10. B

Exercise 3

1. Rhinitis: nose; inflammation—inflammatioin of nose or nasal passages
2. Bronchorrhagia: bronchi; hemorrhage—bronchial hemorrhage
3. Laryngoptosis: larynx; falling—falling or displacement of the larynx from normal position
4. Nasopharyngitis: nose; pharynx; inflammation—inflammation of nose and pharynx
5. Mediastinits: mediastinum; inflammation—inflammation of the mediastinum

SENSE ORGANS

Exercise 1

1. Cornea
2. Retina
3. Lacrimal
4. Rods, cones
5. Sclera
6. External, middle, inner
7. Hearing and equilibrium
8. Malleus, incus, stapes
9. Eardrum
10. Auditory
11. Nose
12. Tongue
13. Epidermis, dermis
14. Touch, heat, cold and pain
15. Sebum

Exercise 2

1. C	6. H
2. E	7. A
3. D	8. G
4. I	9. J
5. F	10. B

Exercise 3

1. Retinoblastoma: retina; germ cell; tumor—tumor arising from retinal blast (germ) cell
2. Belpharitis: eyelid; inflammatioin—inflammation of the eyelid
3. Conjunctivitis: conjunctiva; inflammation—inflammation of the conjunctiva
4. Diplopia: double; see—double vision
5. Dacryoadenectomy: tear; gland; excision or removal—surgical excision of a tear gland
6. Dacryocystitis: tear; sac; inflammation—inflammation of tear, or lacrimal sac
7. Retinitis: retina; inflammation—inflammation of retina
8. Keratitis: cornea; inflammation—inflammation of the cornea
9. Aphakia: absence; lens; congenital anomaly of absence of lens
10. Microophthalmos: small; eye; abnormally small eyes

11. Myringitis: eardrum; inflammation—inflammation of the eardrum
12. Tympanomastoiditis: tympanic membrane; mastoid; inflammation—inflammation of tympanic membrane and mastoid process
13. Otalgia: ear; pain—earache
14. Otorrhea: ear; discharge—discharge from the ear
15. Microtia: small; ear—abnormally small ear
16. Labyrinthectomy—labyrinth; excision— excision of the labyrinth of the ear
17. Stapedectomy: stapes; removal—excision of the stapes
18. Anosmia: absence; smell—absence of the sense of smell
19. Dermatosclerosis: skin; hardening—hardening of the skin
20. Albinism: white; condition—congenital defect in melanin development, causing lack of pigment in skin, hair, and eyes

EXCRETORY SYSTEM

Exercise 1

1. Kidneys (two), ureters (two), bladder, urethra
2. Hilum
3. Nephrons
4. Filter the waste
5. Rugae
6. Glomerulus, Bowman's
7. Medulla
8. Cortex
9. Micturition
10. Adrenal

Exercise 2

1. Anuria: without; urine—complete failure of secretion of urine due to renal failure or blockage of urinary tract
2. Dysuria: difficulty; urine—difficult or painful urination
3. Glomerulonephritis: glomerulus; kidney; inflammation—inflammation of kidney due to injury to the glomeruli due to antigen-antibody reaction
4. Hematuria: blood; urine—blood in urine
5. Pyelitis: renal pelvis; inflammation—inflammation of renal pelvis
6. Urethroplasty: urethra;ureter; plastic repair—plastic repair of the urethra
7. Nephrectomy: kidney; removal—surgical removal of the kidney

8. Nephropexy: kidney; fixation—surgical fixation of a displaced kidney
9. Nephrotomy: kidney; incision—incision into kidney
10. Ureteropyelostomy: urethra; renal pelvis; anastomosis—anastomosis of ureter and renal pelvis.

REPRODUCTIVE SYSTEM

Exercise 1

1. Sperm cell
2. Testosterone
3. Spermatic cord
4. Ova
5. Ovulation, hormonal secretion
6. Menarche
7. Menopause
8. Vagina
9. Embryonic
10. Placenta

Exercise 2

1. E	6. H	11. C
2. N	7. M	12. K
3. F	8. B	13. D
4. A	9. O	14. G
5. I	10. L	15. J

Exercise 3

1. Anarchism: without; testis—absence of testis
2. Hydrocele: water; protrusion—hernia (sac) of fluid in the testes or in the tubes leading from the testes
3. Prostatomy: prostate; incision—incision into the prostate
4. Orchotomy: testis; incision—incision into the testis
5. Hydrosalpinx: water; salpinx—collection of watery fluid in a uterine tube, occurring as the end state of pyosalpinx
6. Mastitis: breast; inflammation—inflammation of the breast
7. Menorrhagia: menses; flow—excessive bleeding
8. Oopheritis: ovary; inflammation—inflammation of the ovary
9. Salpingo-oophorectomy: fallopian tube; ovary; removal—removal of fallopian tube and ovary
10. Vulvectomy: vulva; removal—partial removal of vulva

Index

Page numbers followed by *f* refer to figure and *t* refer to table